# Reviewer

**Jennifer J. Yeager, PhD, RN, APRN**
Assistant Professor and
Director of the Graduate Nursing Program
Tarleton State University
Stephenville, Texas

# Study Guide Student Learning Strategies

## INTRODUCTION

Welcome to the *Pharmacology and the Nursing Process Study Guide*. This study guide is another tool the authors have developed to assist you in learning the key terms, key concepts, and core content of pharmacology. Before you begin to use this book, it is a good idea to revisit some of the learning strategies that will help you be successful in learning and applying pharmacology. The trend in college education today emphasizes active learning and is referred to as *student-centered learning*. This puts you in control of your own learning. For student-centered learning to be beneficial, you need to be provided with tools and techniques to guide you in your journey. You should utilize those student learning strategies that meet your learning style and, thus, maximize your learning. Because everyone learns a little differently, you should check out your learning style in Part 4 of the textbook. In this section of the study guide, you will be provided with additional information and learning tips that will keep you on the road to successfully mastering the pharmacology content.

## TIME MANAGEMENT

As a college student and, in particular, as a student entering the profession of nursing, you will soon realize that you have so much to accomplish. Therefore time cannot be wasted because when it is gone, it cannot be recovered. The amount of time that is required to read your textbooks and attend classes, laboratory sessions, and clinical practice hardly leaves time for studying, work, and family life. So if you do not want your college life to use up all your available time, you need to be organized and learn good time management skills. One of the best ways to accomplish an organized life is to use a planner (refer to Part 6 in the textbook). After you have plotted all your important dates related to your college life, you can see the big picture of how the rest of your life can fit in. Remember that in addition to scheduling your class times, project due dates, and test dates, you should leave blocks of time for reading and reviewing. Reading your textbooks and reviewing what you learned are two major components of active learning. If everything is plotted in your planner, it will be easy to see conflicts ahead of time so that arrangements can be made. It is also helpful if you

make a list on a daily basis. You can prioritize the things that are important to complete that day. Crossing the tasks off the list can be liberating and gives you a sense of organization and accomplishment. It may also be a way to keep yourself on task if you are the type of student who likes to procrastinate. When your life is planned and you are in control, it can actually reduce stress and the feeling of being overwhelmed. You will then be able to see breaks where you can take time for yourself, your family, and your friends. Taking care of yourself and being there for your family makes everything seem a lot more manageable and satisfying. Schoolwork is important, but so is relaxing with family and friends.

## RESOURCES

You are attending college in an age when the learning resources available to you are endless. Your first resource is your pharmacology textbook. Inside this book is a variety of colorful boxes, charts, and case studies to help you further understand and apply the principles you are learning. In each chapter you will find a list of key terms, review of key concepts, and practice questions to quiz yourself. This study guide provides further opportunity for you to check your comprehension in a variety of ways. There are worksheets corresponding to each chapter in the textbook, providing you with more case studies and review questions. There is an overview of key drug calculation concepts because it is imperative that you correctly perform the mathematical problems when calculating drug dosages. You can review dosage calculations with practice problems and a practice quiz. There are even sample drug labels that you can view.

Information technology in the form of downloadable applications for your smartphones and tablets is a great resource for learning, reviewing, and preparing for tests. Don't forget that your student resources for this textbook include interactive review questions and downloadable files of the key points from each chapter to help you study for tests (refer to Part 4 in the textbook).

Another resource that students sometimes neglect to consider is their instructor. Although you are expected to be actively learning on your own, coming to class prepared to discuss what you read, this does not mean that you are alone in your learning process. Your instructor can help you clarify misunderstood concepts and offer suggestions to improve your studying and increase your comprehension. Remember that your instructor is the one who is guiding your learning and can provide you with the blueprint of what is especially important to know. Instructors often provide their students with PowerPoint presentations of their lectures. It is a good idea to use these resources to take good notes so that the PowerPoint presentations can help you review the material. The same is true any of class learning activities and case studies; they are also valuable as learning resources. Many times the instructors are nurses who have a wealth of firsthand experience and will share their life experiences of pharmacology in nursing. This can help you link your learning to real-world practice.

The last resource you should consider is using a study group. When working within a study group, you have the ability and advantage to get another person's perspective on a topic. Sometimes another student can explain something in a way that makes it easier for you to understand. The work can be divided up so that everyone brings something to the table, with everyone learning from one another. Because of technology, these groups do not even need to meet in person because finding a time that everyone is available often poses a problem. Group chat rooms and discussion groups are ways to facilitate meeting with your group off campus (refer to Part 5 in your textbook).

# Contents

# 1 The Nursing Process and Drug Therapy

**Select the best answer for each question.**

1. Which phase of the nursing process requires the nurse to establish a comprehensive baseline of data concerning a particular patient?
   a. Assessment
   b. Planning
   c. Implementation
   d. Evaluation

2. The nurse monitors the fulfillment of goals, and may revise them, during which phase of the nursing process?
   a. Assessment
   b. Planning
   c. Implementation
   d. Evaluation

3. The nurse prepares and administers prescribed medications during which phase of the nursing process?
   a. Assessment
   b. Planning
   c. Implementation
   d. Evaluation

4. When developing a plan of care, which nursing action ensures the goal statement is patient centered?
   a. Considering family input
   b. Involving the patient
   c. Developing the goal first and then sharing it with the patient
   d. Including the physician

5. The nurse includes which information as part of a complete medication profile? *(Select all that apply.)*
   a. Use of "street" drugs
   b. Current laboratory work
   c. History of surgeries
   d. Use of alcohol
   e. Use of herbal products
   f. Family history

6. During which phase of the nursing process does the nurse prioritize the nursing diagnoses?
   a. Assessment
   b. Planning
   c. Implementation
   d. Evaluation

7. The nurse is preparing to administer morning doses of medications to a patient and has just checked the patient's name on the identification band. The patient has stated his name. Which is the nurse's next appropriate action?
   a. Administer the medications.
   b. Ask the patient's wife to verify the patient's identity.
   c. Ask the patient to verify his date of birth.
   d. Ask a second nurse to verify the patient's identity.

8. The nurse is administering a medication, and the order reads: "Give 250 mcg PO now." The tablets in the medication dispensing cabinet are in milligram strength. What is the right dose of the drug in

   milligrams? _____

9. The nurse is administering a medication, and the order reads: "Give 0.125 mg PO now." The tablets in the medication dispensing cabinet are in microgram strength. What is the right dose of the drug in

   micrograms? _____

10. Place the steps of the nursing process in order, with 1 being the first step and 5 being the last step.

    _____ a. Implementation

    _____ b. Planning

    _____ c. Evaluation

    _____ d. Assessment

    _____ e. Formulation of nursing diagnoses

**1**

11. The nurse is attempting to administer the morning dose of the patient's medication. The patient refuses the medication, stating, "It makes me sick to my stomach!" What is the nurse's responsibility?
    a. Document the patient's refusal in the record.
    b. Discard the medication according to hospital policy.
    c. Disguise the medication in food.
    d. Offer the medication again in 30 minutes.

12. Which medication is appropriately administered at the correct time?
    a. Amoxicillin ordered at 0800 and given at 0700
    b. Diltiazem ordered at 0900 and given at 0930
    c. Furosemide ordered at 0730 and given at 0825
    d. Levothyroxine sodium ordered at 1000 and given at 0915

## CRITICAL THINKING AND APPLICATION

**Answer the following questions on a separate sheet of paper.**

13. The following is a list of data gathered during an assessment of Ms. B., a young woman visiting an outpatient clinic with what she describes as "maybe an ulcer." Label each item as either objective data (O) or subjective data (S).

    _____ Ms. B. tells the nurse that she smokes a pack of cigarettes a day.
    _____ She is 5 feet 5 inches tall and weighs 135 lb.
    _____ The nurse finds that Ms. B.'s pulse rate is 68 beats/min, and her blood pressure is 128/72 mm Hg.
    _____ Her stool was tested for occult blood by a laboratory technician; the results were negative.
    _____ Ms. B. says that she does not experience nausea, but she reports pain and heartburn, especially after eating popcorn—something she and her husband have always done while watching TV before bedtime.
    _____ She experiences occasional increases in stomach pain, a "feeling of heat" in her abdomen and chest at night when she lies down, and increased incidents of heartburn.

14. Identify the "nine rights" of drug administration, and specify ways to ensure that each of these rights is addressed.

15. The following fill-in-the-blank items will help in reviewing the nursing process:

    Data are collected during the (a) _____ phase of the nursing process.

    Data can be classified as (b) _____ or (c) _____.
    To formulate the nursing diagnosis, the nurse must first (d) _____ the information collected. The planning phase includes identification of (e) _____ and (f) _____.

    The (g) _____ phase consists of carrying out the nursing care plan.

    The (h) _____ phase is ongoing and includes monitoring the patient's response to medication and determining the status of goals.

16. During a busy night shift, the nurse notices a medication order that reads: "Give amoxicillin, 500 mg PO three times a day." What is the most important thing the nurse must check before giving this medication to the patient?

17. Summarize the nurse's role in the prevention of medication errors. Relate how this role of prevention meets the QSEN requirements for safe practice.

## CASE STUDY

**Read the scenario, and answer the following questions on a separate sheet of paper**

A 75-year-old woman has been admitted to the hospital because of nausea and vomiting. She also has a diagnosis of hepatitis C. She says she stopped drinking 3 years ago but has had increasing problems with peripheral edema and shortness of breath, and has had trouble getting out of bed or a chair by herself. Laboratory results show that her liver enzyme levels are slightly elevated; her sodium and potassium levels are decreased. Her blood pressure is 160/98 mm Hg, her pulse rate is 98 beats/min, and her respiratory rate is 24 breaths/min. She is afebrile and states that she is having slight abdominal pain.

1. From the brief facts given, what information will be important to consider when obtaining a medication profile?

2. From the nursing diagnoses in Box 1-3, choose at least two current and two "risk for" nursing diagnoses for this patient. How would you determine the priority of the nursing diagnoses?
3. The physician wrote the following drug order:

November 4, 2018

Give furosemide now.

Charles Simmons, MD

| Patient's Name: Jane Dow | F | Age: 75 |
| Medical Record No: 1234567 | Date of Birth: 1/16/38 |

What elements, if any, are missing from the medication order? What will you do next?

4. After the order is clarified, the pharmacy sends up furosemide, 80-mg tablets, but the patient is unable to swallow them because of her nausea. Your colleague suggests giving the furosemide to her as an intravenous injection. What will you do next?

5. After the patient receives the dose of furosemide, what will you do?

# 2 Pharmacologic Principles

**Select the best answer for each question.**

1. Number the following drug forms in order of speed of dissolution and absorption, with 1 being the fastest and 5 being the slowest:

   _____ a. Capsules

   _____ b. Enteric-coated tablets

   _____ c. Elixirs

   _____ d. Powders

   _____ e. Orally-disintegrating tablets

2. When considering the various routes of drug elimination, the nurse is aware that elimination occurs mainly by which routes?
   a. Renal tubules and skin
   b. Skin and lungs
   c. Bowel and renal tubules
   d. Lungs and gastrointestinal tract

3. The nurse is aware that excessive drug dosages, impaired metabolism, or inadequate excretion may result in which drug effect?
   a. Tolerance
   b. Cumulative effect
   c. Incompatibility
   d. Antagonistic effect

4. Drug half-life is defined as the amount of time required for 50% of a drug to
   a. be absorbed by the body.
   b. reach a therapeutic level.
   c. exert a response.
   d. be removed by the body.

5. The nurse recognizes that drugs given by which route will be altered by the first-pass effect? *(Select all that apply.)*
   a. Oral
   b. Sublingual
   c. Subcutaneous
   d. Intravenous
   e. Rectal

6. If a drug binds with an enzyme and thereby prevents the enzyme from binding to its normal target cell, it will produce which effect?
   a. Receptor interaction
   b. Enzyme affinity
   c. Enzyme interaction
   d. Nonspecific interaction

7. The nurse is reviewing a list of a patient's medications and notes that one of the drugs is known to have a low therapeutic index. Which statement accurately explains this concept?
   a. The difference between a therapeutic dose and toxic dose is large.
   b. The difference between a therapeutic dose and toxic dose is small.
   c. The dose needed to reach a therapeutic level is small.
   d. The drug has only a slight chance of being effective.

8. The nurse prepares to obtain a patient's blood sample from a central line for a drug level that is to be drawn just before that medication's next dose. What is the timing of this blood draw known as?
   a. Half-life
   b. Therapeutic level
   c. Peak level
   d. Trough level

9. A drug has a half-life of 4 hours. If at 0800 the drug level is measured as 200 mg/L, at what time

   would the drug level be 50 mg/L? _____

10. When drug A functions as an enzyme inhibitor of drug B, the nurse will anticipate which result in drug B?
    a. Levels of drug B could rise to toxicity.
    b. Levels of drug B will remain unchanged.
    c. Levels of drug B will move into the receptor sites more quickly.
    d. Levels of drug B will be eliminated from the tubules with greater ease.

11. When administering a new medication to a patient, the nurse notes the drug is "highly protein bound." The patient's albumin level is normal. When compared to a drug that is not highly protein bound, the nurse would expect the protein-bound drug to
    a. demonstrate quicker renal excretion.
    b. be metabolized more quickly.
    c. have a longer duration of action.
    d. exit the vascular system via osmosis.

12. The nurse administers warfarin to a patient who is concurrently taking a second drug that is highly protein bound. The nurse knows a drug–drug interaction could occur, which would result in
    a. both drugs being rendered useless.
    b. neither drug reaching a therapeutic level.
    c. the second drug increasing the action and toxicity of the first drug.
    d. only the protein-bound drug being able to exit the vascular system.

## MATCHING

**Match each field of study with the corresponding job description of a person working in that field.**

13. _____ Pharmaceutics

14. _____ Pharmacokinetics

15. _____ Pharmacodynamics

16. _____ Pharmacogenomics

17. _____ Pharmacotherapeutics

18. _____ Pharmacognosy

19. _____ Toxicology

20. _____ Pharmacoeconomics

a. Lisa is researching botanical and zoologic sources of drugs to treat multiple sclerosis. She is part of a university research team that is currently experimenting with varying the biochemical composition and therapeutic effects of several possible new drugs.
b. Jeffrey works for a pharmaceutical corporation. One of its new drugs looks very promising, and Jeffrey's company is experimenting with dosage forms for this investigational new drug. He is responsible for measuring the relationship between the physiochemical properties of the dosage form and the clinical therapeutic response.
c. Micah is performing a cost–benefit analysis to compare the effectiveness of two blood pressure medications for a health insurance company.

d. Devon researches various poisons and is particularly concerned with the detection and treatment of the effects of drugs and other chemicals in certain mammals.
e. Diane and Phil have spent the past 3 years gathering family histories, legal case reports, and current clinical data to identify possible genetic factors that influence individuals' responses to meperidine and related drugs.
f. David works on a study that is gathering data on the use of two different drugs for the treatment of rheumatoid arthritis.
g. Leslie's laboratory monitors drug distribution rates between various body compartments from absorption through excretion. Recently, her laboratory was able to suggest a positive change in the dosage regimen for an injectable drug, bringing her firm a prestigious award.
h. Gregory's research unit recently recommended two new contraindications for the use of a newly marketed drug after discovering previously unknown biochemical and physiologic interactions of this drug with another, unrelated drug.

## CRITICAL THINKING AND APPLICATION

**Answer the following questions on a separate sheet of paper.**

21. Mr. C. is to receive a drug that can be given by injection, either intramuscularly or subcutaneously. Mr. C.'s condition dictates that the drug needs to be absorbed quickly. Which route of administration will the prescriber order? How can the nurse further increase absorption?

22. Ms. D. had a thyroidectomy 4 years ago and has been taking the thyroid hormone levothyroxine since the surgery. She visits her primary care provider for periodic laboratory work to check her hormone levels. This is an example of which type of drug therapy: acute, maintenance, supplemental, or palliative? Explain your answer.

23. E.S. has a prescription for an extended-release, enteric-coated tablet. The next day, his wife calls to ask about crushing the tablet, saying, "He just cannot swallow that big pill." What is the nurse's best answer?

24. Identify the advantages of a "biosimilar" drug for the pharmaceutical company and the patient.

**Read the scenario, and answer the following questions on a separate sheet of paper.**

A 65-year-old man with liver cirrhosis is admitted to the medical-surgical unit with nausea and vomiting. He also has a diagnosis of heart failure. You note that his serum albumin (protein) level is low. The physician has written admission orders, and you are trying to make the patient comfortable. He is to take nothing by mouth except for clear liquids. An intravenous (IV) infusion of dextrose 5% in water at 50 mL/hr has been ordered, and the nurses have had difficulty inserting his IV line.

1. One of the drugs ordered is known to reach a maximum level in the body of 200 mg/L and has a half-life of 2 hours. If this maximum level of 200 mg/L is reached at 1600 hours, then what will the drug's level in the body be at 2200?

2. Describe how factors identified in the patient's history would affect the following:
   a. Absorption
   b. Distribution
   c. Metabolism
   d. Excretion

3. Placement of a peripherally inserted central catheter is ordered. The physician writes an order for a dose of an IVPB antibiotic to be given as soon as IV access is established. What is the reason for this order?

4. This patient is also receiving digoxin for heart failure. This drug is known to have a low therapeutic index. Explain this concept and what will be done to monitor the patient's response.

# 3 Lifespan Considerations

## CHAPTER REVIEW AND NCLEX® EXAMINATION PREPARATION

**Select the best answer for each question.**

1. Which physiologic factor is most responsible for the differences in the pharmacokinetic and pharmacodynamic behavior of drugs in neonates and adults?
   a. Infant's stature
   b. Infant's smaller weight
   c. Immaturity of neonatal organs
   d. Adult's longer exposure to toxins

2. Understanding the role of the kidney in the elimination of drugs from the body, which laboratory test assessment is priority in evaluating kidney function?
   a. Albumin level
   b. Red blood cell count
   c. Creatine
   d. Bicarbonate

3. Most drug references provide recommended pediatric dosages based on which of the following?
   a. Total body water content
   b. Fat-to-lean mass ratio
   c. Renal function studies
   d. Body weight in kilograms

4. The nurse recognizes that drug dosages in older adults are based on which factor?
   a. Age
   b. Weight
   c. Total body water
   d. Serum albumin

5. When giving medications to older adults, the nurse will keep in mind the changes that occur as a result of aging. Which statements regarding changes in the older patient are true? *(Select all that apply.)*
   a. The ratio of fat to water is increased.
   b. Gastric pH is less acidic because of reduced hydrochloric acid production.
   c. Protein albumin binding sites are reduced because of decreased serum protein.
   d. Total body water content increases as body composition changes.
   e. The absorptive surface area of the gastrointestinal tract is increased because of flattening and blunting of the villi.

6. Which factor would have the greatest effect on medication response in the newborn?
   a. Immaturity of the organs
   b. Increased muscle mass
   c. Increased protein binding
   d. Less drugs enter the brain

7. A child is to receive a medication that is dosed as 8 mg/kg. The child weighs 40 kg. What is the dose of medication that the nurse will administer to this child? _____

8. A toddler is to receive a daily dose of digoxin 2 mcg/kg/day IV. The toddler weighs 23 lb. Calculate the amount of medication in milligrams that the toddler will receive. _____

9. The medication in Question 7 is available in a vial of 0.1 mg/mL. Calculate how much solution the nurse will draw up into the syringe and then mark the syringe with your answer.

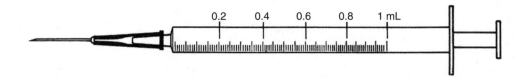

10. Which explanation underpins the nurse's understanding that the greatest risk to the fetus to the exposure of maternal drugs occurs in the first semester?
    a. This is the period of organogenesis.
    b. This is the period of greatest placental blood flow.
    c. This is the period of nutritional interruption because of pregnancy-induced emesis.
    d. This is the period of greatest resistance to insulin receptors throughout the maternal body.

**Match each pregnancy safety category with its corresponding description.**

11. _____ Category A

12. _____ Category B

13. _____ Category C

14. _____ Category D

15. _____ Category X

a. Possible fetal risk in humans is reported; however, consideration of potential benefit versus risk may, in selected cases, warrant use of these drugs in pregnant women.
b. Studies indicate no risk to animal fetuses; information for humans is not available.
c. Fetal abnormalities are reported, and positive evidence of fetal risk in humans is available from animal or human studies.
d. Studies indicate no risk to human fetuses.
e. Adverse effects are reported in animal fetuses; information for humans is not available.

### CRITICAL THINKING AND APPLICATION

**Answer the following questions on a separate sheet of paper.**

16. The nurse works at a community clinic frequented by a number of older patients. Mrs. M. comes to the clinic complaining of dizziness and nausea. As the nurse takes her medication history, she shows the nurse her "pill box." Inside the nurse sees almost a dozen different pills, all to be taken at noon. How could this happen? How could she possibly need so many medications at the same time?

17. The physician confirms that Mrs. M.'s "new symptoms," as she refers to them, are a result of polypharmacy. She protests, telling the nurse, "Honey, I've got news for the doctor. I've had to take lots of drugs at the same time all my life. It never bothered me before. Why would it now when I'm even more used to it?" Explain at least three physiologic changes that occur with aging and the way in which these changes affect pharmacokinetics and pharmacodynamics.

18. A 14-year-old girl has been diagnosed with type 1 diabetes mellitus, and the nurse is preparing to teach her how to test her own blood glucose levels with a glucometer. Describe some strategies that would be effective for this teaching session.

19. A nurse presenting information to new mothers at a community center is asked about the differences among infants, children, and adults in response to medications. What facts regarding these differences should the nurse include in her response?

### CASE STUDY

**Read the scenario, and answer the following questions on a separate sheet of paper.**

You are performing telephone triage in a pediatric clinic. A mother calls about her 28-month-old toddler, who has had chickenpox for 2 days. She wants to give aspirin because the toddler's fever is 101° F (38.3° C) but is unsure because her toddler "hates to take pills."

1. Should the mother use aspirin for this fever? Refer to Chapter 44 as needed for developmental considerations for the use of aspirin.

2. The mother states that her husband is going to the drugstore for some medicine. What advice will you give her regarding the dosage form of an antipyretic for her toddler?

3. When the husband returns from the store, he shows the mother the bottle of generic acetaminophen liquid suspension formula for children that was recommended by the store's pharmacist. He wonders, though, why the pharmacist would need to know the toddler's weight before suggesting this medication. Explain.

4. The toddler receives a dose of 1 tsp per the directions for a child of his weight of 28 lb. Later, when his 5-year-old sister needs a dose, she receives 1.5 tsp because she weighs 45 lb. If the drug contains 160 mg per teaspoon, then how many milligrams of medication did the 5-year-old child receive in her dose?

5. What should the parents look for when evaluating the children's responses to a dose of acetaminophen?

# 4 Cultural, Legal, and Ethical Considerations

## CHAPTER REVIEW AND NCLEX® EXAMINATION PREPARATION

**Select the best answer for each question.**

1. When reviewing drug classifications, the nurse knows that drugs classified as category C-I, which are to be dispensed "only with an approved protocol," include which drugs?
   a. Codeine, cocaine, and meperidine (Demerol)
   b. Heroin, LSD, and marijuana
   c. Phenobarbital, chloral hydrate, and benzodiazepines
   d. Cough preparations and diarrhea-control drugs

2. When a health care provider is writing a prescription for a drug, he or she is not permitted to mark a refill on the prescription if the drug falls into which category?
   a. C-II
   b. C-III
   c. C-IV
   d. C-V

3. The nurse is aware that the ethical principle of "Do no harm" is known by which name?
   a. Autonomy
   b. Beneficence
   c. Confidentiality
   d. Nonmaleficence

4. Which legal act required drug manufacturers to establish the safety and efficacy of a new drug before its approval for use?
   a. Federal Food and Drugs Act of 1906
   b. Federal Food, Drug, and Cosmetic Act of 1938
   c. Kefauver-Harris Amendment of 1962
   d. Durham-Humphrey Amendment of 1951

5. Which is the correct definition of *placebo*?
   a. An investigational drug used in a new drug study
   b. An inert substance that is not a drug
   c. A legend drug that requires a prescription
   d. A substance that is not approved as a drug but is used as an herbal product

6. The nurse is performing an admission assessment. Which finding is considered part of the cultural assessment?
   a. The patient uses aspirin as needed for pain.
   b. The patient has a history of hypertension.
   c. The patient is allergic to shellfish.
   d. The patient does not eat pork products for religious reasons.

7. While reviewing a newsletter about medications, the nurse notices that one drug has a new black box warning from the Food and Drug Administration (FDA). What does this warning entail? *(Select all that apply.)*
   a. The drug is about to be recalled by the FDA.
   b. Serious adverse effects have been reported with the use of this drug.
   c. The drug can still be prescribed, but the warning is present to make sure that the prescriber is aware of the potentially significant risks.
   d. The drug manufacturer has refused to recall the medication despite documented problems.
   e. The drug cannot be prescribed.

8. The nurse is to administer ranitidine (Zantac) 150 mg IV. The available medication is ranitidine 25 mg/mL. How many milliliters will the nurse administer? _____

9. Mark the syringe with the amount of medication the nurse will draw up for Question 8.

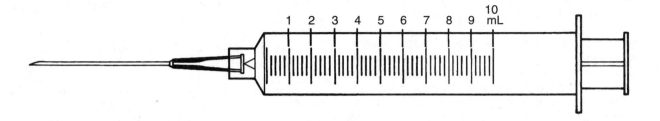

10. Which term applies to differences observed in patients' response to medications based on ethnicity?
    a. Pharmacogenomics
    b. Drug polymorphism
    c. Pharmacodynamics
    d. Drug intolerance

11. Which drug response finding would the nurse expect in patients who are identified as slow acetylators?
    a. No change in bioavailability
    b. Elevated drug concentrations
    c. Enhanced first-pass effect
    d. Absence of protein binding

## MATCHING

**Match each investigational drug study phase with its corresponding description.**

12. _____ Phase I

13. _____ Phase II

14. _____ Phase III

15. _____ Phase IV

a. A study using small numbers of volunteers who have the disease or disorder that the drug is meant to diagnose or treat; subjects are monitored for drug effectiveness and adverse effects
b. Postmarketing studies conducted by drug companies to obtain further proof of the drug's therapeutic and adverse effects
c. A study that involves a large number of patients at research centers designed to monitor for infrequent adverse effects and to identify any associated risks; double-blind, placebo-controlled studies eliminate patient and researcher bias
d. A study that uses small numbers of healthy volunteers, as opposed to volunteers with the target ailment, to determine dosage range and pharmacokinetics

**Match each cultural group with its corresponding cultural practice.**

16. _____ Asian

17. _____ Hispanic

18. _____ Native American

19. _____ African American

a. May believe in herbal remedies; heat; acupuncture
b. May use folk medicine or root doctors; may use herbs, oils, and roots
c. May believe that health is the result of good luck and living right and that illness is a result of doing bad
d. May believe in living in harmony with nature; may believe that ill spirits cause disease

## CRITICAL THINKING AND APPLICATION

**Answer the following questions on a separate sheet of paper.**

20. During morning report, a nurse is asked to work on a transplant unit for the day. The nurse has personal objections to working on that unit for religious reasons. What is the best course of action for the nurse in this situation?

21. Identify a cultural group in the area in which you live, and explore the health belief practices for that group.
    a. Are there any barriers to adequate health care?
    b. What is the attitude toward Western medicines and health treatments?
    c. What questions should you ask in your cultural assessment?

Chapter **4 Cultural, Legal, and Ethical Considerations**

**Read the scenario, and answer the following questions on a separate sheet of paper.**

You work in an outpatient treatment clinic for patients with human immunodeficiency virus (HIV) infection. During a recent staff meeting, the medical director discussed a new drug that has shown good results in clinical trials in another country. This drug has not yet been tested in the United States. She stated that she hopes to start clinical trials of that drug in the HIV clinic.

The following week, you are asked to start a new drug regimen for four patients with HIV infection. One of the drugs is new to you, and when you ask about it, the medical director replies, "Oh, that's the new drug I mentioned last week! One of my colleagues in that country sent me some samples, so we're going to try it here. The Food and Drug Administration has already started trials here in the United States. We will be comparing how these four patients do compared with four other patients who are in the same stages of HIV infection. The patients won't even know about this change."

1. Should you give the drugs as requested? If not, what needs be done to correct the situation?

2. What ethical principles guide your decision?

3. One of the potential study patients, brought in by his brother, seems reluctant to answer questions and says he "doesn't need any drugs." Upon further questioning, you find out that he would prefer to take some home remedies that his mother has made for him. How will you handle this situation?

4. When you meet with potential study patients, several mention that they fear others will find out about their illness if they participate in the study. What will you tell these patients?

# 5 Medication Errors: Preventing and Responding

## CHAPTER REVIEW AND NCLEX® EXAMINATION PREPARATION

**Provide the best answer by filling in the blank for each question.**

1. Any preventable unexpected response to a drug involving inappropriate medication use by a patient or health care professional, which may or may not cause the patient harm, is a(n) _____.

2. A(n) _____ is defined as an unexpected, unintended, or excessive response to a medication given at therapeutic dosages (as opposed to over-dose) and is one type of adverse drug event.

3. A(n) _____ is an immunologic reaction resulting from an unusual sensitivity of a patient to a particular medication.

4. A(n) _____ reaction is any abnormal and unexpected response to a medication, other than an allergic reaction, that is peculiar to an individual patient.

**Provide the answer to each question.**

5. True or false: High-alert medications are involved in more errors than other drugs. Explain your answer.

6. True or false: Allergic reactions are often predictable. Explain your answer.

7. Identify five actions to help prevent medication errors.

8. Identify the four categories of medication errors.

9. Name at least four of the classes of medications that are considered "high-alert" drugs.

10. Outline the process of medication reconciliation.

11. The National Coordinating Council for Medication Error Reporting and Prevention recommends that certain terms be written out in full instead of being abbreviated. Write out the full meaning of each abbreviated word or phrase that appears in bold in the following list.

| | |
|---|---|
| Digoxin 125 mcg PO **now** | |
| Lasix 40 mg IV **qd** | |
| **d/c** all meds | |
| NPH insulin 12 **u** subcut every morning before breakfast | |
| Floxin Otic 1 **gtt** AD bid | |
| Lactulose 30 mL PO **q.o.d.** | |

12. The medication order reads: "Metoprolol 25 mg PO twice a day for high blood pressure. Hold if systolic blood pressure is less than 95 mm Hg." Today the pharmacy supplied 50-mg tablets because there were no 25-mg tablets in stock.
    a. How many tablets will the nurse administer per dose? _____
    b. The nurse gives the patient the entire tablet. How many milligrams does the patient receive? _____
    c. What will the nurse do next? _____

13. The order reads: "Give levothyroxine (Synthroid) 50 mcg PO every morning." Which answer correctly depicts the dose in milligrams?
    a. 0.05 mg
    b. 0.05 mg
    c. 0.050 mg
    d. 50,000 mg

14. The order reads: "Give furosemide 50 mg per gastrostomy tube every morning." The medication is available in liquid form, 10 mg/1 mL. Calculate how much medication the nurse will administer.

    _____

15. Mark the medication cup with the answer you obtained for Question 14.

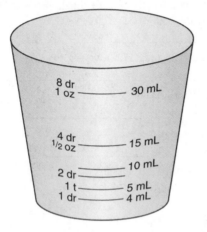

16. The patient develops Stevens-Johnson syndrome after administration of Dilantin. The nurse would recognize this is a(n)
    a. allergic response.
    b. expected outcome.
    c. adverse reaction.
    d. sign of a medication error.

**Read the scenario, and answer the following questions on a separate sheet of paper.**

A nursing student discovers that she has given her patient two aspirin tablets instead of the one-tablet daily dose that was ordered for antiplatelet effects. She is upset and talks to her fellow students, who tell her to keep quiet about it. "One extra aspirin won't hurt your patient," they tell her.

1. What should the nursing student do first? Describe other appropriate actions after the initial action.

2. How could the student have prevented this error?

3. Should the patient be told about it? Explain your answer.

4. If the patient was not hurt by this incident, then is it considered a medication error? Explain.

5. The student has decided to inform her instructor. The instructor helps the student complete a hospital incident report and a report to the US Pharmacopeia Medication Errors Reporting Program (USPMERP). Explain the reason for this report. Will the student's name be reported to the USPMERP?

# 6 Patient Education and Drug Therapy

**Select the best answer for each question.**

1. A nurse is preparing for an education session on safe medication administration. Which is the best example of a learning activity that involves the cognitive domain?
   a. Teaching a patient how to self-administer nasal spray
   b. Teaching a patient how to measure the pulse before taking digoxin
   c. Discussing which foods to avoid while taking oral anticoagulants
   d. Teaching a family member how to give an injection

2. The nurse is developing a discharge plan regarding a patient's medications. When is the ideal time to begin discharge planning?
   a. When family members are present
   b. Just before the patient leaves the hospital
   c. When the patient has been medicated for pain
   d. As soon as possible when the patient is ready

3. The nurse is providing discharge teaching for a patient who has a new colostomy after a partial colectomy. Reading material at which grade level is most useful for patient education materials?
   a. 10th grade
   b. 8th grade
   c. 6th grade
   d. 1st grade

4. A nurse has completed an education session on self-administration of insulin injections. Which statement(s) describe successful learning in the affective domain? *(Select all that apply.)*
   a. The patient states, "I am feeling more confident about insulin self-injection."
   b. The patient states, "It is essential to check my blood sugar before I take the insulin."
   c. The patient states, "Insulin works to lower my blood sugar levels."
   d. The patient measures the correct amount of insulin in the syringe for the injection.
   e. The patient self-injects the insulin using the correct technique.

5. An important first step in developing a teaching plan for a patient is
   a. identifying the patient's readiness to learn and current knowledge level.
   b. establishing the outcomes of the learning experience.
   c. collecting all of the teaching materials.
   d. finding a place where they will be uninterrupted for teaching to occur.

6. Which teaching and learning outcome would best address an objective in the psychomotor domain regarding the application of a nitroglycerin patch?
   a. The patient removes the old patch before placing a new one and chooses an area free of hair and scars.
   b. The patient correctly identifies three of five side effects of Nitro-Dur.
   c. The patient identifies the purpose of the nitroglycerin patch.
   d. The patients relates three fears regarding the use of a nitroglycerin patch.

**15**

7. A patient has been instructed to take 25 mg of diphenhydramine (Benadryl) oral syrup twice a day as treatment for a severe case of poison ivy. The medication comes in a bottle that contains 12.5 mg/5 mL. The nurse will be teaching the patient how to measure a dose of the medication. How many milliliters will the nurse measure for each dose?

_____

8. During a teaching session, the nurse demonstrates how to draw up insulin into a syringe. The patient then provides a return demonstration and draws up 17 units of insulin. Mark on the syringe the correct dose of 17 units.

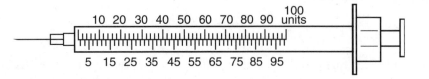

## CRITICAL THINKING AND APPLICATION

**Answer the following questions on a separate sheet of paper.**

9. The nurse is to present information regarding antihypertensive drug therapy to two patients, a 40-year-old patient and a 78-year-old patient. Describe the differences in interventions the nurse would use in his or her teaching strategies related to possible alterations in thought processes and sensory-perceptual status in these two patients.

10. The nurse is to present information to a young mother on how to help her 8-year-old child use a metered-dose inhaler. Neither the mother nor her child speaks English. Discuss strategies the nurse will use in developing a teaching plan for them.

11. The patient has been taking oral hypoglycemics for 1 month, and her blood glucose readings are still very high. On assessment, the nurse discovers a possible reason for these high readings. Develop a nursing diagnosis for this patient based on the following:
    a. The patient says that no one has ever told her about required dietary restrictions.
    b. The patient tells the nurse that she only takes the medication if she feels ill.

12. Develop a measurable outcome with specific measurement criteria related to teaching a patient about the medication therapy for transdermal nitroglycerin patches. Refer to Chapter 23 as needed.

13. Develop a patient teaching plan for a 55-year-old patient who will be receiving warfarin (Coumadin) therapy after discharge. Refer to Chapter 26 for information. Include the following:
    a. Assessment—the objective and subjective data that would be needed
    b. Nursing diagnosis
    c. Planning—a measurable outcome with specific criteria
    d. Implementation—specific educational strategies
    e. Evaluation—means for validating that learning has occurred

## CASE STUDY

**Read the scenario, and answer the following questions on a separate sheet of paper.**

A 77-year-old man, accompanied by his wife, visits the office for a 3-month checkup. He has been treated for hypertension and has a history of angina. While in the office, he pulls a small bottle of sublingual nitroglycerin tablets from his pants pocket and states, "I never go anywhere without these." He says he "gets along okay" with his medicines at home and that it "doesn't hurt anything" if he misses a day or two of his medications. His blood pressure today is 130/92 mm Hg, pulse rate is 88 beats/min, and respiratory rate is 12 breaths/min. Previously, his blood pressure readings have been 160/98, 152/92, and 148/94 mm Hg.

After the patient is evaluated by the physician, new medication orders are written as follows:

- Hydrochlorothiazide, 25-mg tablet, once a day
- Potassium chloride, 20-mEq tablet, once a day
- Diltiazem, 60-mg tablet, three times a day
- Lansoprazole, 15-mg capsule, before breakfast and dinner
- Nitroglycerin sublingual tablets, as needed for chest pain

1. Based on your assessment, what nursing diagnosis would you suggest for this situation?

2. State an outcome with measurable criteria for your nursing diagnosis.

3. Describe the teaching strategies you would use when teaching this patient about how to take his medications correctly.

4. How would you evaluate the effectiveness of the education process in this situation?

# 7 Over-the-Counter Drugs and Herbal and Dietary Supplements

## CRITICAL THINKING CROSSWORD

**Each statement refers to an herbal product that is described in the text. For reference, see the list of Safety: Herbal Therapies and Dietary Supplements boxes on the inside back cover of your text.**

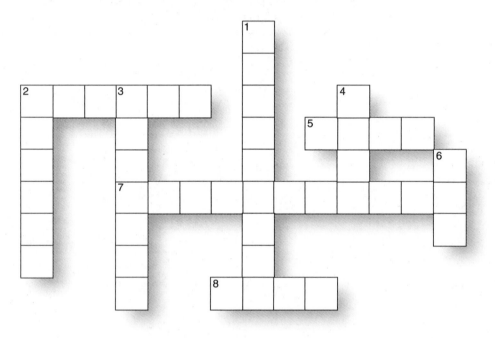

**Across**

2. Used for relief of nausea and vomiting induced by cancer chemotherapy, morning sickness, and motion sickness
5. Both the seed and the oil of this plant are used to reduce high cholesterol levels.
7. Used to relieve the symptoms of benign prostatic hyperplasia (two words)
8. Used to help promote relaxation or sleep; however, prolonged use may cause yellow discoloration of nails and skin and a risk for liver toxicity

**Down**

1. Used for its immunostimulant effect to reduce cold symptoms and recovery time when taken early in the illness
2. The dried leaf of this plant is used by some to prevent organic brain syndrome.
3. Has been used for more than 5000 years to improve physical endurance and concentration and reduce stress
4. The topical application of this plant has been known for years to aid in wound healing.
6. Used by women for relief of menopause symptoms as an alternative to hormonal therapy

**Select the best answer for each question.**

1. Which drug classes are commonly used as over-the-counter (OTC) remedies? *(Select all that apply.)*
   a. Nonsteroidal antiinflammatory drugs (NSAIDs)
   b. Cold remedies
   c. Antibiotics
   d. Smoking deterrent systems
   e. Antihypertensive drugs
   f. Histamine 2 ($H_2$) blockers

2. The nurse is reviewing drug therapy with OTC medications. Which is an advantage of OTC remedies?
   a. Third-party health insurance payers usually cover the costs.
   b. Patients can feel better faster when self-medicating.
   c. There are fewer drug interactions.
   d. Patients can self-treat minor ailments and reduce physician visits.

3. A patient is discussing his wish to use herbal products instead of medications and exclaims, "They work! The government tests them!" How will the nurse respond?
   a. "The U.S. Food and Drug Administration enforces standards of herbal product quality and safety."
   b. "The U.S. Food and Drug Administration requires the manufacturers of herbal products to prove that the herbals are effective."
   c. "The U.S. government sets standards for quality control of herbal products."
   d. "In the United States, herbal products are classified as dietary supplements and do not undergo testing for effectiveness."

4. A patient is asking about side effects of over the counter (OTC) drugs such as NSAIDs. The nurse would be correct in identifying which potential side effects? *(Select all that apply.)*
   a. Gastrointestinal ulceration
   b. Kidney dysfunction
   c. Myocardial infarction
   d. Stroke
   e. Pancreatitis

5. The nurse is admitting a patient who has a diagnosis of right lower lobe pneumonia. Upon assessment, the nurse learns that the patient is wearing an herbal pack on her chest. What will the nurse do first?
   a. Remove the pack immediately.
   b. Report the pack to the physician.
   c. Ask the patient about the herbal pack.
   d. Document the presence of the herbal pack.

6. A construction worker is treating himself with acetaminophen after an injury on the job. After 2 days, he comes to the urgent care facility because he thinks his hand is broken. He tells the nurse that he has been taking two "extra-strength" acetaminophen tablets six times a day, but he still has pain. Each tablet is 500 mg. How many milligrams per day has

   he taken? _____

7. Is there a concern regarding the construction worker's acetaminophen intake as described in Question 6? Explain your answer.

8. A patient is taking paroxetine, a selective serotonin reuptake inhibitor (SSRI), as part of treatment for depression. The patient tells the nurse that he has taken herbal products in the past and shows a list to the nurse. Which herbal product, if taken by the patient who is taking an SSRI, could cause an interaction?
   a. Garlic
   b. Echinacea
   c. St. John's wort
   d. Saw palmetto

9. During a clinic visit for a yearly examination, a patient asks the nurse about medications to take for heartburn. The patient shows the nurse the medication bottles that she had in her medicine cabinet. Which of these would be appropriate to use for the patient's heartburn, after checking for contraindications and other drug interactions? *(Select all that apply.)*
   a. Chlorpheniramine maleate
   b. Famotidine
   c. Clotrimazole
   d. Orlistat
   e. Omeprazole

10. The patient visits the warfarin clinic for follow-up and to get the results of the latest PT-INR. The nurse notes the INR levels indicate a significant risk for hemorrhage caused by prolonged clotting times. In conversation with the patient, the nurse obtains a list of all current medications. Which medication would the nurse suspect is contributing to the prolonged times?
    a. Saw palmetto
    b. St. John's wort
    c. Echinacea
    d. Garlic

11. An older adult patient is eating breakfast. The nurse knows this patient is taking a variety of different types of medications. Which item on the patient's tray would most concern the nurse about possible effects on drug metabolism?
    a. Whole-wheat toast
    b. Scrambled eggs
    c. Whole milk
    d. Grapefruit juice

## CRITICAL THINKING AND APPLICATION

**Answer the following questions on a separate sheet of paper.**

12. Review the Safety: Herbal Therapies and Dietary Supplements boxes for garlic, ginger, ginseng, flax, saw palmetto, ginkgo, and valerian in the appropriate chapters. (To help you locate these boxes, see the list inside the back cover of your textbook.) Which of these herbal products may have serious interactions with anticoagulants such as warfarin (Coumadin) and heparin?

13. List the types of individuals who may have more frequent adverse reactions to OTC drugs.

14. A patient tells the nurse that he has had diarrhea for more than 3 weeks and has been self-treating it at home with over-the-counter (OTC) drugs. "I thought it was something that I ate and that it would go away, but it didn't," he says. He states that he feels tired and weak, and the nurse notes that he shows some signs of dehydration. What concerns are there, if any, with this patient's self-treatment with OTC medications?

15. Identify an OTC product or herbal or dietary supplement that you (or a family member) take, and review the indications, drug interactions, contraindications, and adverse effects. Did you find any concerns?

## CASE STUDY

**Read the scenario, and answer the following questions on a separate sheet of paper. You may need to refer to the list of Safety: Herbal Therapies and Dietary Supplements boxes on the inside back cover of your textbook.**

A 30-year-old woman is in the clinic for her yearly gynecologic checkup. She is not pregnant but would like to have children soon and states that she and her husband are trying to conceive. She says that she is "very concerned" about her health and watches her diet and exercises regularly to stay in shape. She has a family history of heart disease but no other health concerns. Her physical assessment reveals no abnormalities or health problems.

On her medical history sheet, she writes that she takes several drug and herbal products, as follows:

- Echinacea, from September to March, to prevent the flu
- Adult aspirin, one tablet every day, to prevent a heart attack
- Garlic tablets twice a day for her heart
- Kava tea, as needed for relaxation
- One glass of red wine with dinner
- Valerian capsules for sleep, as needed (usually three or four times a week)

1. Does the patient's regimen of drugs and herbal products pose any risk for drug or herbal interactions?

2. Do any of these products have a potential for problems if used long term?

3. Will you focus on any specific information when taking the patient's history or performing an assessment, given that she is using these drugs and herbal products?

4. She tells you that she thinks the herbal products are "safe" because the government would not allow them to be sold if they were not. Is this true?

5. What would you emphasize when teaching her about the use of herbal products and OTC drugs?

# 8 | Gene Therapy and Pharmacogenomics

**Match each definition with its corresponding term. (Note: Not all terms will be used.)**

1. _____ A structure in the nucleus that contains a thread of DNA that transmits genetic information

2. _____ The particular alleles present at a given site on the chromosomes that determine a specific genetic trait for that organism

3. _____ The biologic unit of heredity

4. _____ The complete set of genetic material of any organism

5. _____ The study of genomes, including the way genes and their products work in both health and disease

a. Chromosome
b. Gene
c. Genome
d. Genomics
e. Genetics
f. Genotype
g. Pharmacogenetics

**Select the best answer for each question.**

6. The nurse is reviewing concepts of gene therapy. Which statements correctly describe possible approaches to gene therapy? *(Select all that apply.)*
   a. Replacing a mutated gene with a healthy copy of the gene
   b. Preventing an immature gene from growing into a mature gene
   c. Inactivating a mutated gene that is functioning improperly
   d. Introducing a new gene into the body to help fight a disease
   e. Causing the body to produce new genes

7. The nurse is explaining concepts of ethical issues related to gene therapy in the United States. Which statement is correct?
   a. The U.S. Food and Drug Administration approves all human clinical gene therapy trials.
   b. Gene therapy research poses little risk to the subjects who participate in studies.
   c. Eugenics is currently part of gene therapy research in the United States.
   d. Gene therapy is exempt from approval by an institutional review board.

8. Which bacteria has been employed in the development of the human insulin gene to generate human insulin?
   a. *Escherichia coli*
   b. *Streptococcus aureus*
   c. *Staphylococcus aureus*
   d. *Candida albicans*

## CRITICAL THINKING AND APPLICATION

**Answer the following questions on a separate sheet of paper.**

9. Describe the concept of eugenics as related to gene therapy in the United States.

10. What is recombinant DNA? Give an example of how this technology is useful in pharmacology.

11. A patient asks the nurse, "I read something about gene therapy. Has it been approved in the United States for routine treatment of disease?" How will the nurse answer the patient?

12. During a health history interview before a scheduled surgery, a patient tells the nurse, "Everyone in my family has had a bad reaction to pain medicines. Do you think I will also?" What is the most important action for the nurse at this time? How will the nurse answer this patient's question?

**21**

13. A patient's sister is visiting the patient, who is recovering from breast cancer surgery. As the sister leaves, she takes the nurse aside and asks, "I need to know something. I know they did genetic testing. Does she have the type of breast cancer that is genetic?" How will the nurse answer the patient's sister? Explain your answer.

## CASE STUDY

**Read the scenario, and answer the following questions on a separate sheet of paper.**

Dale, a 32-year-old construction worker, fell off a roof 2 months ago and, as a result, needs to have surgery on his ankle. The nurse is preparing him for the surgery and begins the admission process. During the interview, Dale mentions that he is a bit nervous because his cousin had surgery and had a "terrible reaction" to the medications.

1. Is this information about his cousin significant? Explain.

2. What further questions will the nurse ask?

3. When obtaining a genetic history, how many generations back should the nurse ask about?

4. What will be done concerning Dale's surgery?

# 9 Photo Atlas of Drug Administration

**Select the best answer for each question.**

1. The nurse is preparing to give an intradermal injection and will perform which action?
   a. Massage the site lightly after the injection.
   b. Have the patient massage the site until the pain diminishes.
   c. Avoid massaging the site.
   d. Apply heat to the site after the injection.

2. When giving a medication via intravenous push, how will the nurse correctly occlude the intravenous line?
   a. Pinch or clamp the tubing just above the injection port.
   b. Pinch the tubing at least 2 inches above the injection port.
   c. Fold the tubing just below the injection port.
   d. It is not necessary to occlude the tubing for this procedure.

3. The nurse is adding more than one medication to a solution. What is the priority action at this time?
   a. Use an equal volume of each medication.
   b. Assess the two drugs for compatibility.
   c. Add the drugs at least 1 hour apart.
   d. Use the same needle for both medications.

4. When administering oral medications, the nurse will follow which correct procedure?
   a. If a patient cannot swallow medications, crush all the medications together and administer with applesauce.
   b. Give oral medications with meals to avoid gastrointestinal upset.
   c. Stay with the patient until each medication has been swallowed.
   d. Give all medications on an empty stomach to facilitate absorption.

5. After administering eardrops, which action by the nurse is correct?
   a. Press a cotton ball firmly into the ear canal.
   b. Have the patient sit up and tilt the head for 2 to 3 minutes.
   c. Gently massage the tragus of the ear.
   d. Have the patient remain in the side-lying position for 20 minutes.

6. A nurse assessing the response of a patient to a sublingual or intravenous push medication would evaluate the patient according to which time frame?
   a. 1 hour
   b. 30 minutes
   c. 15 minutes
   d. Less than 5 minutes

7. As a portion of the new nine rights of medication administration, the nurse knows to use two patient identifiers before administering medications. The nurse would be functioning according to policy if which two identifiers were used?
   a. Patient name and city of birth
   b. Patient name and birthday
   c. Patient account number and supervising physician
   d. Confirmation of patient by family member and place of employment

8. Which position is correct when the nurse administers nasal drops for the frontal or maxillary sinuses?
   a. Tilt the patient's head backward and facing toward the left side.
   b. Tilt the patient's head back over the edge of the bed with the head turned toward the side treated.
   c. Place a pillow under the patient's shoulders and tilt back the head.
   d. Tilt the patient's head to the side opposite the side treated.

**23**

9. Which action by the nurse is correct when administering drugs via a nasogastric tube?
    a. Allow the fluid to flow via gravity.
    b. Use gentle but consistent pressure when forcing the fluid into the tube.
    c. Shake the tube gently to facilitate the movement of fluid in the tube.
    d. Confirm the placement of the tube after the medication is given.

10. The nurse is preparing to give a Z-track intramuscular injection. This technique is indicated in which situation?
    a. When there is insufficient muscle mass in the landmarked area
    b. Whenever massaging the area after medication administration is contraindicated
    c. With medications that are known to be irritating, painful, or staining to tissues
    d. With any injection that is given into the dorsogluteal muscle

11. When giving sublingual medications, the nurse recalls that medications given by this route have which advantage?
    a. They are immediately absorbed.
    b. They are excreted rapidly.
    c. They are metabolized immediately.
    d. They are distributed equally.

12. The prochlorperazine rectal suppository is twice the strength of what has actually been ordered. Which is the nurse's best action?
    a. Cut the suppository in half.
    b. Call the physician for clarification.
    c. Administer another type of suppository.
    d. Instruct the patient to retain the suppository for only 5 minutes.

13. During medication administration, which will the nurse consider to be a contraindication to the administration of rectal suppositories?
    a. Vomiting
    b. Fever
    c. Constipation
    d. Rectal bleeding

14. The nurse will apply a transdermal patch to a site that is
    a. over a bone.
    b. nonhairy.
    c. moist.
    d. within a skinfold.

15. What is important for the nurse to teach the patient about the instillation of nasal drops?
    a. Clear the nasal passages by blowing the nose gently before administering the medication.
    b. Clear the nasal passages by blowing the nose gently after administering the medication.
    c. Sit in a semi-Fowler's position for 5 minutes after the instillation of the medication.
    d. Place the nose dropper approximately ½ inch into the nostril when instilling drops.

16. Which interventions are correct regarding the administration of ophthalmic medications? *(Select all that apply.)*
    a. Have the patient look upward while instilling the medication.
    b. Instill the prescribed number of drops into the conjunctival sac.
    c. Have the patient close his or her eyes tightly after the drop has been instilled.
    d. Apply gentle pressure to the patient's nasolacrimal duct for 30 to 60 seconds after instilling the drops.
    e. Apply ointment to the conjunctival sac starting at the outer canthus and working toward the inner canthus.

17. When withdrawing insulin from a vial, the nurse needs to remove 14 units for the medication dosage. How much air will the nurse inject into the vial before removing the medication? Mark the syringe with your answer.

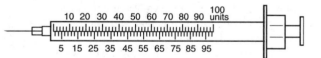

18. A 2-month-old child needs to receive pain medication after surgery. The order reads: "Give morphine sulfate, 0.05 mg/kg IV now." The infant weighs 10.5 lb. Calculate the number of milligrams the infant will receive. Round to hundredths. _____

19. Referring to your answer for Question 18, calculate how many milliliters of medication the nurse will draw up, and then mark the amount on the syringe. The medication comes in a vial of 0.5 mg/mL. _____

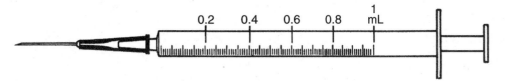

**Answer the following questions on a separate sheet of paper.**

20. Describe how to assess injection sites for each of the following:
    a. Subcutaneous injections
    b. Intramuscular injections
    c. Intradermal injections

21. Describe the proper technique of needle insertion for each of the following:
    a. Subcutaneous injections
    b. Intramuscular injections
    c. Intradermal injections

22. The nurse is administering an intramuscular injection. After the needle enters the site, the nurse grasps the lower end of the syringe barrel with the nondominant hand and slowly pulls back on the plunger to aspirate the drug. Blood appears in the syringe. What is the nurse's best action at this time?

23. The nurse is preparing an oral liquid medication for a patient. How does the usual procedure change when the volume of medication required is less than 5 mL?

24. A patient has been given a new inhaler that contains 100 doses of medication. The order specifies that the patient is to take "one puff four times a day." How many days will this inhaler last before it becomes empty?

## CASE STUDY

**Read the scenario, and answer the following questions on a separate sheet of paper.**

A mother comes to a family practice office with her 2-year-old daughter and 8-month-old son. She is planning a trip abroad and needs to obtain immunizations for herself and her children before she leaves.

1. The mother and the infant each need to be given an intramuscular immunization. Describe the differences in choosing sites and giving an intramuscular injection to the mother and the infant.

2. The 2-year-old daughter has an ear infection, and the physician has prescribed eardrops. What will you teach the mother about giving these eardrops to her daughter?

3. Two days later, the mother brings the infant back to the office because a high fever has developed. You prepare to give the infant a liquid oral antipyretic and note that the dose is 2 mL. How do you measure this medication?

4. The mother wants to add the medication to the baby's bottle. What is the best method for administering the liquid medication to the infant?

# 10 Analgesic Drugs

## CRITICAL THINKING CROSSWORD

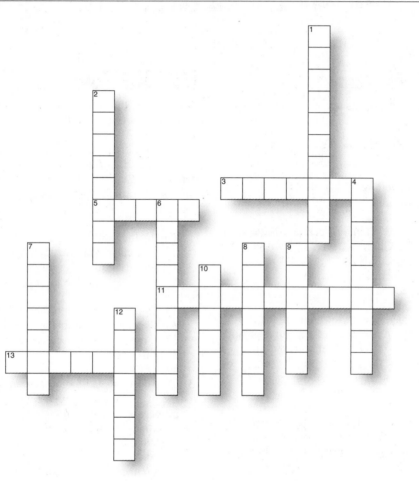

**Across**

3. Any drug that binds to a receptor and causes a

   response has _____ properties.
5. Mrs. M. had breast reduction surgery yesterday and is complaining of pain around her incisions. Mrs. M. is

   experiencing _____ pain.
11. Mrs. G. is experiencing pain and itching as a result of a severe case of poison ivy on the skin of her arms

    and legs. She is experiencing _____ pain.

13. Mr. E. paces the floor all night, holding his side. The pain is so severe that he is nauseated. His wife brings him to the emergency department, where it is quickly discovered that Mr. E. has a kidney stone. The type of pain he has been experiencing is

    _____ pain.

**Down**

1. Mr. D.'s drug binds to a receptor, but the drug prevents, or blocks, a response. He is taking a drug with

   _____ properties.
2. When a second drug is given with a primary analgesic to enhance the analgesic effect, the second drug is

   being used as a(n) _____ drug.
4. Mr. P. is receiving an opioid around the clock for late-stage cancer pain. Lately, he has found that the pain medication is not working as well as it did a week ago. This is an example of opioid

   _____.
6. The level of stimulus needed to produce a painful

   sensation is referred to as the pain _____.
7. Mr. J. twisted his ankle in a friendly basketball game with his peers after work. His wife brings him to the urgent care center several hours later because of the pain. Mr. J. is probably experiencing

   _____ pain.
8. Mrs. H. has experienced back pain "for years." She says that it is worse in the late afternoon and at night but that "really, even when it lessens somewhat, it is there all the time in some form." Mrs. H. is

   experiencing _____ pain.
9. Mr. R. is brought to the emergency department in severe pain. The emergency department team recognizes the need to immediately bring the pain under some control. After assessing that it is not contraindicated, the attending physician initiates administration of a very strong pain reliever. This is no

   doubt a(n) _____ analgesic.
10. This word is often used interchangeably with the term *opioid*.
12. Ms. T. is taking a drug that binds to part of a receptor and causes effects that are not as strong as those of a pure agonist. She is taking a(n)

   _____ agonist.

## CHAPTER REVIEW AND NCLEX® EXAMINATION PREPARATION

**Select the best answer for each question.**

1. During a marathon, a runner had to drop out after 16 miles because of severe muscle spasms. Which type of pain is the runner experiencing?
   a. Chronic pain
   b. Somatic pain
   c. Visceral pain
   d. Superficial pain

2. A young man has been taken to the emergency department because of a suspected overdose of morphine tablets. The nurse prepares to administer which drug?
   a. Atropine
   b. Activated charcoal
   c. Flumazenil
   d. Naloxone

3. An anticonvulsant drug has been ordered as part of a patient's pain management program. The nurse explains to the patient that the purpose of the anticonvulsant is to
   a. produce sleep.
   b. prevent seizures.
   c. relieve neuropathic pain.
   d. reduce anxiety.

4. Moderate to severe pain is best treated with which medication?
   a. Acetaminophen
   b. Aspirin
   c. Alprazolam
   d. Fentanyl

5. The nurse is preparing to administer an opioid analgesic. Which factors should be assessed before the dose is given? *(Select all that apply.)*
   a. Blood clotting times
   b. The level of pain rated on a scale
   c. Prior analgesic use (time, type, amount, and effectiveness)
   d. Dietary history
   e. Allergies

6. When evaluating the patient's drug history, the nurse notes the patient is taking an opioid twice a day for pain. Which additional drug, taken concurrently, would concern the nurse the most?
   a. An antihistamine
   b. A calcium channel blocker
   c. A monoamine oxidase inhibitor
   d. A disease-modifying antirheumatic drug

7. Acetaminophen is similar to nonsteroidal antiinflammatory drugs with the exception that it lacks which effects? *(Select all that apply.)*
   a. Antipyretic
   b. Antiinflammatory
   c. Analgesic
   d. Antiplatelet
   e. GI irritation

8. A patient complaining of severe knee pain visits the clinic. He states that he twisted his knee last week and has been self-medicating with an old prescription of Percocet and extra-strength acetaminophen. He tells the nurse that he takes "two of the acetaminophen four times a day and two Percocets twice a day." The Percocet contains acetaminophen 325 mg and oxycodone 5 mg; the extra-strength acetaminophen contains 500 mg per tablet. How much acetaminophen has he taken per day, and is this a concern? Explain your answer.

9. A postoperative patient is complaining of pain at a level of 7 on a scale of 1 to 10. The nurse checks the medication administration sheet and sees that the patient can receive morphine oral solution (Roxanol) 6 mg PO every 4 hours, and the patient has not had a dose for 8 hours. The medication comes in a 5-mL unit dose container that is labeled 10 mg/5 mL. How many milliliters will the nurse administer to the patient? _____.

10. A patient is to receive fentanyl (Sublimaze) 60 mcg IV stat. The drug is available in vials that contain 50 mcg/mL. How many milliliters will the nurse administer for this dose? _____.

11. Mark the syringe with the answer you obtained for Question 10.

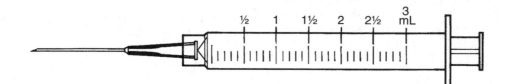

## MATCHING

Match each type of pain with its corresponding description.

12. _____ Acute pain

13. _____ Chronic pain

14. _____ Somatic pain

15. _____ Visceral pain

16. _____ Superficial pain

17. _____ Vascular pain

18. _____ Neuropathic pain

19. _____ Phantom pain

20. _____ Central pain

a. Pain that is thought to account for most migraine headaches
b. Pain that relates to a body part that has been removed
c. Pain that originates from the skin or mucous membranes
d. Pain that occurs with tumors, trauma, or inflammation of the brain
e. Persistent or recurring pain that is often difficult to treat
f. Pain that is sudden and usually subsides when treated
g. Pain that originates from the organs or smooth muscles
h. Pain that originates from the skeletal muscles, ligaments, or joints
i. Pain that results from injury or damage to the peripheral nerve fibers

## CASE STUDY

**Read the scenario, and answer the following questions on a separate sheet of paper.**

A 58-year-old woman has been admitted for a total abdominal hysterectomy. That evening, she asks for pain medication. Upon assessment, you find that she rates her pain level as an 8 on a scale from 1 to 10 and states that her pain is located mainly in the immediate area around her incision. You prepare to give her an intravenous dose of morphine sulfate.

1. What type of pain is she experiencing?

2. Within 1 hour of receiving the morphine, the patient complains that her skin feels "itchy," but she cannot see any hives. What do you tell her?

3. What serious adverse effect is possible if she receives too much morphine sulfate? What, if anything, can be given to treat this?

4. The next day, she is ready to be discharged home. Her physician writes a prescription for hydrocodone–acetaminophen (Vicodin). The patient sees the generic label and asks why the medication contains Tylenol. Explain the purpose of the acetaminophen (Tylenol) in this medication and for her pain treatment.

# 11 General and Local Anesthetics

**Match each term with its corresponding definition or description.**

1. _____ A type of anesthetic that is applied directly to the skin and mucous membranes

2. _____ A rapid- to intermediate-acting nondepolarizing neuromuscular blocking drug (NMBD)

3. _____ The term for anesthetic drugs that alter the central nervous system (CNS), resulting in loss of consciousness and deep muscle relaxation

4. _____ A type of anesthetic drug that reduces pain sensations at the level of the peripheral nerves

5. _____ Drugs used in combination with anesthetics for anesthesia initiation (induction), sedation, reduction of anxiety, and amnesia

6. _____ The term for drugs that depress the CNS; used for surgical procedures

7. _____ The practice of using combinations of drugs to produce general anesthesia rather than using a single drug

8. _____ An anticholinergic drug given preoperatively to dry secretions

9. _____ Generic name for the drug that is most often used for moderate-sedation procedures

10. _____ The only depolarizing neuromuscular blocking drug (NMBD) available; used for endotracheal intubation

a. Anesthetics
b. Midazolam
c. Atropine
d. Adjunctive
e. Local
f. Topical
g. Rocuronium
h. Succinylcholine
i. Balanced
j. General

**Select the best answer for each question.**

11. Which drug classes are used as adjunctive drugs with anesthesia? *(Select all that apply.)*
    a. Sedative-hypnotics
    b. Anticonvulsants
    c. Anticholinergics
    d. Inhaled gases
    e. Opioid analgesics

12. While assisting with a procedure in the emergency department, the nurse prepares lidocaine (Xylocaine) for use with which type of anesthesia?
    a. Moderate sedation
    b. Infiltration
    c. Intravenous
    d. General

13. The nurse monitoring a patient after surgery keeps in mind that the primary concern with the use of a neuromuscular blocking drug is which adverse effect?
    a. Respiratory arrest
    b. Headache
    c. Bradycardia
    d. Hypertension

14. To decrease the possibility of a headache after spinal anesthesia, the nurse will provide which instruction to the patient?
    a. Sit in high Fowler's position.
    b. Maintain strict bedrest.
    c. Limit fluids.
    d. Ambulate in the hall several times a day.

15. The nurse is reviewing a policy for local anesthesia. Local anesthesia is indicated for which procedures? *(Select all that apply.)*
    a. Cardioversions
    b. Suturing a skin laceration
    c. Diagnostic procedures
    d. Long-duration surgery
    e. Dental procedures

16. A patient who has just returned from surgery has suddenly developed a severe elevation in body temperature. The nurse recognizes that this change may indicate which condition?
    a. A normal temperature change after surgery
    b. Malignant hypertension
    c. Malignant hyperthermia
    d. Fever

17. During a procedure, the nurse is monitoring a patient who has received dexmedetomidine (Precedex) for moderate sedation. The nurse will observe for which potential adverse effect?
    a. Respiratory depression
    b. Tachycardia
    c. Dizziness
    d. Hypotension

18. Which of the following is an identified advantage for the use of nitrous oxide?
    a. It demonstrates effectiveness as a single agent.
    b. It has good analgesic properties.
    c. It does not promote postoperative nausea and vomiting.
    d. It offers a parenteral and inhaled route option.

19. When the effects of local anesthetics begin to wear off, which physiologic response is the first to occur?
    a. Memory returns.
    b. Motor activity returns.
    c. Sensory activity returns.
    d. Autonomic activity returns.

20. Which is a new selective relaxant binding agent that is used for reversal of rocuronium or vecuronium?
    a. Sugammadex
    b. Succinylcholine
    c. Rocuronium
    d. Pancuronium

21. A patient is receiving a neuromuscular blocking drug. Indicate the order in which the following areas become paralyzed once this drug is given (1 = first; 3 = last).

    _____ a. Limbs, neck, trunk muscles

    _____ b. Intercostal muscles and diaphragm

    _____ c. Small, rapidly moving muscles, such as those of the fingers and eyes

22. A patient has an order to receive atropine sulfate, 0.4 mg IM, as a preoperative medication. The vial contains atropine sulfate, 1 mg/mL. How many milliliters of medication will the nurse draw up for this injection? _____

23. In preparation for a colonoscopy, a patient is to receive midazolam, 0.05 mg IV push over 2 minutes. The medication comes in a strength of 1 mg/mL. How much medication will the nurse draw up into the syringe for this dose? _____

## CRITICAL THINKING AND APPLICATION

**Answer the following questions on a separate sheet of paper.**

24. Henry is a student nurse who has assisted the nurse anesthetist in surgery on prior occasions. Today, however, he is nervous because it is a child who will undergo general anesthesia. Why might this make Henry more nervous than usual?

25. Mr. S. is being administered a neuromuscular blocking drug while he is receiving mechanical ventilation. What is the most important thing the nurse needs to remember when working with him during this therapy?

26. Mrs. E. will undergo cardioversion this afternoon, and the nurse anesthetist has explained to her that she will not be asleep but that she will not remember the procedure. Mrs. E. asks, "How can this be?" What is the nurse anesthetist's explanation?

27. A patient is in the emergency department because he accidentally put a nail into his arm with a nail gun. The emergency provider requests "lidocaine with epinephrine," but the only type available in the supply cart is "plain" lidocaine. What is the difference, and why does it matter which one is used?

## CASE STUDY

**Read the scenario, and answer the following questions on a separate sheet of paper.**

You are a nursing student, and today you are assigned to an observation day in the operating room, with a certified registered nurse anesthetist (CRNA) as your contact for the day. The first case is a patient undergoing a right lower lung lobectomy because of lung cancer. The patient has a history of paraplegia from an old automobile accident. The patient's blood pressure has been maintained at 120/72 mm Hg, and the pulse has ranged from 100 to 110 beats/min during the surgery. The patient's body temperature has lowered to 96.2° F (35.7° C) after surgery. The patient's respirations have been maintained by ventilator.

1. Before the surgery, the CRNA explains that the patient will undergo "balanced anesthesia." What is meant by this term?

2. What is the purpose of administering the drug succinylcholine (Anectine) during anesthesia?

3. As your patient goes to the postanesthesia care unit (PACU), the CRNA asks you to monitor for signs of succinylcholine toxicity. Why would this be of concern at this time?

4. What can be done if the patient has received too much succinylcholine?

5. Another patient is undergoing a procedure performed using local anesthesia. Are there advantages of this type of anesthesia over general anesthesia?

6. In the PACU, what are the main concerns of the nurse monitoring the patient recovering from anesthesia?

# 12 Central Nervous System Depressants and Muscle Relaxants

**Select the best answer for each question.**

1. When reviewing actions of drugs, the nurse recognizes that a hypnotic is a drug that performs which action?
   a. Produces sleep
   b. Stops seizures
   c. Prevents nausea and vomiting
   d. Relieves pain

2. A patient who has been taking a benzodiazepine for 5 weeks has been instructed to stop the medication. Which instruction will the nurse provide to the patient on how to discontinue the medication?
   a. Stop taking the drug immediately.
   b. Plan a gradual reduction in dosage.
   c. Overlap this medication with another drug.
   d. Take the medication every other day for a number of weeks.

3. A patient will be undergoing a brief surgical procedure to obtain a biopsy from a superficial mass on his arm. The nurse expects that which type of barbiturate will be used at this time?
   a. Ultrashort
   b. Short
   c. Intermediate
   d. Long

4. While monitoring a patient who took an overdose of barbiturates, the nurse keeps in mind that a potential cause of death would be which of these?
   a. Tachycardia
   b. Hypertension
   c. Dyspnea
   d. Respiratory arrest

5. A patient with back muscle spasms is being treated with a skeletal muscle relaxant. To ensure that these drugs are most effective, the nurse will make sure what other treatment is ordered?
   a. Benzodiazepines
   b. Moist heat
   c. Physical therapy
   d. Aspirin

6. The nurse is providing care for a patient who has accidentally taken an overdose of benzodiazepines. Which drug would be used to treat this patient?
   a. Methamphetamine
   b. Flumazenil
   c. Epinephrine
   d. Naloxone

7. Which drug represents the only drug that acts directly on skeletal muscle?
   a. Diazepam
   b. Dantrolene
   c. Baclofen
   d. Methocarbamol

8. In which time frame should the nurse expect the greatest risk for hypotension after administration of muscle relaxants?
   a. 10 minutes after administration
   b. 60 minutes after administration
   c. 2 hours after administration
   d. 4 hours after administration

9. A patient will be receiving the barbiturate phenobarbital as part of treatment for seizures. The nurse assesses the patient's current list of medications. Which medications are known to cause interactions with barbiturates? *(Select all that apply.)*
   a. Benzodiazepines
   b. Proton pump inhibitors
   c. Oral contraceptives
   d. Anticoagulants
   e. Monoamine oxidase inhibitors (MAOIs)

10. A child will be receiving PO midazolam as preoperative sedation. The child weighs 33 lb. The dose ordered is 0.5 mg/kg, and the medication is available as a syrup, with a concentration of 2 mg/mL.
    a. What will be the dosage for this child?

    _____

    b. How much is the PO dose for this child in milliliters? _____

11. A patient is to receive diazepam 10 mg twice a day via a PEG tube. The medication comes in a liquid, with a concentration of 5 mg/5 mL. How many milliliters will the nurse administer with each dose? _____

12. Mark the medication cup with the amount of medication the nurse will administer for Question 11.

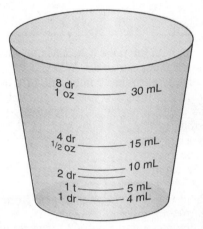

## CRITICAL THINKING AND APPLICATION

**Answer the following questions on a separate sheet of paper.**

13. A 19-year-old college freshman is brought into the emergency department with a suspected barbiturate overdose. What symptoms would you expect to see? How is overdose treated?

14. Jackie is taking benzodiazepines to treat her insomnia. Today she visits your clinic and states that she is going to Europe for 2 months and wants a prescription that will allow her to take enough medication along for her entire stay. The physician declines. Jackie is a little insulted and asks you why the physician refused her request. "Does my doctor think I'm an addict or something?" What do you explain to her? What other options are possible for her?

15. Mrs. A., who is 81 years of age, weighs significantly more than her 47-year-old daughter, yet she is given a lower dosage of a benzodiazepine for insomnia of a similar degree. Explain the rationale for the lower dose.

16. You have been asked to take a patient history for William, who will be given a benzodiazepine.
    a. What conditions or disorders will you ask about?
    b. What drug intake will you be most concerned about?
    c. What if William were an infant? A great-grandfather? Would this additional information matter? Why or why not?

17. Mr. P. is recovering from an automobile accident and has received a prescription for cyclobenzaprine for painful muscle spasms.
    a. What patient teaching will he need about this medication?
    b. What other measures should be included in addition to this drug therapy?

## CASE STUDY

**Read the scenario, and answer the following questions on a separate sheet of paper.**

A 54-year-old woman has had problems with insomnia "off and on for a few years" and has tried over-the-counter medications, herbal remedies, and prescription drugs. She likes to drink a glass of wine each night before going to bed. Today she is visiting the clinic for a checkup and asks for a prescription for secobarbital because that was the last drug she tried several years ago. The physician prescribes zaleplon instead. She says she can't understand why the doctor won't refill her prescription for secobarbital.

1. Why did the physician change her prescription?

2. What are the consequences of long-term use of barbiturates?

3. What interactions should she be cautioned about while she is taking zaleplon?

4. What other patient teaching is important for this patient?

Chapter **12** **Central Nervous System Depressants and Muscle Relaxants**

# 13 Central Nervous System Stimulants and Related Drugs

**Select the best answer for each question.**

1. The nurse is reviewing a patient's medication administration record. Which best describes a common use for doxapram?
   a. To control increased respiration caused by other drugs
   b. To treat drug-induced respiratory depression
   c. To treat postoperative respiratory excitation
   d. To stimulate respirations in a patient with a head injury

2. The nurse is administering a stimulant drug and expects which responses from stimulation of the central nervous system (CNS)? *(Select all that apply.)*
   a. Increased fatigue
   b. Decreased drowsiness
   c. Increased respiration
   d. Bradycardia
   e. Euphoria

3. A patient has asked for a cup of coffee. The nurse keeps in mind that patients with a history of which condition need to avoid caffeine?
   a. Cardiac dysrhythmias
   b. Asthma
   c. Diabetes mellitus
   d. Gallbladder disease

4. The physician has ordered orlistat. The nurse recognizes that this drug is used to treat which condition?
   a. Anorexia
   b. Malnutrition
   c. Narcolepsy
   d. Obesity

5. When a child is taking drugs for attention-deficit/hyperactivity disorder (ADHD), what will the nurse instruct the caregivers to closely monitor in the child?
   a. Blood glucose levels
   b. Physical growth, especially weight
   c. Grades at school
   d. Respiratory rates

6. A patient with migraine headaches is being treated with a serotonin antagonist. Which condition would cause the nurse to question the use of this class of medication to treat the patient's migraines? *(Select all that apply.)*
   a. Asthma
   b. Hypertension
   c. Glaucoma
   d. Diabetes mellitus

7. A patient will be taking sumatriptan (Imitrex) as part of treatment for migraine headaches. Before beginning therapy, the nurse reviews the patient's current list of medications. Which medications may have an interaction with sumatriptan? *(Select all that apply.)*
   a. Opioids
   b. Ergot alkaloids
   c. Selective serotonin reuptake inhibitors (SSRIs)
   d. Monoamine oxidase inhibitors (MAOIs)
   e. Nonsteroidal antiinflammatory drugs (NSAIDs)

8. In which patient population would the nurse expect to see the use of analeptics in the treatment of respiratory depression?
   a. Neonates
   b. Children
   c. Adults
   d. Older adults

9. A child will be taking amphetamine/dextroamphetamine for ADHD. He weighs 88 lb, and the initial dose ordered is 2.5 mg/kg daily. How many milligrams will the nurse administer with each dose? _____

10. The medication order reads: "Give doxapram 0.5 mg/kg IV STAT." The patient weighs 165 lb. How much medication will the patient receive? _____

**Answer the following questions on a separate sheet of paper.**

11. Stacey, age 35 years, reports that she falls asleep unexpectedly at work, in class, and even while singing in her city's choir.
    a. Which condition might Stacey have?
    b. What might be the drug of choice for Stacey?
    c. Describe the therapeutic effects of such drugs.
    d. Draw up a patient teaching plan for Stacey. Offer guidelines for substances she might be wise to avoid.

12. Five-year-old Jeffrey is taking atomoxetine (Strattera) for ADHD. What specific precautions must be taken with children who are taking ADHD drugs? Why?

13. What nutritional counseling is needed for patients taking orlistat (Xenical)?

14. Sadie experiences migraine headaches about four times a year and has a new prescription for a serotonin receptor agonist. She tells you that she hopes that the medication will prevent her "awful headaches." What is the best response to Sadie's comments?

15. George, a 14-year-old student, has been taking a medication for ADHD for 6 months. At today's follow-up visit, the physician suggests that George take a "drug holiday" on the weekends and during the school's spring break. Explain the reasoning behind drug holidays.

**Read the scenario, and answer the following questions on a separate sheet of paper.**

Nancy, a 44-year-old accountant, has had an increasing number of headaches in the past year. When she has these headaches, she often is nauseated and vomits. She has been to her physician, who has ordered several diagnostic tests. As a result, Nancy has been diagnosed with migraine headaches and will be given a prescription for a serotonin receptor agonist.

1. How do serotonin receptor agonists work in the treatment of migraine headaches?

2. What dosage form(s) would be helpful for Nancy's situation?

3. If the physician decides to write a prescription for sumatriptan (Imitrex), Nancy's history should be assessed for which conditions?

4. What foods may be associated with the development of migraine headaches?

5. What else should be included in the treatment regimen for Nancy's migraine headaches?

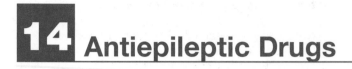 

**CRITICAL THINKING CROSSWORD**

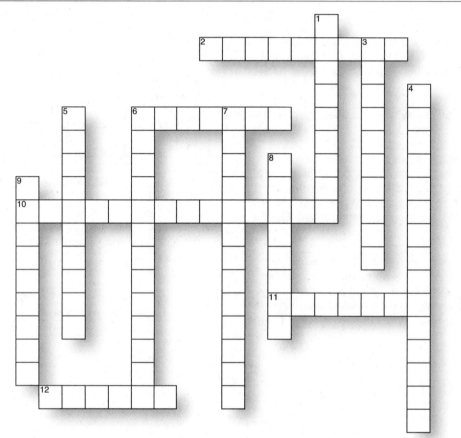

**Across**

2. Status epilepticus is considered a life-threatening

   medical _____.
6. A type of epilepsy with an unknown cause
10. A potential adverse effect of valproic acid
11. A brief episode of abnormal electrical activity in the nerve cells of the brain
12. Intravenously administered antiepileptic drugs are

   given _____ to avoid serious adverse effects.

**Down**

1. A type of epilepsy with a distinct cause
3. An involuntary spasmodic contraction of voluntary muscles throughout the body

4. This class of drugs is one of the first-line drugs used to treat status epilepticus.
5. Another term for 6 Across
6. A barbiturate used primarily to control tonic-clonic and partial seizures
7. The metabolic process that occurs when the metabolism of a drug increases over time, which leads to lower-than-expected drug concentrations.
8. Recurrent episodes of convulsive seizures
9. Generic name of a first-line antiepileptic drug that can cause gingival hyperplasia with long-term use

## CHAPTER REVIEW AND NCLEX® EXAMINATION PREPARATION

**Select the best answer for each question.**

1. A patient has been taking antiepileptic drugs for 1 year. The nurse is reviewing the patient's recent history and will monitor for which condition that may develop during this time?
   a. Loss of appetite
   b. Jaundice
   c. Weight loss
   d. Suicidal thoughts or behavior

2. A patient is experiencing a seizure that has lasted for several minutes, and he has not regained consciousness. The nurse recognizes that this is a life-threatening emergency known as
   a. status epilepticus.
   b. tonic-clonic convulsion.
   c. epilepsy.
   d. secondary epilepsy.

3. The nurse is giving an intravenous dose of phenytoin. Which guidelines will the nurse follow for administration? *(Select all that apply.)*
   a. Inject phenytoin into a smaller vein.
   b. Inject phenytoin slowly.
   c. The injection of phenytoin is followed by an injection of sterile saline.
   d. Do not infuse phenytoin continuously.
   e. Mix the phenytoin with $D_5W$ (5% dextrose and water) for the infusion.

4. The nurse is administering phenobarbital and will monitor the patient for which possible adverse effect?
   a. Constipation
   b. Gingival hyperplasia
   c. Drowsiness
   d. Dysrhythmias

5. A patient has been admitted to the emergency department with status epilepticus. The nurse knows that which of these drugs is considered the drug of choice for this condition?
   a. Phenobarbital
   b. Diazepam
   c. Valproic acid
   d. Phenytoin

6. A patient who is experiencing neuropathic pain tells the nurse that the physician is going to start him on a new medication that is generally used to treat seizures. The nurse anticipates that which drug will be ordered?
   a. Phenobarbital
   b. Phenytoin
   c. Gabapentin
   d. Tiagabine

7. Phenytoin is prescribed for a patient. The nurse checks the patient's current list of medications and notes that interactions may occur with which drugs or drug classes? *(Select all that apply.)*
   a. Proton pump inhibitors
   b. Warfarin
   c. Sulfonamide antibiotics
   d. Corticosteroids
   e. Oral contraceptives

8. The nurse is providing discharge instruction to the patient who will be taking phenytoin. With an understanding of the side effects of phenytoin, which instruction is most important?
   a. Drink plenty of fluids throughout the day.
   b. Perform mouth care at least twice a day.
   c. Limit intake of spinach.
   d. Use sunscreen liberally.

9. Which drug is considered first-line treatment for partial and tonic-clonic seizures?
   a. Carbamazepine
   b. Diazepam
   c. Oxcarbazepine
   d. Ethosuximide

10. A patient is unable to take oral medications and has received a loading dose of phenytoin intravenously. The orders call for him to receive phenytoin 5 mg/kg/day in three divided doses. The medication comes in a vial with 50 mg/mL. The patient weighs 90 kg.
    a. How many milligrams will the patient receive each day? For each dose? _____
    b. How many milliliters of medication will be drawn up for each dose? _____

11. Indicate on the syringe the amount of medication the nurse will draw up for each dose of the medication in Question 10.

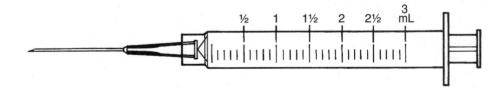

## CRITICAL THINKING AND APPLICATION

**Answer the following questions on a separate sheet of paper.**

12. What is meant by *autoinduction* in a drug? Identify at least one antiepileptic drug that undergoes autoinduction.

13. Jeremy, an 8-year-old boy, has resisted his oral doses of topiramate, which has made compliance with the drug regimen difficult. His mother calls and says that she has found a way to get him to take it: she crushes the tablet and sprinkles it on flavored gelatin. She is delighted. How will the nurse respond?

14. Rosie, a 24-year-old paralegal, has been taking antiepileptic drugs for several years, with her seizures well controlled with the drug therapy. She is in the clinic for an annual checkup and tells the nurse, "I want to stop all my medicines because we want to have a baby. I've always read that these drugs are unsafe for the unborn baby. What do I need to do?" What is the nurse's best response?

## CASE STUDY

**Read the scenario, and answer the following questions on a separate sheet of paper.**

Four-year-old Mattie has started preschool. Today the teacher calls Mattie's mother to tell her that she noticed that Mattie seems to have a problem with "daydreaming." She explains that Mattie seemed inattentive during group work and was staring out into space several times during the day. She is also worried because she saw Mattie's eyes move back and forth rapidly during these episodes. These "spells" lasted a minute or two, and then Mattie seemed fine. Mattie's mother has brought her to the pediatric office to have her checked. The health care provider suspects that Mattie is experiencing a type of seizure disorder and has ordered some diagnostic testing.

1. What type of seizure is Mattie experiencing?

2. Mattie's mother is given a prescription for a liquid antiepileptic drug for Mattie. What is important to teach the mother regarding administration of this type of medication?

3. What will the nurse teach Mattie's mother to monitor for during Mattie's drug therapy with this medication?

4. After a year, Mattie's mother is pleased that the seizures have "disappeared" and wants to take Mattie off the medication. What is the best response by the nurse?

# 15 Antiparkinson Drugs

**Select the best answer for each question.**

1. A patient with Parkinson's disease has difficulty performing voluntary movements. What is the correct term for this symptom?
   a. Akinesia
   b. Dyskinesia
   c. Chorea
   d. Dystonia

2. Which drug may be used early in the treatment of Parkinson's disease but eventually loses effectiveness and must be replaced by another drug?
   a. Amantadine
   b. Levodopa
   c. Selegiline
   d. Tolcapone

3. Which drug may be used as monotherapy or in conjunction with levodopa to treat Parkinson's disease?
   a. Bromocriptine
   b. Benztropine
   c. Carbidopa
   d. Selegiline

4. A patient who is newly diagnosed with Parkinson's disease and beginning medication therapy with entacapone, a COMT inhibitor, asks the nurse, "How soon will improvement occur?" What is the nurse's best response?
   a. "That varies from patient to patient."
   b. "You should discuss that with your physician."
   c. "You should notice a difference in a few days."
   d. "It may take several weeks before you notice any degree of improvement."

5. A patient asks the nurse why a second drug is given with his drugs for Parkinson's disease. The nurse notes that this drug, an anticholinergic, is given to control or minimize which symptom?
   a. Constipation
   b. Muscle rigidity
   c. Bradykinesia
   d. Dry mouth

6. Which are expected side effects of the anticholinergic drugs used to treat Parkinson's disease? *(Select all that apply.)*
   a. Dry mouth and decreased salivation
   b. Urinary retention
   c. Decreased GI motility and constipation
   d. Pupillary constriction
   e. Smooth muscle relaxation

7. The nurse is providing teaching on COMT inhibitors to a patient with a new prescription. The nurse will be sure to educate the patient on the possibility of which adverse effect?
   a. Insomnia
   b. Urine discoloration
   c. Leg edema
   d. Visual changes

8. Carbidopa–levodopa is prescribed for a patient with Parkinson's disease. The nurse will inform the patient of which possible adverse effects? *(Select all that apply.)*
   a. Palpitations
   b. Insomnia
   c. Hypotension
   d. Urinary frequency
   e. Depression

9. Which statement describes the rationale for combining carbidopa with levodopa in the treatment of Parkinson's disease?
   a. The combination eliminates the side effects of both medications.
   b. The combination decreases the liver's first-pass effect on dopamine.
   c. The combination decreases the level of acetylcholine at the synapses.
   d. The combination allows lower levels of dopamine to be used with the same effect on alleviation of symptoms.

10. The medication order reads: "Give benztropine 2.5 mg PO every morning." The medication is available in 1-mg tablets. How many tablets will the nurse administer? _____

**Answer the following questions on a separate sheet of paper.**

11. Mr. H. is about to have levodopa added to his carbidopa treatment regimen.
    a. Why must dopamine be administered in the form of levodopa?
    b. What problems are avoided when carbidopa is given with levodopa?
    c. How does the carbidopa work when given with levodopa?
    d. What foods should Mr. H limit in the amount consumed?

12. Mrs. R., a 35-year-old new mother, has experienced slowing movements, cogwheel rigidity, and pill-rolling tremor. She has been diagnosed with Parkinson's disease, a somewhat rare occurrence in someone her age. In addition to the usual history questions, what must the nurse ask in anticipation of dopaminergic therapy in Mrs. R.'s specific situation?

13. Jane, age 45 years, is taking benztropine in addition to a dopaminergic drug for Parkinson's disease. Her 76-year-old neighbor comments that he cannot take benztropine because it is too risky for him. Jane calls and asks why this is not a concern in her case. What do you say?

14. Explain the difference between the concepts of the "on–off phenomenon" and the "wearing-off phenomenon."

## CASE STUDY

**Read the scenario, and answer the following questions on a separate sheet of paper.**

Alexander, a 54-year-old man, has been diagnosed with Parkinson's disease and is about to start drug therapy. His symptoms are mild, yet he has some akinesia that interferes with his ability to type at work. The physician explains that Alexander may have to take a variety of drugs as the disease progresses.

1. What is the underlying pathologic defect in Parkinson's disease?

2. What is the aim of drug therapy for Parkinson's disease?

3. The first drugs prescribed for Alexander are amantadine along with levodopa–carbidopa. What is the purpose of taking the amantadine at this time?

4. The physician tells Alexander that the amantadine may be helpful in the early stages but will need to be changed at a later date. Why is this true?

5. How does the carbidopa affect the "on–off phenomenon" that may occur with the use of levodopa?

# 16 Psychotherapeutic Drugs

**Select the best answer for each question.**

1. The nurse is administering the antipsychotic drug clozapine (Clozaril) and should monitor the patient for what long-term problems associated with this drug? *(Select all that apply.)*
   a. Mood swings
   b. Agranulocytosis
   c. Weight gain
   d. Photosensitivity
   e. Increased appetite

2. During therapy for depression with a selective serotonin reuptake inhibitor (SSRI), it is most important for the nurse to instruct the family to monitor for which adverse effect?
   a. Suicidal thoughts
   b. Visual disturbances
   c. Tardive dyskinesia
   d. Bleeding tendencies

3. The wife of a patient who has started taking antidepressant therapy asks, "How long will it take for him to feel better?" What is the nurse's best response?
   a. "Well, depression rarely responds to medication therapy."
   b. "He should be feeling better in a few days."
   c. "It may take 4 to 6 weeks before you see an improvement."
   d. "You may not see any effects for several months."

4. When administering certain antipsychotic drugs, the nurse monitors for which extrapyramidal effects? *(Select all that apply.)*
   a. Tremors
   b. Elation and a sense of well-being
   c. Painful muscle spasms
   d. Motor restlessness
   e. Bradycardia

5. The nurse instructs a patient who is undergoing therapy with monoamine oxidase inhibitors (MAOIs) to avoid tyramine-containing foods. What medical emergency may occur if the patient eats these foods while taking MAOIs?
   a. Gastric hemorrhage
   b. Toxic shock
   c. Cardiac arrest
   d. Hypertensive crisis

6. A patient has been taking antipsychotic medication for years, and his wife has noticed that he has had some new physical symptoms. She describes him as having odd facial movements, sticking out his tongue, and having movements of his arms that he cannot seem to control. The nurse suspects that the patient is exhibiting signs of which condition?
   a. Hypomania
   b. Serotonin syndrome
   c. Tardive dyskinesia
   d. Neuroleptic malignant syndrome

7. Which outcome represents the most serious adverse effect of lithium?
   a. Renal failure
   b. Hyponatremia
   c. Respiratory depression
   d. Cardiac dysrhythmia

8. Primary side effects of the SSRIs include which symptoms?
   a. Rash and alopecia
   b. Gastritis and diarrhea
   c. Weight gain and sexual dysfunction
   d. Photosensitivity and discoloration of the skin

9. A patient will be receiving benztropine (Cogentin) 1.5 mg PO daily. The medication comes in 0.5-mg tablets. How many tablets will the nurse administer per dose? _____

10. A patient is to receive lithium carbonate, 1800 mg/day in two divided doses. The medication is available in 300-mg capsules. How many milligrams of lithium will the patient receive for each dose? How many capsules per dose? _____

## MATCHING

**Match each term with its corresponding definition or description.**

11. _____ Buspirone (BuSpar)

12. _____ Tyramine

13. _____ Tricyclics

14. _____ Psychosis

15. _____ Mania

16. _____ Diazepam (Valium)

17. _____ Amitriptyline (Elavil)

18. _____ Risperidone (Risperdal)

19. _____ Benzodiazepines

20. _____ Lithium (Eskalith)

21. _____ Anxiety

22. _____ Affective disorders

23. _____ Depression

24. _____ Bipolar affective disorder

25. _____ Extrapyramidal

a. The unpleasant state of mind in which real or imagined dangers are anticipated or exaggerated

b. A state characterized by an expansive emotional state (including symptoms of extreme excitement and elation) and hyperactivity

c. A group of psychotropic drugs prescribed to alleviate anxiety

d. Emotional disorders characterized by changes in mood

e. A major psychologic disorder characterized by episodes of mania or hypomania cycling with depression

f. Patients taking MAOIs need to be taught to avoid foods that contain this substance.

g. An older class of antidepressant drugs

h. An abnormal emotional state characterized by exaggerated feelings of sadness, melancholy, and worthlessness out of proportion to reality

i. A long-acting benzodiazepine

j. The most widely used tricyclic antidepressant

k. An atypical antipsychotic drug used to treat schizophrenia

l. A nonbenzodiazepine drug used to treat anxiety

m. Term for the symptoms or adverse effects that often occur with antipsychotic medications

n. Medication used to treat mania

o. A type of serious mental illness that can take several different forms and is associated with being truly out of touch with reality

## CRITICAL THINKING AND APPLICATION

**Answer the following questions on a separate sheet of paper.**

26. Carl, a 26-year-old unemployed electrician, is brought to the emergency department by his sister. He is extremely drowsy and confused, and his breathing is slow and shallow. The sister tells you that Carl has been seeing a psychiatrist for his "anxiety" and had a prescription for "nerve pills."
   a. What do you suspect might be wrong with Carl?
   b. How will he likely be treated?

27. Mr. D., a 49-year-old restaurant owner, has been prescribed the MAOI phenelzine (Nardil). After the physician leaves the room but before you have a chance to discuss Mr. D.'s medication regimen with him, he turns to his wife and says, "I'm sure this medicine will work. Let's have a bottle of wine tonight to celebrate our anniversary."
   a. What teaching is necessary in this situation?
   b. A few weeks later, Mr. D. is brought to the emergency department with a severe headache, stiff neck, sweating, and elevated blood pressure. His wife says his symptoms started a few minutes after they ate at their favorite restaurant. What is wrong with Mr. D., and what has probably caused it?

28. Beth has been diagnosed with depression. Why might the physician prescribe a second-generation antidepressant instead of a first-generation antidepressant?

29. A young adult has been admitted to the emergency department with a suspected overdose of a tricyclic antidepressant. The physicians are monitoring his cardiac status closely. Why is this monitoring necessary?

**Read the scenario, and answer the following questions on a separate sheet of paper.**

Gene, a 38-year-old businessman, mentions during a checkup that he has felt very anxious and upset over the past few months. He discusses the pressures of his business and states that he has had trouble sleeping at night, which makes him more irritable. Lately he has been very worried over a contract proposal presentation that will take place in a few months. The physician gives him a prescription for the benzodiazepine alprazolam (Xanax), 0.25 mg three times a day.

1. Gene is concerned about potential adverse effects of this group of medications. What will you tell him?

2. What other measures will be taken for Gene at this time?

3. After 3 months, Gene is back in the office for a follow-up appointment. He is upset because a friend told him about another friend who was taking the same medication and died because of an overdose. Gene wants to stop taking the alprazolam immediately. Is this recommended for this class of medications? If not, why not?

4. What are the symptoms of benzodiazepine overdose, and what is the antidote, if any?

5. Six months later, Gene is no longer taking alprazolam but comes back to the office because he still feels anxious. The physician gives him a prescription for buspirone (BuSpar), 15 mg twice a day. Gene questions why he is given a different drug. What are the advantages, if any, of taking buspirone instead of alprazolam?

# 17 Substance Use Disorder

**Match each drug with its corresponding description.**

1. _____ Cocaine

2. _____ Ecstasy

3. _____ Flumazenil

4. _____ Heroin

5. _____ Disulfiram

6. _____ Nicotine

7. _____ Naltrexone

8. _____ Bupropion

9. _____ Methamphetamine

10. _____ "Roofies"

a. A nicotine-free treatment for nicotine dependence
b. Known as the "date rape" drug
c. This substance is commonly manufactured from the over-the-counter decongestant pseudoephedrine.
d. The addictive chemical in tobacco products
e. An opioid that is injected by "mainlining" or "skin popping"
f. Used to antagonize the action of benzodiazepines and reverse sedation
g. Used to deter the use of alcohol during alcohol abuse treatment
h. A stimulant that is either "snorted" through the nasal passages or injected intravenously
i. A stimulant that is popular at "raves" with college-age students
j. An opioid antagonist used for opioid abuse or dependence

**Select the best answer for each question.**

11. A patient who has been taking disulfiram therapy for 3 months has been off the therapy for 2 days. He decides to go out with friends to have a beer. What effects may he experience? *(Select all that apply.)*
    a. Diaphoresis
    b. Diarrhea
    c. Vomiting
    d. Euphoria
    e. Drowsiness
    f. Facial flushing

12. During an information session about drug abuse, the nurse relates that the most common drug effect that leads to abuse of opioids is
    a. hallucinations.
    b. sleepiness.
    c. stimulation.
    d. euphoria.

13. The nurse is assisting a patient who is experiencing opioid withdrawal and anticipates the possible use of which medications to lessen the symptoms of withdrawal? *(Select all that apply.)*
    a. Disulfiram
    b. Clonidine
    c. Methadone
    d. Bupropion
    e. Naloxone

14. When teaching a patient about drug interactions, the nurse is aware that combining benzodiazepines with ethanol or barbiturates may lead to death from
    a. cardiac dysrhythmia.
    b. convulsions.
    c. respiratory arrest.
    d. stroke.

15. A patient with a known history of chronic excessive ingestion of ethanol has developed memory problems and comes to the health clinic with hard-to-believe stories of what has happened to him. The nurse recognizes that these symptoms are associated with which disorder?
    a. Cerebrovascular accident
    b. Korsakoff's psychosis
    c. Encephalopathy
    d. Bipolar disorder

16. The nurse is teaching a class to high school students regarding the negative effects of nicotine on the body. The nurse would include which effects? *(Select all that apply.)*
    a. Stimulation followed by depression
    b. Increased heart rate and blood pressure
    c. Constipation
    d. Vomiting
    e. Insomnia

17. A patient is to receive flumazenil 0.2 mg, IV push over 30 seconds as initial treatment for a possible benzodiazepine overdose. The medication is available in a 0.1-mg/mL vial. How many milliliters of medication will the nurse draw up into the syringe for this dose?_____

## CRITICAL THINKING AND APPLICATION

**Answer the following questions on a separate sheet of paper.**

18. Describe how nicotine is used to ease withdrawal from nicotine use. Compare the use of bupropion and varenicline in smoking cessation programs.

19. How is medication therapy different for mild, moderate, and severe alcohol withdrawal?

20. A woman brings her teenage daughter into the emergency department. The teen is lethargic and dizzy and has been vomiting. While the teen is being examined and stabilized, the mother tells the nurse that her daughter told her that she and her friends used cough syrup to get high. The mother states, "How could cough syrup do this?" What is the nurse's best answer?

21. Explain why the decongestant pseudoephedrine is restricted.

## CASE STUDY

**Read the scenario, and answer the following questions on a separate sheet of paper.**

A 19-year-old man, Mr. C., is admitted to the emergency department after he collapsed at a fraternity party. The paramedics state that there were beer-drinking contests at the party, and it is unknown how much Mr. C. had to drink. His friend says that Mr. C. was upset over breaking up with a girlfriend and that he is worried about how heavily Mr. C. has been drinking in the past 2 weeks.

Mr. C. is semiconscious but unable to answer questions coherently, and his speech is slurred. His blood pressure is 100/58 mm Hg, his pulse rate is 110 beats/min, and his breathing is heavy with a respiratory rate of 16 breaths/min. He vomited on the way to the hospital.

1. Is ethanol considered a central nervous system stimulant or depressant?

2. What are the effects of severe alcoholic intoxication on the cardiovascular and respiratory systems?

3. The patient is admitted to the medical unit for observation. For what will you observe at this time?

4. The next evening, Mr. C. is more alert but still unsteady in his gait. He says he wants to go home, but you notice fine tremors of his hands. Should he be discharged at this time? Explain.

5. If Mr. C. continues the pattern of heavy drinking, what effects could the chronic ingestion of ethanol have on his body?

# 18 Adrenergic Drugs

**Select the best answer for each question.**

1. What is another name for an adrenergic drug?
   a. Anticholinergic drug
   b. Parasympathetic drug
   c. Central nervous system drug
   d. Sympathomimetic drug

2. The nurse is administering an adrenergic drug and will monitor for which possible effect?
   a. Hypotension
   b. Tachycardia
   c. Decreased respiratory rate
   d. Diarrhea

3. The nurse is aware that adrenergic drugs may be used to treat which conditions? *(Select all that apply.)*
   a. Asthma
   b. Open-angle glaucoma
   c. Hypertension
   d. Nasal congestion
   e. Seizures
   f. Nausea and vomiting

4. A woman who is allergic to bees has just been stung while out in her garden. She reaches for her bee-sting kit, which would most likely contain which drug?
   a. Epinephrine
   b. Phenylephrine
   c. Formoterol
   d. Norepinephrine

5. A 13-year-old girl was diagnosed with asthma 2 years ago. Today her physician wants to start her on salmeterol administered via inhaler. The nurse needs to remember to include which statement when teaching the girl and her family about this drug?
   a. "It should be taken at the first sign of an asthma attack."
   b. "The dosage is two puffs every 4 hours or any time needed for asthma attacks."
   c. "This inhaler is for prevention of asthma attacks, not for an acute attack."
   d. "Be sure to take your steroid inhaler first."

6. Which instruction should the nurse provide to the patient taking salmeterol by inhaler?
   a. Increase fluid intake.
   b. Rinse mouth after use.
   c. Monitor heart rate.
   d. Remain upright for 30 minutes.

7. The nurse is reviewing the medication orders of a newly admitted patient who has an infusion of the adrenergic drug dopamine. Which of these drugs or drug classes, if also given to the patient, may cause an interaction? *(Select all that apply.)*
   a. Tricyclic antidepressants
   b. Monoamine oxidase inhibitors (MAOIs)
   c. Anticoagulants
   d. Corticosteroids
   e. Antihistamines

8. The nurse is administering dopamine to the patient in cardiogenic shock after a motor vehicle accident. Which assessment finding indicates the dopamine is achieving its desired effect? *(Select all that apply.)*
   a. Blood pressure of 90/60 mm Hg
   b. Hyperactive bowel sounds
   c. Decreased in heart rate to 100 beats/min
   d. Presence of adventitious lung sounds
   e. Increase in urine output to 30 mL/hr

9. During pharmacology class, a nursing student asks about the use of beta$_2$ agonists in pregnancy. The most appropriate response by the nursing faculty member would be which of the following?
   a. They lower blood pressure in pregnancy-induced hypertension.
   b. They increase milk production during lactation.
   c. They interrupt premature labor contractions.
   d. They facilitate uterine involution.

10. An infant is having an allergic reaction and is to receive two doses of epinephrine 10 mcg/kg subcutaneously. The infant weighs 11 lb. How many micrograms of medication will the infant receive

    with each dose?_____

11. The nurse is to administer epinephrine 0.5 mg subcutaneously. The ampule contains 1 mL of medication and is labeled "Epinephrine 1:1000—1 mg." How many milliliters of epinephrine will the nurse give? _____

12. Mark the syringe with the amount of medication the nurse will draw up for Question 10.

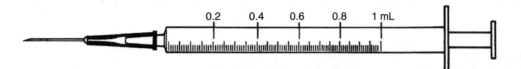

**Answer the following questions on a separate sheet of paper.**

13. The mother of 3-year-old Kyle is giving him phenylephrine drops as a nasal decongestant.
    a. How does this medication help with nasal congestion?
    b. Kyle's mother comes back to the clinic and complains that after 1 week, his congestion is worse, not better. What possible explanation can the nurse offer?

14. Mr. D., who has had a history of problems with a hormonal imbalance, has been admitted for septic shock, and the physician prescribes dopamine. However, the nurse double-checks the patient's history before administering the drug. What condition may be a contraindication to dopamine?

15. Mr. G. and Mr. C. are both on dopamine infusions. Mr. G.'s infusion is being administered at a low rate, and Mr. C.'s at a high rate. Why might these infusion rates be different?

16. A patient in the intensive care unit has received too high a dose of epinephrine. The nurse will monitor for what effects? What will the nurse expect to do for this patient?

17. Greg, a 49-year-old construction worker, is in the urgent care center for treatment of a leg laceration. Just after a dose of intravenous penicillin is started, he begins to wheeze and says, "Oh, I just remembered. I'm allergic to penicillin!"
    a. What is happening?
    b. What will the nurse do first?
    c. What drug will be given in this situation?

## CASE STUDY

**Read the scenario, and answer the following questions on a separate sheet of paper.**

Sixteen-year-old Maureen, who plays soccer on her high school team, has been treated for asthma for 1 year. Her symptoms have been controlled with an inhaled steroid and occasional use of an albuterol metered-dose inhaler. This afternoon, though, her mother brings her into the urgent care center because Maureen has had trouble "getting her breath" after a particularly rough game. Maureen complains of a feeling of "tightness" in her chest and wants to sit up. She appears anxious and has a nonproductive cough. Her respiratory rate is 28 breaths/min, and her peak expiratory flow is 70% of normal. Chest auscultation reveals a short inspiratory period with prolonged expiratory wheezes in both lungs.

1. The physician orders albuterol to be given through a nebulizer. What should you assess before giving this medication? During and after administration?

2. Why is the albuterol given via inhalation rather than orally?

3. After the nebulizer medication treatment is completed, Maureen complains of feeling "shaky and jittery." What do you tell her?

4. The physician gives Maureen a prescription for a salmeterol inhaler. What is important to teach Maureen and her mother about this medication?

**47**

# 19 Adrenergic-Blocking Drugs

**Select the best answer for each question.**

1. Adrenergic blockade at the alpha-adrenergic receptors leads to which effects? *(Select all that apply.)*
   a. Vasodilation
   b. Decreased blood pressure
   c. Increased blood pressure
   d. Constriction of the pupil
   e. Tachycardia

2. The nurse discovers that the intravenous infusion of a patient who has been receiving an intravenous vasopressor has infiltrated. The nurse will expect which drug to be used to reverse the effects of the vasopressor in the infiltrated area?
   a. Phentolamine
   b. Prazosin
   c. Epinephrine
   d. Metoprolol

3. A patient has a new prescription for a beta blocker as part of treatment for hypertension. The nurse is reviewing the patient's current medications and notes that there may be a concern regarding interactions with which medication?
   a. Thyroid hormone supplement
   b. Antibiotic for a sinus infection
   c. Oral hypoglycemic for type 2 diabetes mellitus
   d. Oral contraceptive

4. A patient has been given an alpha blocker as treatment for benign prostatic hyperplasia. Which instruction is important to include when the nurse is teaching him about the effects of this medication?
   a. Avoid foods and drinks that contain caffeine.
   b. Change to sitting or standing positions slowly to avoid a sudden drop in blood pressure.
   c. Watch for weight loss of 2 lb within 1 week.
   d. Take extra supplements of calcium.

5. A patient who has been taking a beta blocker for 6 months tells the nurse during a follow-up visit that she wants to stop taking this medication. She is wondering if there is any problem with stopping the medication today. What is the nurse's best response?
   a. "No, there are no ill effects if this medication is stopped."
   b. "There should be only minimal effects if you stop this medication."
   c. "You may experience orthostatic hypotension if you stop this medication abruptly."
   d. "If you stop this medication suddenly, there is a possibility you may experience chest pain or rebound hypertension."

6. A patient has been taking tamsulosin for about 1 year. During today's office visit, he asks the physician about taking a drug for erectile dysfunction. How does the nurse expect the physician to respond?
   a. "These drugs are safe to take together."
   b. "You can take them together, but the dosage of the Flomax will need to be reduced."
   c. "Taking these two drugs together may lead to dangerously low blood pressure."
   d. "You will be able to try taking these two drugs together, but watch for side effects."

7. Which instruction should take priority in teaching patients how to manage the adverse effects of alpha blockers?
   a. Avoid the intake of grapefruit or grapefruit juice.
   b. Drink plenty of fluids throughout the day.
   c. Eat plenty of green leafy vegetables.
   d. Change positions slowly.

8. Which statement correctly describes the method of action of the drug in treating benign prostatic hypertrophy?
   a. It reduces smooth muscle contraction of the bladder neck and the urethra, decreasing resistance to urine outflow.
   b. It reverses prostatic hypertrophy, reducing the size of the prostate gland.
   c. It inhibits production of prostate-specific antigen, decreasing gland size.
   d. It enhances the diameter of the urinary meatus, improving urine flow.

9. Which of the following drug orders should alert the nurse to the possibility of drug error?
   a. Tamsulosin for a 65-year-old woman
   b. Inderal for a 35-year-old patient with asthma
   c. Carvedilol for a 50-year-old with hypertension
   d. Metoprolol for a 55-year-old woman with hypertension

10. An admission order reads, "Start IV of 0.9% normal saline and infuse 1 L over the next 12 hours." The nurse will set the infusion pump to what rate?

    _____

11. A patient is to receive labetalol (Trandate) 20 mg IV push over 10 minutes, STAT. The medication is available in a vial that contains 5 mg/mL. How many milliliters will the nurse administer for this

    dose? _____

## CRITICAL THINKING AND APPLICATION

**Answer the following questions on a separate sheet of paper.**

12. Mrs. W., a patient on a cardiac step-down unit, is receiving a dopamine intravenous infusion. When the nurse first comes on the late-night shift, Mrs. W. seems just fine. However, the next time the nurse checks on her, the intravenous line has dislodged, and the infusion has infiltrated. What could happen as a result? Is this serious? What treatment will the nurse expect to see ordered? Describe the procedure and provide the rationale.

13. Mr. C. has had a myocardial infarction (MI). He is told that he will be prescribed a "cardioprotective drug." He asks the nurse to explain. How can some beta blockers be said to "protect" the heart?

14. Ms. M. has been prescribed a beta blocker. She is about to be released from the hospital, but first her nurse gives her instructions about taking her blood pressure and her apical pulse for 1 full minute. Why? What should she be looking for? Is there anything she should be instructed to report to her physician?

15. Mr. S., a 78-year-old widower, has a new prescription for tamsulosin because of a new diagnosis of benign prostatic hyperplasia. What concern, if any, is there with this drug? What teaching will he need?

## CASE STUDY

**Read the scenario, and answer the following questions on a separate sheet of paper.**

Bruce, a 58-year-old accountant, is in the hospital after having an MI. The physician has told him that the damage to his heart was minimal, and Bruce has started post-MI rehabilitation and education. In addition to the MI, he has had asthma for years that has been managed poorly. The physician discusses starting Bruce on a beta blocker to "protect his heart" and gives him a prescription for atenolol (Tenormin).

1. What type of beta blocker is appropriate for Bruce? Why?

2. Discuss how atenolol helps in this situation.

3. What adverse effects will you teach Bruce to expect when taking this medication?

4. At his 3-month checkup, Bruce tells you that he wants to stop taking this medication. Should this medication be stopped abruptly? What do you think may be the reason that Bruce wants to stop taking the atenolol?

**49**

# 20 Cholinergic Drugs

**Match each definition with its corresponding term. (Note: Not all terms will be used.)**

1. _____ Antidote for overdose of a cholinergic drug

2. _____ Cholinergic drugs that act by making more acetylcholine (ACh) available at the receptor site, thus allowing ACh to bind to and stimulate the receptor

3. _____ Cholinergic drugs that bind to cholinergic receptors and activate them

4. _____ Receptors located postsynaptically in the effector organs (smooth muscle, cardiac muscle, glands) supplied by the parasympathetic fibers

5. _____ Receptors located in the ganglia of the parasympathetic nervous system (PSNS) and the sympathetic nervous system (SNS)

6. _____ A description of the action of the PSNS

7. _____ The neurotransmitter responsible for the transmission of nerve impulses to the effector cells in the PSNS

8. _____ The enzyme responsible for breaking down ACh

a. Cholinesterase
b. Muscarinic
c. Catecholamine
d. "Fight or flight"
e. "Rest and digest"
f. Direct-acting cholinergic drugs
g. Indirect-acting cholinergic drugs
h. Atropine
i. Acetylcholine
j. Nicotinic

**Select the best answer for each question.**

9. The desired effects of cholinergic drugs come from stimulation of which receptors?
a. Cholinergic
b. Nicotinic
c. Muscarinic
d. Ganglionic

10. The undesirable effects of cholinergic drugs come from stimulation of which receptors?
a. Cholinergic
b. Nicotinic
c. Muscarinic
d. Ganglionic

11. The patient mentions bethanechol when asked about his medication history. The nurse recognizes that this drug is used for the treatment of which condition?
a. Diarrhea
b. Urinary retention
c. Urinary incontinence
d. Bladder spasms

12. Which existing condition in a patient would cause the nurse to question an order for bethanechol? *(Select all that apply.)*
a. Asthma
b. Peptic ulcer disease
c. Pernicious anemia
d. Hyperthyroidism
e. Diabetes

13. When caring for a patient with a diagnosis of myasthenia gravis, the nurse can expect to see which drug ordered for the symptomatic treatment of this disease?
a. Bethanechol
b. Tacrine
c. Donepezil
d. Pyridostigmine

14. A 62-year-old woman has started taking donepezil for early-stage Alzheimer's disease. Her daughter expresses relief that "there is finally a pill to cure Alzheimer's disease." What is the nurse's best response?
    a. "She can expect reversal of symptoms within a few days."
    b. "The dosage will need to be increased if no improvement is noted."
    c. "This drug may help to improve symptoms, but it is not intended as a cure."
    d. "Yes, it has been a great help for many patients."

15. A patient has received an inadvertent overdose of a cholinergic drug. The nurse will monitor for which early signs of a cholinergic crisis? *(Select all that apply.)*
    a. Dry mouth
    b. Salivation
    c. Flushing of the skin
    d. Abdominal cramps
    e. Constipation
    f. Dyspnea

16. The nurse will prepare to give which drug to a patient who is experiencing a cholinergic crisis?
    a. Atropine
    b. Tacrine
    c. Donepezil
    d. Physostigmine

17. Which of the following patients would benefit from administration of atropine?
    a. A patient with a blood pressure of 218/110 mm Hg and complaining of headache
    b. A patient with a heart rate of 40 beats/min and complaining of lightheadedness
    c. A patient who is 3 hours postoperative and has not voided.
    d. A patient with glaucoma and complaining of eye pain.

18. The nurse is monitoring a patient who has been receiving bethanechol after abdominal surgery. Which of these are therapeutic outcomes for this medication? *(Select all that apply.)*
    a. Decreased heart rate
    b. Passage of flatus
    c. Decreased temperature
    d. A bowel movement
    e. Decreased respiratory secretions

19. An intravenous piggyback medication is ordered to infuse over 1 hour. The volume of the medication bag is 100 mL; the tubing drop factor is 10 gtt/mL. What is the rate for a gravity infusion of this

    medication? _____

20. The order reads: "Give pyridostigmine (Mestinon) 0.25 mg/kg IV now." The patient weighs 235 lb. How many milligrams of medication will the patient receive? *(Record answer using one decimal place.)*

_____

## CRITICAL THINKING AND APPLICATION

**Answer the following questions on a separate sheet of paper.**

21. List the effects of cholinergic poisoning by using the acronym SLUDGE.

22. Mrs. S. has recently had abdominal surgery, and she is resting well except that she is unable to void her urine. She has some distention in her lower abdomen over the symphysis pubis.
    a. What is likely to be the drug of choice?
    b. Mrs. S. is still unable to void her urine. Her urinary retention worsens and becomes painful, and she begins to exhibit signs of a renal stone, which is confirmed by radiography. How much can the physician increase her dosage?

23. Mr. K. has been determined to have a high potential for a negative reaction to the cholinergic prescribed to him. However, his physician believes that the potential benefits are worth the risk.
    a. The nurse will closely monitor Mr. K. for what reaction?
    b. In addition to close monitoring, what else can the nurse do to prepare?

24. Ms. B. has recently been diagnosed with myasthenia gravis and is taking medication for the treatment of symptoms associated with the disease. She asks the nurse, "How much success can I expect?"
    a. How should the nurse respond?
    b. What kind of negative effects should Mrs. B. report to her physician?

## CASE STUDY

**Read the scenario, and answer the following questions on a separate sheet of paper.**

Arthur, a 68-year-old retired banker, has been diagnosed with early-stage Alzheimer's disease. He has remained active in his church and likes to golf every week. He is in the office today with his son and is asking about the "new drugs that are available to reverse Alzheimer's disease." His son is concerned because Arthur was diagnosed with Parkinson's disease 6 months ago, but it has been controlled well with medications.

1. What drugs are available to "reverse Alzheimer's disease?" Explain.

2. The physician is considering either galantamine or rivastigmine for Arthur. Is there anything in his history that may influence the choice of medication?

3. Describe the different mechanisms of action of direct- and indirect-acting cholinergic-blocking drugs.

4. Arthur is given a prescription for rivastigmine. What are the possible adverse effects, and what should he and his son be told regarding ways to manage these adverse effects?

5. A few months later, Arthur's son reports that Arthur has trouble swallowing tablets. What is a possible solution to this problem?

# 21 Cholinergic-Blocking Drugs

**Select the best answer for each question.**

1. Before giving an anticholinergic drug, the nurse will check the patient's history for which conditions? *(Select all that apply.)*
   a. Glaucoma
   b. Osteoporosis
   c. Acute asthma
   d. Thyroid disease
   e. Diabetes mellitus
   f. Benign prostatic hyperplasia

2. The nurse will monitor for which adverse effects of anticholinergic drugs? *(Select all that apply.)*
   a. Dilated pupils
   b. Hypertension
   c. Dry mouth
   d. Urinary retention
   e. Dysphagia
   f. Diarrhea

3. In reviewing the medication orders for a newly admitted patient, the nurse recognizes that which is an indication for atropine sulfate?
   a. Myasthenia gravis
   b. Sinus bradycardia
   c. Pitting edema
   d. Narrow-angle glaucoma

4. During patient teaching for a 70-year-old man who will be taking an anticholinergic drug, the nurse will reinforce that this medication places the patient at higher risk for which problem?
   a. Angina
   b. Fluid overload
   c. Delirium
   d. Hypothermia

5. A 28-year-old woman is preparing to take a cruise and has asked for a prescription drug to prevent motion sickness. The physician orders scopolamine transdermal patches. The nurse will include which statement when teaching the patient about this drug?
   a. "The patch can be applied anywhere on the upper body."
   b. "Apply the patch 4 to 5 hours before travel."
   c. "Apply the patch just before boarding the ship."
   d. "Be sure to change the patch daily."

6. Patient teaching regarding scopolamine transdermal patches should include which side effects? *(Select all that apply.)*
   a. Drowsiness
   b. Blurred vision
   c. Constipation
   d. Dry mouth
   e. Bradycardia

7. A patient has a new prescription for tolterodine. Which condition, if present, would make it necessary to reduce the usual dosage of this drug?
   a. Coronary artery disease
   b. Diabetes mellitus
   c. Hypertension
   d. Cirrhosis of the liver

8. The preoperative orders read, "Give atropine 0.6 mg IV push, 30 minutes before the procedure." The medication comes in a 1-mg/mL vial. How much medication will the nurse

   administer? _____

9. A 14-month-old toddler is in the preoperative area, and the order reads: "Give glycopyrrolate 4 mcg/kg IV now." The toddler weighs 22 lb.
   a. How many micrograms of medication will the

      toddler receive for this dose? _____
   b. The medication is available in a vial that contains 0.2 mg/mL. How many milliliters will the nurse draw up into the syringe for this dose?

      _____

**53**

**Answer the following questions on a separate sheet of paper.**

10. A patient is given atropine sulfate before surgery. Describe how this drug is helpful during the perioperative period. What other drug can be used for this purpose?

11. Mr. M. is brought into the emergency department with an overdose of a cholinergic blocker. He is still conscious.
    a. Describe how Mr. M. will be treated.
    b. How will the nurse respond if Mr. M. begins having hallucinations related to the overdose?

12. Mr. H. is taking dicyclomine for irritable bowel syndrome. He calls the clinic and tells the nurse that he would like to get his doctor's permission to take an antihistamine for his cold. What drug interactions might he expect?

13. How does atropine work in the following situations?
    a. A patient is experiencing severe bradycardia, with a heart rate of 38 beats/min, and he is losing consciousness.
    b. A crop-duster pilot has been exposed to an organophosphate insecticide in an industrial accident.

**Read the scenario, and answer the following questions on a separate sheet of paper.**

Mrs. W., age 63 years, is in the outpatient clinic today for a physical examination. During history taking, she admits to having a "terrible problem" with her bladder. She describes having sudden urges to urinate and is "ashamed to say" that, at times, she has lost control of her bladder. She has had no other health issues except for "some eye problems" off and on for the past year. The provider is considering starting Mrs. W. on tolterodine.

1. What are the contraindications for this medication? Are there any potential concerns given Mrs. W.'s history?

2. What are the advantages of using tolterodine rather than other drugs with similar actions?

3. Mrs. W. enjoys working outside in her yard. What special precautions does she need to take?

4. After a week of therapy, she calls the clinic to complain of a dry mouth. She said she didn't think this was supposed to happen with this drug. What advice do you give to her?

# 22 Antihypertensive Drugs

**CRITICAL THINKING CROSSWORD**

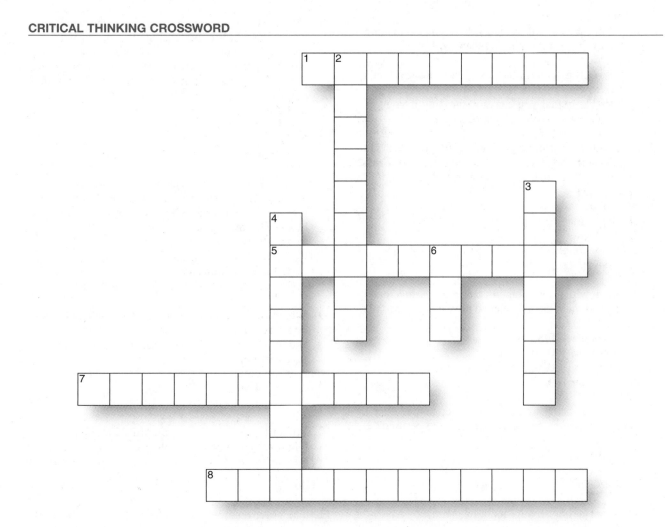

**Across**

1. High blood pressure associated with renal, pulmonary, endocrine, and vascular diseases is known as

   _____ hypertension.
5. Another term for 3 Down
7. A common adverse effect of adrenergic drugs involving a sudden drop in blood pressure when

   patients change position is known as _____ hypotension.
8. These drugs are used in the management of hypertensive emergencies.

**Down**

2. Another term for 3 Down
3. Elevated systemic arterial pressure for which no

   cause can be found is known as _____ hypertension.
4. The primary effect of these drugs is to decrease plasma and extracellular fluid volumes.
6. Drugs that are often used as first-line drugs in the treatment of both heart failure and hypertension are

   known by the acronym _____ inhibitors.

**55**

**Select the best answer for each question.**

1. A 46-year-old man has been taking clonidine for 5 months. For the past 2 months, his blood pressure has been normal. During this office visit, he tells the nurse that he would like to stop taking the drug. What is the nurse's best response?
   a. "I'm sure the doctor will stop it—your blood pressure is normal now."
   b. "Your doctor will probably have you stop taking the drug for a month, and then we'll see how you do."
   c. "This drug should not be stopped suddenly; let's talk to your doctor."
   d. "It's likely that you can stop the drug if you exercise and avoid salty foods."

2. When administering angiotensin-converting enzyme (ACE) inhibitors, the nurse keeps in mind that which are possible adverse effects? *(Select all that apply.)*
   a. Diarrhea
   b. Fatigue
   c. Restlessness
   d. Headaches
   e. A dry cough
   f. Tremors

3. A patient with type 2 diabetes mellitus has developed hypertension. What is the blood pressure goal for this patient?
   a. Less than 110/80 mm Hg
   b. Less than 130/80 mm Hg
   c. Less than 130/84 mm Hg
   d. Less than 140/90 mm Hg

4. A patient is being treated for a hypertensive emergency. The nurse expects which drug to be used?
   a. Sodium nitroprusside
   b. Losartan
   c. Captopril
   d. Prazosin

5. A patient in her eighth month of pregnancy has preeclampsia. Her blood pressure is 210/100 mm Hg this morning. This is classified as which type of hypertension?
   a. Primary
   b. Idiopathic
   c. Essential
   d. Secondary

6. A beta$_1$ blocker is prescribed for a patient with heart failure and hypertension. Which adverse effects, if present, may indicate a serious problem is developing while the patient is taking this medication? *(Select all that apply.)*
   a. Edema
   b. Nightmares
   c. Shortness of breath
   d. Nervousness
   e. Constipation

7. The nurse is obtaining a drug history on a patient being treated for hypertension. The prescriber has chosen the angiotensin receptor blocker losartan to treat the patient's hypertension. Which drug on the patient's current drug list would most concern the nurse?
   a. Furosemide
   b. Albuterol
   c. Ibuprofen
   d. Augmentin

8. Given the nurse's knowledge of the side effects of alpha blockers, which instruction should the nurse provide to the patient with a new order for an alpha blocker to treat hypertension?
   a. Drink plenty of fluids.
   b. Wear sunscreen outside.
   c. Change positions slowly.
   d. Increase intake of potassium-rich foods.

9. Which finding in the patent taking Lisinopril would be an indication to discontinue the drug immediately and avoid taking it in the future?
   a. Heart failure
   b. Albuminuria
   c. Angioedema
   d. Cough

10. The order reads, "Give captopril 25 mg PO every 8 hours." The available tablets are 12.5-mg strength. How many tablets will the nurse administer per dose? _____

11. The order reads, "Give enalapril (Vasotec) 5 mg IV push over 5 minutes now." The medication is available in a vial with the strength of 1.25 mg/mL. How many milliliters will the nurse administer for this dose? _____

**Answer the following questions on a separate sheet of paper.**

12. Mr. Q., 61 years of age, comes to the emergency department with symptoms of a severe hypertensive emergency. The emergency department resident on call initiates therapy with sodium nitroprusside. The patient is transferred to the intensive care unit and monitored. Hours later, his blood pressure falls to 100/60 mm Hg, and he is lethargic and complaining of feeling dizzy. What will the nurse do?

13. Indicate which ACE inhibitor would be best for the following patients. Explain your answers.
    a. Irene, who has liver dysfunction, has high blood pressure, and is seriously ill
    b. Kory, who has a history of poor adherence to his medication regimen

14. Mr. B. will be starting prazosin for hypertension. What will he be taught before he takes even the first dose of this medication?

15. White and African-American patients are known to respond differently to antihypertensive agents.
    a. Which antihypertensives are considered more effective in white patients than in African-American patients?
    b. Which antihypertensives are considered more effective in African-American patients than in white patients?

**Read the scenario, and answer the following questions on a separate sheet of paper.**

John, a 44-year-old African-American man, has been seen twice in the past month for "blood pressure problems." At the first visit, his blood pressure was 144/90 mm Hg; at the second visit, his blood pressure was 154/96 mm Hg. The provider is preparing to start antihypertensive therapy. John has no other medical conditions.

1. What initial drug therapy would be appropriate for him? What factors are considered when choosing which drug to use?

2. John tells you that he hopes this medication will not "slow him down" because he likes to "jump out of bed and get started" with his day. What teaching will you provide for him to help him adjust to his blood pressure medication?

3. John also mentions that he likes to go the gym three times a week and visit with his friends in the sauna after a good workout. What teaching will you emphasize for this patient?

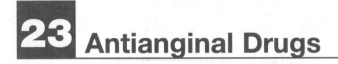

# 23 Antianginal Drugs

**Select the best answer for each question.**

1. What is the purpose of antianginal drug therapy?
   a. To increase myocardial oxygen demand
   b. To increase blood flow to peripheral arteries
   c. To increase blood flow to ischemic cardiac muscle
   d. To decrease blood flow to ischemic cardiac muscle

2. The nurse will teach a patient who will be taking nitroglycerin about which common adverse effect of this drug?
   a. Blurred vision
   b. Dizziness
   c. Headache
   d. Weakness

3. The nurse is reviewing dosage forms of nitroglycerin. This drug can be given by which routes? *(Select all that apply.)*
   a. Continuous intravenous drip
   b. Intravenous bolus
   c. Sublingual spray
   d. Oral
   e. Topical ointment
   f. Rectal suppository

4. For a patient using transdermal nitroglycerin patches, the nurse knows that the prescriber will order which procedure for preventing tolerance?
   a. Leave the old patch on for 2 hours when applying a new patch.
   b. Apply a new patch every other day.
   c. Leave the patch off for 24 hours once a week.
   d. Remove the patch at night for 8 hours, and then apply a new patch in the morning.

5. Patients who are taking beta blockers for angina need to be taught which information?
   a. These drugs are for long-term prevention of angina episodes.
   b. These drugs must be taken as soon as angina pain occurs.
   c. These drugs will be discontinued if dizziness is experienced.
   d. These drugs need to be carried with the patient at all times in case angina occurs.

6. The nurse would recognize which of the following symptoms as descriptive of a side effect of nitrates?
   a. Reflex tachycardia
   b. Hypertension
   c. Nausea
   d. Cough

7. Which of the following describes the rationale for the administration of nitroglycerin by the sublingual route?
   a. The first-pass effect is avoided.
   b. Side effects are lessened.
   c. Patients can self-administer.
   d. It can be used in patients with swallowing problems.

8. A patient with coronary artery spasms will be most effectively treated with which type of antianginal medication?
   a. Beta blockers
   b. Calcium channel blockers
   c. Nitrates
   d. Nitrites

9. During his morning walk, a man begins to experience chest pain. He sits down and takes one nitroglycerin sublingual tablet. After 5 minutes, the chest pain is worsening. What action would be the priority in this situation?
   a. Call 911 (emergency medical services).
   b. Take another nitroglycerin tablet.
   c. Take two more nitroglycerin tablets at the same time.
   d. Sit quietly to wait for the pain to subside.

10. The nurse is preparing for administration of a nitrate to a patient. After reviewing the patient's current medications, the nurse holds the nitrate and contacts the provider. Which medication concerned the nurse?
    a. Furosemide
    b. Sildenafil
    c. Digoxin
    d. lisinopril

11. The order reads: "Give isosorbide dinitrate 80 mg twice a day." The medication is available in 40-mg capsules. How many capsules will the patient receive for each dose? _____

**Answer the following questions on a separate sheet of paper.**

12. The order reads: "Nitroglycerin transdermal patch, 0.2 mg/hr; apply one patch in the morning and remove every evening at 10 PM." The pharmacy has supplied a transdermal patch that supplies 0.4 mg/hr. What will the nurse do to administer this drug?

13. The nurse is playing racquetball at a community center when he notices a commotion at a gathering of senior citizens in a nearby room. The nurse rushes in to find a man lying unconscious on the floor. Several people say that he is having a "heart attack." One man hands the nurse a pill bottle and asks, "Would it help to give him one of my heart pills?" A woman agrees, saying, "Yes! Can't you put it under his tongue?" The nurse sees that the medication bottle is labeled isosorbide dinitrate. What does the nurse know about this medication, and what needs to be done next?

14. Ms. V. is a 70-year-old patient seen in the emergency department for a laceration to her thumb. During the assessment, Ms. V. tells the nurse that she has been "tired and depressed" and has been having "nightmares" since her physician prescribed heart medicine for her angina. Which drug does the nurse suspect Ms. V. is taking? Why?

15. During a home visit with Theresa, she shows the nurse a journal entry describing the duration, time of onset, and severity of a recent angina attack. She reports no adverse effects to her nitroglycerin and shows the nurse where she keeps the tablets—in a clear plastic pillbox on the kitchen windowsill. What will the nurse discuss with Theresa?

## CASE STUDY

**Read the scenario, and answer the following questions on a separate sheet of paper.**

While playing handball, 59-year-old Gideon experiences chest pain. He has had angina before and has sublingual nitroglycerin in his gym bag.

1. What type of angina is he experiencing?

2. What should he do to treat this episode of angina?

3. After Gideon takes the nitroglycerin tablet, the chest pain does not subside. He wants his handball partner to drive him to the hospital. Is this appropriate? Explain your answer.

4. Other than nitroglycerin, which class of drugs is typically used for this type of angina?

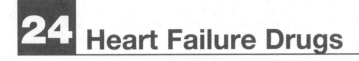

# 24 Heart Failure Drugs

**Select the best answer for each question.**

1. As part of treatment for early heart failure, a patient is started on an angiotensin-converting enzyme (ACE) inhibitor. The nurse will monitor the patient's laboratory work for which potential effect?
   a. Agranulocytosis
   b. Proteinuria
   c. Hyperkalemia
   d. Hypoglycemia

2. Before giving oral digoxin, the nurse discovers that the patient's radial pulse is 52 beats/min when assessed apically for 1 minute. What will be the nurse's next action?
   a. Give the dose.
   b. Delay the dose until later.
   c. Hold the dose and notify the physician.
   d. Obtain a blood pressure reading.

3. Which statement regarding digoxin therapy and potassium levels is correct?
   a. Low potassium levels increase the chance of digoxin toxicity.
   b. High potassium levels increase the chance of digoxin toxicity.
   c. Digoxin reduces the excretion of potassium in the kidneys.
   d. Digoxin promotes the excretion of potassium in the kidneys.

4. When infusing milrinone, the nurse will keep which consideration in mind?
   a. The patient must be monitored for hyperkalemia.
   b. The patient's cardiac status must be monitored closely.
   c. The drug may cause reddish discoloration of the extremities.
   d. Hypertension is the primary effect seen with excessive doses.

5. The nurse would identify the most serious side effect of milrinone as
   a. cardiac dysrhythmias.
   b. hypotension.
   c. heart failure.
   d. liver toxicity.

6. When caring for a patient who is taking digoxin, the nurse will monitor for which signs and symptoms of toxicity? *(Select all that apply.)*
   a. Anorexia
   b. Diarrhea
   c. Visual changes
   d. Nausea and vomiting
   e. Headache
   f. Bradycardia

7. A patient who has heart failure will be started on an oral ACE inhibitor. While monitoring the patient's response to this drug therapy, which laboratory tests would be a priority? *(Select all that apply.)*
   a. White blood cell count
   b. Platelet count
   c. Serum potassium level
   d. Serum magnesium level
   e. Creatinine level
   f. Blood urea nitrogen (BUN)

8. The nurse would recognize that a rise in human B-type natriuretic peptide (BNP) would indicate which of the following?
   a. Increases in myocardial damage
   b. Decreased renal perfusion
   c. Increases in sodium retention
   d. Worsening of heart failure

9. Adverse effects of nesiritide include which of the following? *(Select all that apply.)*
   a. Hypotension
   b. Cardiac dysrhythmias
   c. Insomnia
   d. Headache
   e. Abdominal pain
   f. Photosensitivity

10. The nurse is preparing to administer the initial dose of ivabradine. The nurse will monitor the patient for which adverse effect?
    a. Hypotension
    b. Bradycardia
    c. Hyperkalemia
    d. Asthma

11. A patient is to receive an initial dose of digoxin, 0.5 mg IV push, followed by an oral maintenance dose of 0.25 mg PO daily, starting the next day. The medication is available in ampules that contain 0.25 mg/mL. How many milliliters will he receive for the IV dose? _____

12. Mark the syringe with the correct amount of digoxin the patient will receive for the IV dose in Question 11.

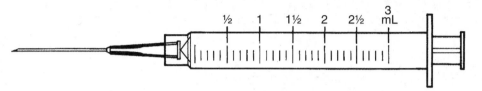

13. Convert the 0.25-mg dose to micrograms.

## CRITICAL THINKING AND APPLICATION

**Answer the following questions on a separate sheet of paper.**

14. The nurse is caring for Mrs. C., who is undergoing cardiac glycoside therapy. She begins to vomit and complains of a headache and fatigue. Diagnostic studies reveal short episodes of ventricular tachycardia on the ECG and a serum potassium level of 6 mEq/L. What action might the nurse expect to be taken?

15. Explain the limitations of nesiritide therapy for heart failure.

16. While monitoring Mr. F. after oral digoxin administration, the nurse notes increased urinary output, decreased dyspnea and fatigue, and constipation. Mr. F. complains that if he were allowed to eat bran as often as he used to, he wouldn't be constipated. What do the nurse's findings indicate? How will the nurse respond to Mr. F.?

17. Mr. M. is experiencing heart failure that has not responded well to diuretic and digoxin therapy. The physician changes his medication to milrinone.
    a. What effect does milrinone have on cardiac muscle contractility and the blood vessels?
    b. What advantage does this phosphodiesterase inhibitor have over the cardiac glycosides?
    c. What is the primary adverse effect of milrinone?

## CASE STUDY

**Read the scenario, and answer the following questions on a separate sheet of paper.**

A 68-year-old woman is admitted to the hospital with a diagnosis of mild left-sided heart failure. At rest, she is comfortable, but she has noticed that she has symptoms when she tries to get dressed or do simple housework. She becomes short of breath with activity, tires easily but cannot sleep at night, and feels "generally irritable." She also has diffuse bilateral crackles that do not clear with coughing and a third heart sound. She has slight pedal edema. The physician has ordered therapy with intravenous digoxin.

1. Digoxin has several effects. Explain the meaning of each of the following:
   a. Positive inotropic effect
   b. Negative chronotropic effect
   c. Negative dromotropic effect

2. As a result of these effects, what would you expect to see with regard to each of the following?
   a. Stroke volume
   b. Venous blood pressure and vein engorgement
   c. Coronary circulation
   d. Diuresis

3. After 3 days of therapy, the patient complains of feeling nauseated and has no appetite. She also wonders why the lights are so bright and blurry. Her radial pulse rate is 52 beats/min. When you check the results of her laboratory work, you note that her digoxin level from that morning is 3.5 ng/mL. What will you do?

# 25 Antidysrhythmic Drugs

**Select the best answer for each question.**

1. The nurse notes in the patient's medication history that the patient is receiving a lidocaine infusion. Based on this finding, the nurse interprets that the patient has which disorder?
   a. Atrial fibrillation
   b. Bradycardia
   c. Complete heart block
   d. Ventricular dysrhythmias

2. When monitoring a patient who is taking quinidine, the nurse recognizes that possible adverse effects of this drug include which conditions? *(Select all that apply.)*
   a. Weakness
   b. Tachycardia
   c. Gastrointestinal upset
   d. Tinnitus
   e. Ventricular ectopic beats

3. The nurse is administering amiodarone and should monitor for which potential adverse effect?
   a. Pulmonary toxicity
   b. Hypertension
   c. Urinary retention
   d. Constipation

4. The nurse is caring for a patient receiving amiodarone. Which drug, if added to the patient's current medication regimen, would cause the nurse concern?
   a. Lidocaine
   b. Ibuprofen
   c. Warfarin
   d. Lasix

5. The nurse would be correct in identifying which condition as a major complication of atrial fibrillation?
   a. Myocardial infarction (MI)
   b. Stroke
   c. Pulmonary edema
   d. Pneumonia

6. A patient is about to receive a dose of verapamil. The nurse notes that this medication is used to treat which condition?
   a. Cardiac asystole
   b. Heart block
   c. Ventricular dysrhythmia, including premature ventricular contraction
   d. Recurrent paroxysmal supraventricular tachycardia (PSVT)

7. A patient is experiencing a rapid dysrhythmia, and the nurse is preparing to administer adenosine. Which is the correct administration technique for this drug?
   a. It should be given as a fast intravenous push.
   b. It should be given intravenously slowly over at least 5 minutes.
   c. It should be taken with food or milk.
   d. It should be given as an intravenous drip infusion.

8. If a drug has a prodysrhythmic effect, then the nurse must monitor the patient for which effect?
   a. Decreased heart rate
   b. New dysrhythmias
   c. A decrease in dysrhythmias
   d. Reduced blood pressure

9. A patient will be starting therapy with quinidine. Which of these drugs, if also on the patient's medication list, may cause a potential drug interaction? *(Select all that apply.)*
   a. Cimetidine
   b. Amiodarone
   c. Digoxin
   d. Warfarin
   e. Erythromycin

10. Which medication has recently been approved for the treatment of atrial fibrillation?
    a. Lidocaine
    b. Propafenone
    c. Adenosine
    d. Bretylium

11. A patient with sustained ventricular tachycardia will be receiving a lidocaine infusion after a bolus dose. The order reads, "Give a bolus of 1.5 mg/kg, then start a drip at 2 mg/min." The lidocaine is available as 20 mg/mL, and the patient weighs 220 lb. How many milligrams of lidocaine will be given in the

bolus dose? _____

12. A patient is to receive adenosine as initial treatment for PSVT. The dose is 6 mg IV push. The medication is available in a vial that contains 3 mg/mL. How many milliliters will the nurse draw up into the

syringe for this dose? _____

13. Match the site to its correct intrinsic rate.
    a. Sinoatrial node
    b. Atrioventricular node
    c. Purkinje fibers
       (1) 40 to 60 beats/min
       (2) 40 or fewer beats/min
       (3) 60 to 100 beats/min

## CRITICAL THINKING AND APPLICATION

**Answer the following questions on a separate sheet of paper.**

14. Mr. K., who has been diagnosed with hypertension, is hospitalized after a myocardial infarction (MI).
    a. To reduce the risk for sudden cardiac death in Mr. K., the physician prescribes a drug from which class? Why?
    b. How would a history of asthma in Mr. K. affect the drug choice?

15. Mr. N. has a life-threatening ventricular tachycardia that has been resistant to treatment. What drug will the nurse expect to be used, and what precautions are necessary with this drug?

16. Mr. M. is a 50-year-old schoolteacher being treated with lidocaine after an MI.
    a. He is very upset and says that he hates injections; he wants to know why he can't just take a pill. What will the nurse tell him?
    b. If Mr. M. has a history of cirrhosis, how would the dosage of the lidocaine be affected?

17. Alicia calls the health clinic complaining of diarrhea and lightheadedness. She says she cannot remember whether she took her quinidine yesterday and wants to know whether she should take two doses today, especially because she is feeling so bad. What will the nurse tell Alicia?

## CASE STUDY

**Read the scenario, and answer the following questions on a separate sheet of paper.**

Jack, age 39 years, has a new prescription for verapamil as part of his treatment for occasional PSVT. This is the first time he has taken this medication. He states he has no previous history of heart problems but that he does smoke one pack of cigarettes a day.

1. How do calcium channel blockers such as verapamil work?

2. What therapeutic effects are expected?

3. What may be a concern regarding his health history?

4. After 4 months of therapy, Jack experiences dizziness, dyspnea, and a very rapid heart rate and is taken to the emergency department. He is diagnosed with sustained PSVT, and intravenous diltiazem (Cardizem) does not help. What drug may be tried next?

# 26 Coagulation Modifier Drugs

**Match each definition with its corresponding term. (Note: Not all terms will be used; terms may be used more than once.)**

1. _____ A drug that prevents the lysis of fibrin, thereby promoting clot formation

2. _____ The termination of bleeding by mechanical or chemical means

3. _____ A substance that prevents platelet plugs from forming

4. _____ The general term for a drug that dissolves thrombi

5. _____ The general term for a substance that prevents or delays coagulation of the blood

6. _____ A laboratory test used to measure the effectiveness of heparin therapy

7. _____ Two tests used to monitor the effects of drug therapy with warfarin sodium *(Select two choices.)*

8. _____ A standardized measure of the degree of coagulation achieved by drug therapy with warfarin sodium

9. _____ A substance that reverses the effect of heparin

10. _____ A substance that reverses the effect of warfarin sodium

11. _____ A pharmaceutically available tissue plasminogen activator (tPA) that is created through recombinant DNA techniques

12. _____ A blood clot that dislodges and travels through the bloodstream

   a. Prothrombin time (PT)
   b. Activated partial thromboplastin time (aPTT)
   c. International normalized ratio (INR)
   d. Rivaroxaban
   e. Alteplase

   f. Thrombus
   g. Embolus
   h. Vitamin K
   i. Protamine sulfate
   j. Antiplatelet drug
   k. Antifibrinolytic
   l. Thrombolytic drug
   m. Anticoagulant
   n. Hemostasis

**Select the best answer for each question.**

13. The nurse is reviewing the use of anticoagulants. Anticoagulant therapy is appropriate for which conditions? *(Select all that apply.)*
   a. Atrial fibrillation
   b. Thrombocytopenia
   c. Myocardial infarction
   d. Presence of mechanical heart valve
   e. Aneurysm
   f. Leukemia

14. Which statement is true regarding enoxaparin and dalteparin?
   a. Their method of action is to interrupt vitamin K–dependent clotting factors.
   b. They do not require clotting-time monitoring.
   c. They are administered deep IM.
   d. They have thrombolytic properties.

15. During the teaching of a patient who will be taking warfarin sodium at home, which statement by the nurse is correct regarding over-the-counter drug use?
   a. "Choose nonsteroidal antiinflammatory drugs as needed for pain relief."
   b. "Aspirin products may result in increased bleeding."
   c. "Vitamin E therapy is recommended to improve the effect of warfarin."
   d. "Mineral oil is the laxative of choice while taking anticoagulants."

16. A patient is at risk for a stroke. Which drug is recommended to prevent platelet aggregation for stroke prevention by the American Stroke Society?
    a. Aspirin
    b. Warfarin sodium
    c. Heparin
    d. Alteplase

17. When administering subcutaneous heparin, the nurse will remember to perform which action?
    a. Use the same sites for injection to reduce trauma.
    b. Use a 1-inch needle for subcutaneous injections.
    c. Inject the medication without aspirating for blood return.
    d. Massage the site after the injection to increase absorption.

18. During thrombolytic therapy, the nurse monitors for bleeding. Which symptoms may indicate a serious bleeding problem? *(Select all that apply.)*
    a. Hypertension
    b. Hypotension
    c. Decreased level of consciousness
    d. Increased pulse rate
    e. Restlessness

19. Which drug is most often used for the prevention of deep vein thrombosis (DVT) after major orthopedic surgery, even after the patient has gone home?
    a. Antiplatelet drugs, such as aspirin
    b. Adenosine diphosphate (ADP) inhibitors, such as clopidogrel
    c. Anticoagulants, such as warfarin sodium
    d. Low-molecular-weight heparins, such as enoxaparin

20. Which of the following findings would the nurse expect to observe in the patient experiencing heparin-induced thrombocytopenia?
    a. Red blood cell count of 3.0/mL
    b. White blood cell count of less than 5000/mL
    c. Platelet count of 50,000/mL
    d. Creatine kinase of 230 U/L

21. The nurse would recognize which drug as the recommended drug for thrombotic stroke prevention?
    a. Warfarin
    b. Clopidogrel
    c. Enoxaparin
    d. Aspirin

22. The nurse is preparing a patient's morning medications and, upon reviewing the list of drugs, notes that the patient is to receive heparin 5000 units and enoxaparin, both subcutaneously. What is the nurse's priority action at this time?
    a. Administer the drugs in separate sites.
    b. Hold the drugs, and clarify the order with the prescriber.
    c. Administer the enoxaparin and hold the heparin.
    d. Check the patient's aPTT.

23. Idarucizumab is a specific antidote for which drug?
    a. Heparin
    b. Dabigatran
    c. Warfarin
    d. Enoxaparin

24. A patient is to receive a bolus dose of heparin 8000 units via IV push. The vial contains heparin 10,000 units/mL. How many milliliters of medication will the nurse draw up to administer the ordered dose?

    _____

25. A patient who weighs 165 lb is to receive daily doses of fondaparinux (Arixtra). According to the accompanying dosage chart for the drug, how many milligrams will this patient receive per dose?

| Patient weight less than 50 kg | 5 mg/day |
|---|---|
| Patient weight 50–100 kg | 7.5 mg/day |
| Patient weight more than 100 kg | 10 mg/day |

## CRITICAL THINKING AND APPLICATION

**Answer the following questions on a separate sheet of paper.**

26. The nurse is preparing to administer a new order of enoxaparin (Lovenox) to a patient. Upon checking the patient, the nurse notes that the patient has an epidural catheter. What is the priority action of the nurse at this time?

27. During cardiopulmonary bypass for heart surgery, Mr. J. was intentionally given a large dose of heparin. The surgeon then determines that the effects of the heparin need to be reversed quickly.
    a. How will this be done?
    b. How will the amount of antidote be determined?
    c. What is the most commonly used test for determining the effects of heparin therapy?

**65**

28. A patient is experiencing warfarin toxicity from accidentally taking too many warfarin tablets.
    a. What will be used as an antidote?
    b. How will the dose of the antidote be determined?
    c. After 4 days, the patient requires anticoagulation again. What drug will be ordered?

29. After surgery, Mr. T. has a chest tube in place. The site has been bleeding excessively. What type of drug might the physician prescribe in this situation? Why?

30. William, a 38-year-old writer who has von Willebrand's disease, has undergone emergency surgery after an automobile accident. What drug is used in the management of bleeding in patients like William? What is its effect?

31. Tobias has been given alteplase (Activase) during his treatment for acute myocardial infarction. A few minutes later, he suffers a reinfarction. What drug does the nurse expect Tobias to receive now?

32. Ursula, an inpatient on the nurse's unit, is on anticoagulant therapy. The nurse enters her room to find that she is restless and confused.
    a. Why are these findings significant?
    b. What other problems might the nurse expect to find?
    c. What will the nurse do?

33. Sara is receiving subcutaneous heparin 5000 units twice a day for DVT prevention. Will her anticoagulation be monitored by laboratory work? Explain.

**Read the scenario, and answer the following questions on a separate sheet of paper.**

After experiencing transient ischemic attacks, Doug has been started on clopidogrel (Plavix). He has had a history of atherosclerotic heart disease and has had problems with peptic ulcer disease.

1. He asks, "Why am I taking this fancy medicine? Why can't I just take an aspirin a day, like they say on television?" What do you tell him?

2. What should he be taught to report to his health care provider while he is taking this drug?

3. What precautions should he follow while he is taking this drug?

4. What herbal products should he avoid while he is taking this drug?

# 27 Antilipemic Drugs

**Select the best answer for each question.**

1. Patients taking cholestyramine may experience which adverse effects?
   a. Blurred vision and photophobia
   b. Drowsiness and difficulty concentrating
   c. Diarrhea and abdominal cramps
   d. Belching and bloating

2. The nurse will instruct the patient who is taking antilipemic drugs about which dietary measures? *(Select all that apply.)*
   a. Taking supplements of fat-soluble vitamins
   b. Taking supplements of B vitamins
   c. Increasing fluid intake
   d. Choosing foods that are lower in cholesterol and saturated fats
   e. Increasing the intake of raw vegetables, fruit, and bran

3. In reviewing the history of a newly admitted cardiac patient, the nurse knows that the patient would have a contraindication to antilipemic therapy if which condition is present?
   a. Phenylketonuria
   b. Renal disease
   c. Coronary artery disease
   d. Diabetes mellitus

4. A woman is being screened in the cardiac clinic for risk factors for coronary artery disease. Which would be considered a negative (favorable) risk factor for her?
   a. High-density lipoprotein (HDL) cholesterol level of 30 mg/dL
   b. HDL cholesterol level of 75 mg/dL
   c. Low-density lipoprotein (LDL) level of 25 mg/dL
   d. History of diabetes mellitus

5. A patient who has started taking niacin complains that he "hates the side effects." Which statement by the nurse is most appropriate?
   a. "You will soon build up tolerance to these side effects."
   b. "You need to take niacin on an empty stomach."
   c. "You can take niacin every other day if the side effects are bothersome."
   d. "Try taking a small dose of ibuprofen 30 minutes before taking niacin."

6. A patient asks, "What is considered the 'good cholesterol'?" How will the nurse answer?
   a. Very low-density lipoprotein (VLDL)
   b. LDL
   c. HDL
   d. Triglycerides

7. A patient taking a statin calls the office to report an increase in muscle pain. Which information takes priority as the nurse communicates with the patient?
   a. "This could be the sign of a serious side effect; stop taking the medication immediately."
   b. "You should take a dose of ibuprofen for the next few days."
   c. "This is an expected occurrence; continue the dose as prescribed."
   d. "Did you pull a muscle or injure yourself?"

8. The nursing student would be correct in identifying which of the following as features of metabolic syndrome? *(Select all that apply.)*
   a. Waist circumference greater than 40 inches in men
   b. Serum triglycerides greater than 150 mg/dL
   c. HDL greater than 80 mg/dL in men and women
   d. Normal blood pressure
   e. Fasting serum glucose of 110 mg/dL or higher

9. The nurse is preparing to administer a newly ordered statin drug to a patient and is reviewing the patient's list of current medications. Which medications may cause an interaction with the statin drug? *(Select all that apply.)*
   a. Warfarin
   b. Metformin
   c. Erythromycin
   d. Cyclosporine
   e. Gemfibrozil

10. Which route will the nurse select for the administration of alirocumab?
    a. Oral
    b. Rectal
    c. Subcutaneous
    d. Intramuscular

11. The medication order reads, "Give lovastatin (Mevacor) 30 mg daily at bedtime, PO." The medication is available in 20-mg tablets. How many tablets will the nurse administer to the patient?

    _____

12. A patient is to receive niacin (Niaspan), 1.5 g/day in 2 divided doses. The medication is available in 250-mg extended-release tablets. How many milligrams will the patient receive for each dose?

    How many tablets per dose? _____

### CRITICAL THINKING AND APPLICATION

**Answer the following questions on a separate sheet of paper.**

13. For each of the following drugs, name the antilipemic category and briefly describe how the drug lowers lipid levels.
    a. Gemfibrozil (Lopid)
    b. Niacin
    c. Lovastatin (Mevacor)
    d. Cholestyramine (Questran)

14. Mr. H. is a 46-year-old business executive who travels frequently. He is slightly overweight "from all that room service," but he did quit smoking 6 years ago. He has no history of coronary heart disease (CHD) or any family history of CHD. During a routine checkup, Mr. H. is found to have an LDL cholesterol level of 170 mg/dL. He says, "I'm a busy man! Just give me some pills. I've got a plane to catch!" Will the physician prescribe an antilipemic for Mr. H.? Explain your answer.

15. Mrs. K. has been treated with cholestyramine (Questran) for type IIa hyperlipidemia for the past 2 months. She tells the nurse that she "can't stand being so irregular" and that she has developed another "embarrassing problem" as well. What does the nurse suspect is wrong with Mrs. K., and how can the nurse help her?

16. Justus is a 55-year-old attorney being treated with lovastatin (Mevacor) for hyperlipidemia. His current health status includes mild hypertension and a peptic ulcer. The nurse knows that niacin is frequently prescribed as an adjunct to other antilipemic drugs. Would niacin be helpful for Justus? Explain your answer.

17. You are visiting Mrs. N., a homebound patient who is being treated for hyperlipidemia and hypertension. During your visit, Mrs. N. takes her antihypertensive medication and then begins to mix her dose of cholestyramine into a glass of orange juice. What patient teaching does Mrs. N. require?

### CASE STUDY

**Read the scenario, and answer the following questions on a separate sheet of paper.**

Mr. M. has been diagnosed with type IIa hyperlipidemia and has been given a prescription for atorvastatin (Lipitor). He acts thrilled with the news, and says, "Great! Now I don't have to worry about watching my diet because I'm on this medicine!"

1. Is he right? What type of dietary guidelines should he follow while on this therapy?

2. What therapeutic effects do you hope to see as a result of his taking this medication?

3. After 2 months of therapy, you note that Mr. M.'s liver enzyme levels are slightly elevated. Is this a concern? What other laboratory values will be monitored while Mr. M. is taking atorvastatin?

4. Mr. M. calls the office to complain about some muscle pain. He thought he had pulled a muscle during a tennis match, but the pain has not lessened in 3 days. Is this a concern?

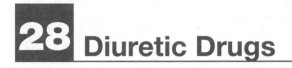

# 28 Diuretic Drugs

**Match each term with its corresponding definition.**

1. _____ Diuretics

2. _____ Potassium-sparing diuretics

3. _____ Loop of Henle

4. _____ Osmotic diuretics

5. _____ Thiazides

6. _____ Ascites

7. _____ CAIs

8. _____ Loop diuretics

9. _____ Nephron

10. _____ GFR

a. Potent diuretics that act along the ascending limb of the loop of Henle; furosemide is an example
b. Abbreviation for the term that describes a gauge of how well the kidneys are functioning as filters
c. A general term for drugs that accelerate the rate of urine formation
d. The main structural unit of the kidney
e. Part of the kidney structure located between the proximal and distal convoluted tubules
f. Diuretics that result in the diuresis of sodium and water and the retention of potassium; spironolactone is an example
g. Diuretics that act on the distal convoluted tubule, where they inhibit sodium and water resorption; hydrochlorothiazide (HCTZ) is an example
h. Abbreviation for a class of diuretics that inhibit the enzyme carbonic anhydrase; acetazolamide is an example
i. Drugs that induce diuresis by increasing the osmotic pressure of the glomerular filtrate, which results in rapid diuresis; mannitol is an example
j. An abnormal intraperitoneal accumulation of fluid

**Select the best answer for each question.**

11. Which are indications for the use of diuretics? *(Select all that apply.)*
    a. To increase urine output
    b. To reduce uric acid levels
    c. To treat hypertension
    d. To treat open-angle glaucoma
    e. To treat edema associated with heart failure

12. When providing patient teaching to a patient who is taking a potassium-sparing diuretic such as spironolactone, the nurse will include which dietary guidelines?
    a. The patient needs to drink grapefruit with the diuretic.
    b. The patient needs to consume foods high in potassium, such as bananas and orange juice.
    c. The patient needs to avoid excessive intake of foods high in potassium.
    d. The patient needs to drink 1 to 2 L of fluid per day.

13. When teaching a patient about diuretic therapy, which would the nurse indicate as the best time of day to take these medications?
    a. Morning
    b. Midday
    c. Bedtime
    d. The time of day does not matter.

14. When monitoring a patient for hypokalemia related to diuretic use, the nurse looks for which possible symptoms?
    a. Nausea, vomiting, and anorexia
    b. Diarrhea and abdominal pain
    c. Orthostatic hypotension
    d. Muscle weakness and lethargy

15. A patient with severe heart failure has been started on therapy with a carbonic anhydrase inhibitor (CAI), but the nurse mentions that this medication may be stopped in a few days. What is the reason for this short treatment?
    a. CAIs are not the first choice for treatment of heart failure.
    b. Metabolic acidosis develops in 2 to 4 days after therapy is started.
    c. It is expected that CAIs will dramatically reduce the fluid overload related to heart failure.
    d. Allergic reactions to CAIs are common.

16. Which diuretic remains effective when creatinine clearance drops below 25 mL/min?
    a. Loop
    b. Thiazide
    c. Osmotic
    d. Potassium sparing

17. The greatest volume of diuresis is produced by which class of diuretics?
    a. Loop
    b. Thiazide
    c. Osmotic
    d. Potassium sparing

18. Which diuretic class has its action at the end point of the nephron?
    a. Loop
    b. Thiazide
    c. Osmotic
    d. Potassium sparing

19. A patient has a new order for daily doses of spironolactone. Which conditions, if present, may be a contraindication to this drug therapy? *(Select all that apply.)*
    a. Heart failure
    b. Renal failure
    c. Diabetes mellitus
    d. Deep vein thrombosis
    e. Hyperkalemia

20. A patient is to receive furosemide 120 mg every morning via PEG tube. The medication is available in a liquid form, 40 mg/5 mL. Mark on the medication cup how many milliliters the patient will receive for this dose.

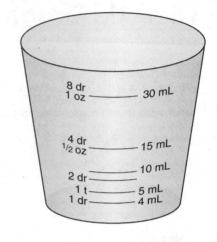

21. A patient is to receive 30 g of mannitol intravenously. The medication on hand is mannitol 20% in a 500-mL bag. How many milliliters will the patient receive?

## CRITICAL THINKING AND APPLICATION

**Answer the following questions on a separate sheet of paper.**

22. Ms. A. is a 62-year-old retired teacher who is being treated for diabetes and open-angle glaucoma. The health care provider has prescribed a diuretic as an adjunct drug in the management of Ms. A.'s glaucoma.
    a. Which diuretic drug was probably prescribed?
    b. What undesirable effect of the drug does the provider need to consider?

23. The nurse is about to administer mannitol to Arthur, who is in early acute renal failure.
    a. What is the significance of Arthur's renal blood flow and glomerular filtration in this situation?
    b. By what means will the nurse administer the mannitol? What special guidelines will be followed?
    c. Arthur later complains of a headache and chills. Should the mannitol therapy be ended? Explain your answer.

24. Mr. F. has been admitted for treatment of ascites. He also has some renal impairment and a history of heavy drinking.
    a. Which diuretic drug will the nurse expect to be administered to Mr. F.?
    b. What monitoring will be performed frequently? Why?

25. Brendan, a 39-year-old bricklayer, is taking a thiazide diuretic for hypertension. During a follow-up visit, he tells the nurse that he thinks the drug is affecting his "love life."
    a. To what adverse effect of thiazide therapy is Brendan probably referring?
    b. While the nurse is talking, she notices a package of licorice in Brendan's coat pocket. He tells her that he eats the candy "for energy," especially because he has been feeling so tired the past couple of days. What will the nurse tell Brendan?

26. The nurse receives a call from Mrs. H., who recently started diuretic therapy for hypertension. Mrs. H. is concerned because her neighbor, who also takes medication for hypertension, has told her not to eat a lot of bananas or other foods containing potassium. "But you told me to eat foods high in potassium," Mrs. H. says to the nurse, "What's going on?" How will the nurse respond to Mrs. H.?

27. Mrs. P. will be started on diuretic therapy for hypertension, but she also has moderate renal failure. Which diuretic—a loop diuretic or a thiazide diuretic—would be more effective for Mrs. P.? Explain your answer.

## CASE STUDY

**Read the scenario, and answer the following questions on a separate sheet of paper.**

Lily has been taking furosemide for 3 months as part of her treatment for heart failure. At this time, she is complaining that she is feeling tired and has muscle weakness and no appetite; her blood pressure is 100/50 mm Hg.

1. What do her symptoms suggest? How did this happen?

2. What dietary measures could she have taken to prevent this problem?

3. The physician switches her medication to spironolactone. How does this drug differ from furosemide?

4. You will check for what drug interactions before she begins taking the spironolactone?

# 29 Fluids and Electrolytes

**Select the best answer for each question.**

1. Which are common uses of crystalloids? *(Select all that apply.)*
   a. Fluid replacement
   b. Promotion of urinary flow
   c. Transport of oxygen to cells
   d. Replacement of electrolytes
   e. As maintenance fluids
   f. Replacement of clotting factors

2. The intravenous order for a newly admitted patient calls for "Normal saline to run at 100 mL/hr." The nurse will choose which concentration of normal saline?
   a. 0.33%
   b. 0.45%
   c. 0.9%
   d. 3.0%

3. A patient has been admitted with severe dehydration after working outside on a very hot day. The nurse expects which intravenous product to be ordered?
   a. Albumin
   b. Hetastarch
   c. Fresh frozen plasma
   d. 0.9% sodium chloride

4. When giving intravenous potassium, which is important for the nurse to remember?
   a. Intravenous doses are preferred over oral dosage forms.
   b. Intravenous solutions should contain at least 50 mEq/L.
   c. Potassium must always be given in diluted form.
   d. It is given by slow intravenous bolus.

5. The nurse monitors for which signs of a possible transfusion reaction when a patient is receiving blood products?
   a. Subnormal temperature and hypertension
   b. Apprehension, restlessness, fever, and chills
   c. Decreased pulse and respirations and fever
   d. Headache, nausea, and lethargy

6. A patient with a blood disorder needs a replacement product that contains clotting factors. The nurse expects which product to be given?
   a. Albumin
   b. Fresh frozen plasma
   c. Packed red blood cells
   d. 0.9% normal saline

7. A patient is receiving conivaptan. Which action by the nurse is appropriate?
   a. Administer the drug by slow IV push over 10 minutes.
   b. Report serum sodium levels of 149 mEq/L.
   c. Monitor for hyperkalemia.
   d. Implement measures to prevent constipation.

8. Administration of a hypertonic intravenous fluid would result in which of the following?
   a. Cellular shrinkage
   b. Cellular swelling
   c. Dependent edema
   d. Dehydration

9. The nurse would anticipate the administration of which of the following in the patient with a potassium level of 5.9 mEq?
   a. Furosemide
   b. Sodium chloride
   c. Magnesium sulfate
   d. Sodium polystyrene sulfonate

10. Which of the following outcomes would be appropriate for the patient receiving patiromer?
    a. Increased serum sodium
    b. Decreased serum potassium
    c. Increased serum magnesium
    d. Decreased serum calcium

11. The following IV is to be given: 1000 mL $D_5W$ with 20 mEq potassium chloride (KCl) over the next 24 hours. The tubing drop factor is 15.
    a. At what rate will the KCl be administered?

    _____

    b. What will the gtt/min be? _____

12. An IVPB antibiotic needs to infuse over 30 minutes. The IVPB bag contains 50 mL. Calculate the setting for the infusion pump. _____

## CRITICAL THINKING AND APPLICATION

**Answer the following questions on a separate sheet of paper.**

13. Name the advantages and disadvantages of using crystalloids to replace fluid in patients with dehydration.

14. Some fluids are known as *oxygen-carrying resuscitation fluids*.
    a. Which class of fluids is given this designation?
    b. Why are these fluids able to carry oxygen?
    c. Why is their origin a potential problem for a recipient?

15. Tanya, a 16-year-old student, is brought to the clinic by her mother, who says that Tanya has been on "some sort of fad diet." The mother is concerned because Tanya is tired and weak. During the nurse's assessment, Tanya admits that she has been using laxatives and eating very little during the past few weeks. Her sodium level is 136 mEq/L, and her potassium level is 2.8 mEq/L. What electrolyte imbalance is Tanya probably experiencing? How can it be corrected?

16. Mr. S., a 45-year-old mail carrier, has come to the emergency department sweating profusely and complaining of stomach cramps and diarrhea. He says that he has been "miserable" from the heat the past few days. His serum sodium level is 128 mEq/L.
    a. What electrolyte imbalance does the patient have?
    b. The health care provider prescribes oral sodium tablets. What adverse effect of sodium may be of special concern for Mr. S.?

17. Victor is receiving a transfusion of a blood product.
    a. The nurse observes Victor, knowing that an adverse reaction to the transfusion may be manifested by what signs and symptoms?
    b. Victor's wife is crying and says, "People get AIDS from transfusions. What happens if Victor gets AIDS?" What will the nurse tell her?
    c. Forty-five minutes after the transfusion was started, Victor is restless, and his pulse rate has increased. Explain the nurse's next actions, including the priority action.

## CASE STUDY

**Read the scenario, and answer the following questions on a separate sheet of paper.**

An older man was admitted to the unit with hypoproteinemia caused by chronic malnutrition. You note that he has some edema over his body, and his total protein level is 4.8 g/dL.

1. What is the relationship between his serum total protein level and the edema you have noted?

2. You are preparing to give him 1 unit of 5% albumin. How does albumin work in this situation?

3. What advantages does albumin have over crystalloids in this situation?

4. You will monitor for what adverse effects while he is receiving albumin?

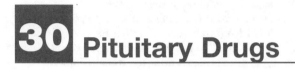

# 30 Pituitary Drugs

**1. Complete the following table.**

| Hormone | Function | Mimicking Drug(s) |
|---|---|---|
| Adrenocorticotropic hormone (ACTH, corticotropin) | Targets adrenal gland; mediates adaptation to stressors; promotes synthesis of the following three hormones:<br>a. *(List three.)* | b. |
| Growth hormone | c. | d. *(List two.)* |
| e. | Increases water resorption in distal tubules and collecting duct of nephron; concentrates urine; potent vasoconstrictor | f. *(List two.)* |
| Oxytocin | g. | h. |

**Select the best answer for each question.**

2. When administering vasopressin, what is the priority vital sign for the nurse to monitor?
   a. Temperature
   b. Pulse
   c. Respirations
   d. Blood pressure

3. A nurse is administering octreotide to a patient who has a metastatic carcinoid tumor. The patient asks about the purpose of this drug. What is the nurse's best response?
   a. "This drug helps reduce the size of your tumor."
   b. "This drug works to prevent the spread of your tumor."
   c. "This drug helps control the flushing and diarrhea that you are experiencing."
   d. "This drug reduces the nausea and vomiting you are having from the chemotherapy."

4. Which nursing diagnosis is most appropriate for a patient who is receiving a pituitary drug?
   a. Constipation
   b. Disturbed body image
   c. Impaired physical mobility
   d. Impaired skin integrity

5. The nurse will instruct a patient taking desmopressin acetate as a nasal spray for the treatment of diabetes insipidus to perform which action to obtain maximum benefit from the drug?
   a. Clear the nasal passages before spraying the medication.
   b. Blow his nose after taking the medication.
   c. Take an over-the-counter preparation to control mucus if nasal congestion occurs.
   d. Press on the pump once to prime it before delivering the dose.

6. During vasopressin therapy, which is the priority nursing action?
   a. Check blood glucose levels regularly.
   b. Monitor the electrocardiogram for changes.
   c. Monitor the IV site for signs of infiltration.
   d. Watch for hyperthermia.

7. Which drug antagonizes the effects of natural growth hormone?
   a. Octreotide
   b. Vasopressin
   c. Somatropin
   d. Cyclosporin

8. When assessing a patient who is receiving octreotide therapy, the nurse will closely monitor which assessment finding?
   a. Blood glucose levels
   b. Pulse
   c. Weight
   d. Serum potassium levels

9. When monitoring for the therapeutic effects of intranasal desmopressin (DDAVP) in a patient who has diabetes insipidus, which assessment finding will the nurse look for as an indication that the medication therapy is successful?
   a. Increased insulin levels
   b. Decreased diarrhea
   c. Improved nasal patency
   d. Decreased urine output

10. A child who weighs 44 lb and is experiencing growth failure is to receive growth hormone therapy. The dosage ordered is 0.3 mg/kg per week, to be given as a series of one injection per day for 6 days.
    a. What is the total dose per week that this child will receive? _____
    b. What is the dose per injection? _____

11. The order reads: "Give octreotide 50 mcg IV bid." The medication is available in a strength of 0.1 mg/mL. How many milliliters will the nurse draw up for this dose? Indicate your answer on the syringe.

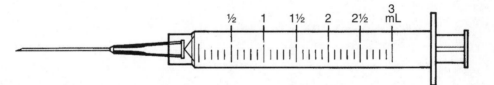

**Answer the following questions on a separate sheet of paper.**

12. The nurse has recently begun working in a specialized endocrinology clinic. Her first patient, Patricia, a second grader, is not growing at the expected rate. The physician has determined that Patricia is a candidate for somatropin therapy. What will be emphasized when the nurse is teaching her parents about giving this drug?

13. A patient is being assessed for possible adrenocortical insufficiency. The physician orders a dose of cosyntropin. The patient, upon hearing that he will be receiving an injection, states "Oh, good! The doctor has already found something to cure me!" How will the nurse respond?

**Read the scenario, and answer the following questions on a separate sheet of paper.**

Mr. C. has been experiencing severe thirst, which he reports "makes me go to the bathroom all the time, it seems." He is also dehydrated despite the large amounts of water he has been drinking. He is diagnosed with diabetes insipidus.

1. What two drugs may be used to treat diabetes insipidus?

2. What are the possible cautions to the use of these drugs?

3. The physician decides that Mr. C. should do well with vasopressin therapy. Indicate how you would describe the treatment and its therapeutic effects (i.e., how it mimics the natural hormone) to the patient.

4. After your explanation, Mr. C. says, "Okay, okay, but what does it do for me?" Explain the physical improvements Mr. C. should be able to see.

# 31 Thyroid and Antithyroid Drugs

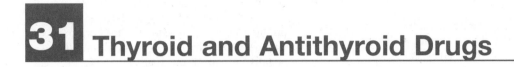

## CRITICAL THINKING CROSSWORD

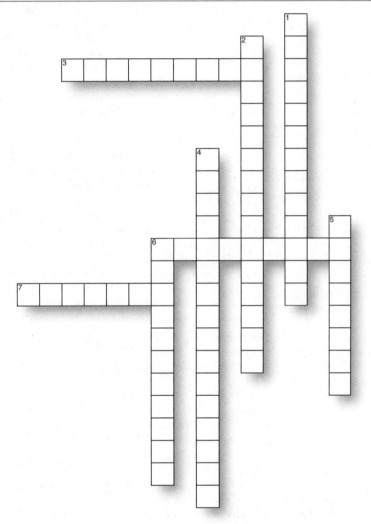

### Across

3. The type of hypothyroidism that results from insufficient secretion of thyroid-stimulating hormone (TSH) from the pituitary gland
6. The principal thyroid hormone that influences the metabolic rate
7. The type of hypothyroidism that is caused by the inability of the thyroid gland to perform a function

### Down

1. The most commonly prescribed synthetic thyroid hormone
2. Excessive secretion of thyroid hormones
4. A drug used to treat hyperthyroidism
5. The type of hypothyroidism that stems from reduced secretion of thyrotropin-releasing hormone from the hypothalamus
6. Another name for TSH

**Select the best answer for each question.**

1. A patient who is beginning therapy with levothyroxine asks the nurse when the medication will start working. What is the nurse's best answer?
   a. Immediately
   b. Within a few days
   c. Within a few weeks
   d. Within a few months

2. A patient wants to switch brands of levothyroxine. What is the nurse's best response?
   a. "If you do this, you should reduce the dosage of your current brand before starting the new one."
   b. "Levothyroxine has been standardized, so there is only one brand."
   c. "It shouldn't matter if you switch brands; they are all very much the same."
   d. "You should check with your provider before switching brands."

3. Patient teaching for a patient taking antithyroid medication will include the need to avoid which foods?
   a. Soy products and seafood
   b. Bananas and oranges
   c. Dairy products
   d. Processed meats and cheese

4. Which information needs to be included in the nurse's teaching of patients taking thyroid medications? *(Select all that apply.)*
   a. Keeping a log or journal of individual responses and a graph of pulse rate, weight, and mood would be helpful.
   b. The medication will be discontinued if the adverse effects become too strong.
   c. The medication needs to be taken at the same time every day.
   d. Nervousness, irritability, and insomnia may be a result of a dosage that is too high.
   e. Take thyroid replacement drugs after meals.

5. A patient is scheduled for a radioactive isotope study. The scheduling nurse notes that he takes levothyroxine daily. Which medication order needs to be made before the radioactive isotope study is scheduled?
   a. Continue to take the levothyroxine as ordered.
   b. Do not take the levothyroxine on the morning of the test.
   c. Stop the levothyroxine about 4 weeks before the test.
   d. Reduce the levothyroxine dosage by one-half 1 week before the test.

6. Which statement is accurate regarding the method of action of I-131?
   a. Radioactive iodine works by decreasing the synthesis of thyroid hormone.
   b. Radioactive iodine works by decreasing the production of thyroid-stimulating hormone.
   c. Radioactive iodine works by inhibiting the negative feedback mechanism.
   d. Radioactive iodine works by destroying the thyroid gland.

7. Which statement is accurate regarding the method of action of methimazole?
   a. Radioactive iodine works by decreasing the synthesis of thyroid hormone.
   b. Radioactive iodine works by decreasing the production of thyroid-stimulating hormone.
   c. Radioactive iodine works by inhibiting the negative feedback mechanism.
   d. Radioactive iodine works by destroying the thyroid gland.

8. The nurse has been providing patient education regarding thyroid hormone replacement therapy. Which statement by the patient reflects a need for further teaching?
   a. "I will take this pill in the mornings."
   b. "Sometimes this medicine can make my heart skip beats, but that's a normal side effect."
   c. "I need to take this pill on an empty stomach and wait about 30 to 60 minutes before eating."
   d. "I will be sure to go to the clinic to have my thyroid levels tested regularly."

9. A patient who is beginning therapy with propylthiouracil (PTU) asks the nurse when the medication will start working. What is the nurse's best answer?
   a. Immediately
   b. Within a few days
   c. Within 2 weeks
   d. Within a few months

10. Levothyroxine (Synthroid) 88 mcg PO is ordered.

    What is 88 mcg expressed as mg? _____

11. The order reads, "Give levothyroxine 150 mcg IV now." The vial of medication, after it is reconstituted, contains 0.1 mg/mL. How many milliliters will

    the nurse draw up for this dose? _____

## CRITICAL THINKING AND APPLICATION

**Answer the following questions on a separate sheet of paper.**

12. Mrs. W., age 43 years, comes into the clinic complaining of hair loss, lethargy, and constipation. "I just can't eat anything," she says. As the nurse takes her blood pressure, he notices that her skin feels thickened. She also seems to have a lump in her neck. The primary care provider makes a diagnosis of hypothyroidism. Suggest several possible appropriate medications. Which of those is generally preferred? Why?

13. After undergoing a thyroidectomy as treatment for a thyroid tumor that turned out to be benign, Rebecca is given a prescription for levothyroxine. "I thought I would be cured after this surgery!" she exclaimed. "Why do I have to take a pill every day?" What will the nurse explain to Rebecca?

14. The nurse is examining changes in a medication administration record after new orders were written. One new medication order reads, "levothyroxine (Levothroid), 200 mg, once a day." The nurse suspects an error. What is wrong with this order?

15. Rory, age 32 years, has been given a prescription for PTU as part of treatment for Graves' disease. What laboratory tests are important to assess before she begins this medication?

## CASE STUDY

**Read the scenario, and answer the following questions on a separate sheet of paper.**

Goldie, a 38-year-old teacher, has come to the clinic complaining of having "no energy or appetite," yet her weight has increased by 15 lb in the past month. You note that her hair is thin, and her skin is dull. Laboratory work reveals an elevated level of thyroid-stimulating hormone (TSH). A diagnosis of hypothyroidism is made.

1. What medication do you expect to be ordered for Goldie?

2. Explain the concept of "euthyroid" as it would relate to Goldie's condition.

3. One month after therapy has begun, Goldie calls the office to complain that she "can't sleep at all" since she started taking the medication. She says she tries to take it at the same time every morning but often forgets and takes it at dinnertime. What teaching, if any, does she need to help her with this problem?

Chapter **31** **Thyroid and Antithyroid Drugs**

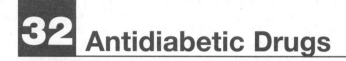

# 32 Antidiabetic Drugs

**Select the best answer for each question.**

1. When administering insulin, the nurse must keep in mind that which is the most immediate and serious adverse effect of insulin therapy?
   a. Hyperglycemia
   b. Hypoglycemia
   c. Bradycardia
   d. Orthostatic hypotension

2. A dose of long-acting insulin has been ordered for bedtime for a patient with diabetes. The nurse expects to give which type of insulin?
   a. Regular
   b. Lispro
   c. NPH
   d. Glargine

3. A patient is to be given an insulin drip to control his high blood glucose levels. The nurse knows that the type of insulin that would be used for this intravenous infusion would be which of these?
   a. Regular
   b. Lispro
   c. NPH
   d. Glargine

4. While monitoring a patient who is receiving insulin therapy, the nurse observes for which signs of hypoglycemia?
   a. Decreased pulse and respiratory rates and flushed skin
   b. Increased pulse rate and a fruity, acetone breath odor
   c. Irritability, sweating, and confusion
   d. Increased urine output and edema

5. When will the nurse administer the drug acarbose?
   a. With the first bite of a meal
   b. 15 minutes before a meal
   c. 30 minutes before a meal
   d. 1 hour after eating

6. A patient taking glipizide asks the nurse, "How does my insulin pill work, anyway?" Which information will the nurse provide to the patient regarding the mechanism of action of glipizide?
   a. "It increases insulin production."
   b. "It helps the body use insulin."
   c. "It decreases the amount of glucose made by the liver."
   d. "It decreases the amount of glucose the body takes in from food."

7. The nurse is reviewing the history of a patient who will be taking the amylin mimetic drug pramlintide. Which condition is a contraindication to the use of this drug?
   a. Hypertension
   b. Coronary artery disease
   c. Hypothyroidism
   d. Gastroparesis

8. The nurse will monitor for significant interactions if sitagliptin is given with which drug class?
   a. Corticosteroids
   b. Sulfonylureas
   c. Thyroid drugs
   d. Nonsteroidal antiinflammatory drugs

9. Which is a major risk factor for the development of type 2 diabetes?
   a. Kidney disease
   b. Liver disease
   c. Obesity
   d. Hypercholesteremia

10. Which A1C level represents the desired level for the glycemic goal for patients with diabetes?
    a. 10
    b. 9
    c. 8
    d. 7

11. Which patient condition would the nurse identify as being a contraindication for the use of Afrezza?
    a. Kidney disease
    b. Chronic lung disease
    c. Chronic liver disease
    d. Psoriasis

12. The duration of action of insulin glargine is
    a. 30 minutes.
    b. 1 hour.
    c. 6 to 8 hours.
    d. 24 hours.

13. The sliding-scale insulin order reads, "Do bedside glucose testing before meals. For glucose results over 150 mg/dL, give regular insulin, 1 unit for every 20 mg/dL over 150 mg/dL." If the blood glucose level is 238 mg/dL, the patient will receive

    _____ unit(s) of insulin.

14. A patient will be receiving NPH insulin 30 units combined with 7 units of regular insulin. Mark the insulin syringe at the line that indicates the combined dose of insulin.

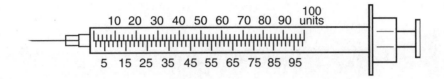

**Answer the following questions on a separate sheet of paper.**

15. What is the mechanism of action of each drug?
    a. Pramlintide
    b. Metformin

16. Alice occasionally experiences hypoglycemia as a result of her diabetes drug therapy.
    a. The nurse will teach Alice about what signs and symptoms of hypoglycemia?
    b. The nurse knows that one of the early signs of hypoglycemia is irritability. Why is this true?
    c. If Alice experiences hypoglycemia at home, what are the treatment options?

17. The newly graduated nurse is preparing a dose of Novolin-R insulin to administer to a patient.
    a. Before the nurse administers the medication, how will the nurse's coworker verify the order?
    b. After examining the syringe, the nurse's coworker tells the graduate nurse that the syringe must be discarded because the insulin is cloudy. The new graduate states, "Insulin is supposed to look this way." Who is right, the new nurse or the coworker?
    c. The nurse examines the vial. A date on the label indicates that it has been on the shelf in this room for 2 months. Is this a problem?

18. Mrs. F. is 5 feet tall and weighs 180 lb. During a routine physical examination, laboratory studies indicate an elevated fasting blood glucose level and a hemoglobin A1C level of 6.6%. The nurse's assessment of Mrs. F. reveals that she is a smoker with mild hypertension. The physician suspects type 2 diabetes. What initial treatment is indicated for Mrs. F.? Explain your answer.

19. Dennis takes glipizide. He comes to the emergency department late one Sunday evening complaining that he feels weak. He vomited earlier, he has a headache, and his face "feels hot." You note that Dennis has profound flushing and is sweating.
    a. What do Dennis's signs and symptoms indicate?
    b. What will you assess immediately?
    c. What may have caused this?

20. A patient who has been taking metformin for type 2 diabetes mellitus needs to have a radiology examination with contrast dye. What is the nurse's best action regarding the metformin?

21. For each listed symptom, specify whether it is associated with hyperglycemia or hypoglycemia.
    a. Irritability
    b. Fatigue
    c. Polydipsia
    d. Tremors
    e. Sweating

Chapter **32 Antidiabetic Drugs**

**Read the scenario, and answer the following questions on a separate sheet of paper.**

The physician is planning to prescribe glipizide for Mr. D., a 50-year-old financial advisor with a history of renal failure and type 2 diabetes. In particular, Mr. D. requires treatment for the short- term elevation in blood glucose level that occurs after he eats.

1. Are there specific guidelines for when this drug needs to be taken?

2. At a visit 3 months later, during a blood draw for fasting laboratory work, Mr. D. tells the nurse, "I've been good for the past few days, so I'm sure my fasting levels are okay. But thankfully, the doctor won't know how I've been sneaking snacks." What laboratory test will be ordered to monitor Mr. D.'s diabetes, and what will this test indicate?

3. A few weeks later, Mr. D. comes down with gastroenteritis. He is vomiting and has been unable to eat all day. What should he do? Why?

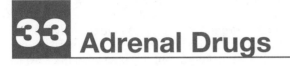

# 33 Adrenal Drugs

**Select the best answer for each question.**

1. A 50-year-old man has been taking prednisone as part of treatment for bronchitis. He notices that the dosage of the medication decreases. During a follow-up office visit, he asks the nurse why he must continue the medication and why he cannot just stop taking it now that he feels better. What is the rationale behind the tapering dosages?
   a. Sudden discontinuation of this medication may result in adrenal insufficiency.
   b. The patient would experience withdrawal symptoms if the drug were discontinued abruptly.
   c. Cushing's syndrome may develop as a reaction to a sudden drop in serum cortisone levels.
   d. When the symptoms have started to disappear, lower dosages are needed.

2. The nurse is reviewing the use of oral glucocorticoids. Which of these is the preferred oral glucocorticoid for antiinflammatory or immunosuppressant purposes?
   a. Fludrocortisone
   b. Dexamethasone
   c. Prednisone
   d. Hydrocortisone

3. When monitoring a patient who is taking corticosteroids, the nurse observes for which adverse effects? *(Select all that apply.)*
   a. Fragile skin
   b. Hyperglycemia
   c. Nervousness
   d. Hypotension
   e. Weight loss
   f. Drowsiness

4. A patient has Cushing's syndrome. The nurse expects which drug to be used to inhibit the function of the adrenal cortex in the treatment of this syndrome?
   a. Dexamethasone
   b. Aminoglutethimide
   c. Hydrocortisone
   d. Fludrocortisone

5. A patient who has been taking corticosteroids has developed a "moon face" and facial redness, and she has many bruises on her arms. Which of these is the most appropriate nursing diagnosis?
   a. Risk for infection
   b. Imbalanced nutrition: less than body requirements
   c. Deficient fluid volume
   d. Disturbed body image

6. Because corticosteroids may cause sodium retention, the nurse will closely monitor patients with which condition when administering corticosteroids?
   a. Diabetes mellitus
   b. Seizure disorders
   c. Heart failure
   d. Hyperthyroidism

7. The nurse would recognize which potential side effect of glucocorticoid therapy in young children?
   a. Arthritis
   b. Growth suppression
   c. Constipation
   d. Iron-deficiency anemia

8. The nurse is administering aminoglutethimide to a patient and will monitor for which adverse effects? *(Select all that apply.)*
   a. Constipation
   b. Dizziness
   c. Anorexia
   d. Hypertension
   e. Lethargy

9. To assist in counteracting the adverse effects of glucocorticoid therapy, the nurse would encourage the patient to increase levels of which nutrient in the diet?
   a. Vitamin K
   b. Vitamin D
   c. Magnesium
   d. Phosphorous

10. The order reads, "Give dexamethasone 1.5 mg, twice a day." The medication is available in 3-mg tablets. How many tablets will the nurse give for each dose?

_____

11. An infant is to receive methylprednisolone (Solu-Medrol) 0.5 mg/kg IV every 6 hours. The infant weighs 14 lb. How many milligrams of medication will this infant receive per dose? *(Record answer using one decimal place.)* _____

## CRITICAL THINKING AND APPLICATION

**Answer the following questions on a separate sheet of paper.**

12. Ms. R., a 30-year-old hospital receptionist, is receiving glucocorticoid therapy after a kidney transplant. The nurse is reviewing her drug regimen with her when she says that she frequently uses aspirin or ibuprofen to treat problems such as headaches and menstrual cramps. She also mentions that she enjoys walking for exercise and likes to visit sick children on the hospital's pediatric ward when she has time. What issues will the nurse discuss with Ms. R.?

13. Peter has developed a severe skin rash after a camping trip. The health care provider is planning to prescribe prednisone (Deltasone). The nursing assessment reveals that Peter has type 1 diabetes.
    a. Does that finding affect Peter's treatment? Explain your answer.
    b. To help minimize gastrointestinal effects, what advice will the nurse have for someone taking an oral form of a systemic glucocorticoid?

14. The nurse is watching a student nurse prepare to apply a topical glucocorticoid to a patient's skin rash. After donning gloves, she places some of the medication on her finger. Should the nurse intervene, or is the student nurse doing fine so far? What other consideration is involved in determining the technique for applying a topical drug?

15. Nina has been prescribed a steroid drug delivered via inhaler. What special instructions will the nurse give her?

# 34 Women's Health Drugs

**Select the best answer for each question.**

1. When reviewing the health history of a patient who wants to begin taking oral contraceptives, the nurse recalls that which conditions are contraindications to this drug therapy? *(Select all that apply.)*
   a. Multiple sclerosis
   b. Pregnancy
   c. Thrombophlebitic disorders
   d. Hypothyroidism
   e. Estrogen-dependent cancers

2. When the nurse is teaching patients about postmenopausal estrogen replacement therapy, which statement is correct?
   a. "It is not recommended in patients with a history of endometrial cancer."
   b. "Use is recommended and beneficial in older women."
   c. "Estrogen therapy should be long term to prevent menopausal symptoms."
   d. "If estrogen is taken, supplemental calcium will not be needed."

3. The most serious side effects of progestins include which of the following?
   a. Menopause
   b. Liver dysfunction
   c. Myocardial infarction
   d. Pancreatic insufficiency

4. When combination oral contraceptives are given to provide postcoital emergency contraception, the nurse must remember which fact?
   a. They are not effective if the woman is already pregnant.
   b. They should be taken within 12 hours of unprotected intercourse.
   c. They are given in one dose.
   d. They are intended to terminate pregnancy.

5. When reviewing an order for dinoprostone cervical gel, the nurse recalls that this drug is used for which purpose?
   a. To induce abortion during the third trimester
   b. To improve cervical ripening near term for labor induction
   c. To soften the cervix in women who are experiencing infertility problems
   d. To reduce postpartum uterine atony and hemorrhage

6. A pregnant woman is experiencing contractions. The nurse remembers that pharmacologic measures to stop contractions are used during which time frame?
   a. Before the 20th week of gestation
   b. Between the 20th and 37th weeks
   c. After the 37th week
   d. At any time during the pregnancy if delivery is not desired

7. What patient teaching is appropriate for a patient taking alendronate? *(Select all that apply.)*
   a. Take with food.
   b. Take at night just before going to bed.
   c. Take with an 8-oz glass of water.
   d. Take with a sip of water.
   e. Take first thing in the morning upon arising.
   f. Do not lie down for at least 30 minutes after taking.

8. A patient is beginning a new prescription of raloxifene. The nurse will teach the patient to expect which potential adverse effects? *(Select all that apply.)*
   a. Leg cramps
   b. Loss of appetite
   c. Diarrhea
   d. Hot flashes
   e. Drowsiness

**85**

9. The nurse at the clinic is taking a health history when the patient tells the nurse intercourse has been painful for the past 3 months. The nurse would anticipate the provider would order which medication?
   a. Ospemifene
   b. Flibanserin
   c. Estrogen
   d. Progesterone

10. The patient is to receive medroxyprogesterone 500 mg weekly on Mondays for 4 weeks. The medication is available in vials of 400 mg/mL. How many milliliters will the nurse administer with each injection? *(Record answer using one decimal place.)* _____

Mark the syringe with the correct amount the nurse will draw up for this injection.

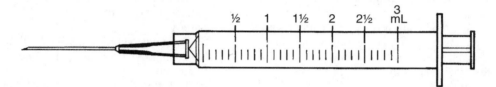

11. A patient is to receive megestrol 400 mg each morning as an appetite stimulant. The medication is available in an oral suspension with a concentration of 40 mg/mL. How many milliliters will the nurse administer for this dose? _____

## CRITICAL THINKING AND APPLICATION

**Answer the following questions on a separate sheet of paper.**

12. Isabelle is a 48-year-old woman exhibiting symptoms of menopause. Assessment of Isabelle reveals a history of depression and mild arthritis.
    a. What will the nurse need to ask Isabelle? Why?
    b. The health care provider decides to prescribe estrogen therapy. At this time, what does the nurse know about the dose and the length of time it will be administered?

13. Ms. K., age 25 years, has type 2 diabetes that is controlled by oral medications. She is at the clinic today because her menstrual periods have ceased. The nurse practitioner has decided to prescribe a hormonal drug.
    a. Which drug will the nurse practitioner likely prescribe?
    b. How will this hormone therapy potentially affect Ms. K.'s diabetes? What will she need to do?

14. Jacklyn receives a prescription for norethindrone and ethinyl estradiol for birth control. At a follow-up visit 4 months later, she tells the nurse practitioner, "I'm really messing up. I take the pills for 3 weeks, but when I'm off them for a week, sometimes I don't remember to start again!"
    a. What might the nurse practitioner suggest to help Jacklyn?
    b. Jacklyn then expresses concern that her menstrual bleeding, now that she is taking birth control pills, is "nothing compared with what it used to be." She asks the nurse practitioner whether she is okay. What will the nurse practitioner tell Jacklyn?

15. Ms. J., a sales associate in a bookstore, is being treated for fertility problems. She is currently on a drug regimen that includes human chorionic gonadotropin and clomiphene (Clomid). Why is she taking two fertility drugs?

16. Mrs. I. has been taking estrogen therapy for several weeks. During a routine checkup, she tells the nurse that she has not been able to quit smoking yet. She also mentions that she is going to Aruba for a vacation the next month. What patient teaching does Mrs. I. require?

17. Mrs. S., age 33 years, comes in for her yearly gynecologic examination, and the provider recommends alendronate (Fosamax), 5 mg daily. Mrs. S. experienced early menopause last year and asks the nurse, "Why did my doctor wait until now to start me on estrogen? I didn't need it before." What will the nurse explain about the purpose of this medication?

18. Mr. G. is receiving 400 mg of megestrol. This drug is a progestin, a female hormone. Why is a male patient receiving this medication?

**Read the scenario, and answer the following questions on a separate sheet of paper.**

J.Q., age 24 years, has decided that she wants to try oral birth control and is in the nurse practitioner's office today for an evaluation. During the health history, she tells the nurse that she has never used oral contraceptives but that she is currently sexually active. She also states that she takes no other medications or herbal products. After a physical assessment, the nurse practitioner prescribes norethindrone and ethinyl estradiol (Ortho-Novum 7/7/7) oral contraceptive.

1. What laboratory test is most important to check before J.Q. starts the oral contraceptive?

2. The nurse needs to assess for what other potential risk factors before J.Q. begins the oral contraceptive?

3. After 6 months, J.Q. calls the office and states, "I forgot to take my birth control pills 3 days in a row. What do I do now?" How does the nurse respond?

# 35 Men's Health Drugs

**Select the best answer for each question.**

1. A 19-year-old college football player asks a nurse about taking steroids to help him "beef up" his muscles. Which statement is true?
   a. There should be no problems as long as he does not exceed the recommended dosage.
   b. Long-term use may cause a life-threatening liver condition.
   c. He would need to be careful to watch for excessive weight loss.
   d. These drugs also tend to increase the male's sperm count.

2. In which situations would androgens be prescribed for a woman? *(Select all that apply.)*
   a. Development of secondary sex characteristics
   b. Fibrocystic breast disease
   c. Ovarian cancer
   d. Treatment of endometriosis
   e. Postmenopausal osteoporosis prevention
   f. Inoperable breast cancer

3. A patient will be receiving testosterone therapy for male hypogonadism and has a new prescription for transdermal testosterone. The nurse needs to include which teaching point about the use of this medication?
   a. Apply the patch only to the scrotum.
   b. Apply the patch to the chest, back, or shoulders.
   c. Apply the patch and then tape it in place.
   d. The patch should be applied to a different area of the upper body each day.

4. Before a patient begins therapy with finasteride, the nurse should make sure that which laboratory test has been performed?
   a. Blood glucose level
   b. Complete blood count
   c. Urinalysis
   d. Prostate-specific antigen (PSA) level

5. A male patient tells the nurse he has been taking finasteride for 3 months and has seen little relief of symptoms. Which is the best response by the nurse?
   a. "You will need surgical intervention."
   b. "Tell me how you are taking your medication."
   c. "It may take up to 6 months for full effect."
   d. "A second drug will need to be added to your medications."

6. In addition to many effects on body systems, the nurse would be correct in identifying which effect as an outcome of androgen therapy?
   a. Increased sperm production and enhanced fertility
   b. Increased red blood cell production
   c. Weight loss
   d. Bone resorption

7. A patient is taking finasteride for the treatment of benign prostatic hyperplasia. His wife, who is 3 months pregnant, is worried about the adverse effects that may occur with this drug. Which statement by the nurse is the most important at this time?
   a. "Gastric upset may be reduced if he takes this drug on an empty stomach."
   b. "He should notice therapeutic effects of increased libido and erection within 1 month."
   c. "This medication should not even be handled by pregnant women because it may harm the fetus."
   d. "He may experience transient hair loss while taking this medication."

8. A male patient wants to know if there are any drugs that can be used for baldness. The nurse knows that which drug, in low dosages, is used for androgenetic alopecia in men?
   a. Finasteride
   b. Vardenafil
   c. Danazol
   d. Oxandrolone

9. A patient has asked for a new prescription for sildenafil. As the nurse reviews the current medications, which drug, if taken by the patient, would cause a significant interaction?
   a. Warfarin, an oral anticoagulant
   b. Amoxicillin, an antibiotic
   c. Esomeprazole, a proton pump inhibitor
   d. Isosorbide dinitrate, a nitrate

10. A patient has a new prescription for finasteride. The nurse will instruct the patient about which potential adverse effects? *(Select all that apply.)*
    a. Loss of erection
    b. Gynecomastia
    c. Headaches
    d. Increased libido
    e. Ejaculatory dysfunction

11. A patient is to receive testosterone cypionate 300 mg every 2 weeks as an intramuscular injection. The medication is available in two strengths: 100 mg/mL and 200 mg/mL.
    a. Which is the most appropriate strength?

    _____

    b. How many milliliters will the nurse administer

    per injection? _____

## CRITICAL THINKING AND APPLICATION

**Answer the following questions on a separate sheet of paper.**

12. Mr. M. is being treated for hypogonadism. He has been taking intramuscular injections of testosterone cypionate but has complained about the pain caused by the injections. Today he will be switched to an oral dosage form. He expects to get "testosterone pills." However, the nurse remembers the poor performance of the drug when given via that route, and she tells him that it will probably not be testosterone itself.
    a. Mr. M. is skeptical of switching drugs and asks for more information. Explain specifically why oral testosterone does not work well.
    b. What does the nurse predict Mr. M. will receive instead?
    c. Discuss potential contraindications that might apply to this patient.

13. Mr. M. is prescribed methyltestosterone buccally. He reports that he gets "tired" of waiting for the buccal tablet to dissolve and asks whether he can swallow or chew it, at least after it is mostly dissolved.
    a. If Mr. M. allows most of the tablet to dissolve on its own, is it acceptable to compromise, for the sake of patient compliance, by letting him chew or swallow the rest?
    b. "And while we're on the subject," Mr. M. says, "I'm going on a fishing trip next week. I'd like not to have to bother with the pills. Can we work something out so that I stop temporarily and pick back up with the treatment as soon as I get back?" What is the best answer for Mr. M.?

14. Mr. H. has been prescribed finasteride for benign prostatic hyperplasia. He asks, "How does it work?" The nurse explains that it will cause his prostate to decrease in size and alleviate discomfort. He is concerned about taking this new drug. What are the most important things for the nurse to include in his patient teaching plan?

15. Compare the application methods for the following forms of testosterone: Testoderm patch, Androderm patch, and AndroGel.

## CASE STUDY

**Read the scenario, and answer the following questions on a separate sheet of paper.**

Mr. E., age 72 years, has asked the physician for "help with a private matter." He tells the health care provider that he would like to try Viagra, "that drug that helps with a certain problem."

1. What assessment findings may contraindicate the use of sildenafil (Viagra) by Mr. E.?

2. If he is a candidate for therapy with Viagra, what patient teaching should he receive?

3. What concerns would there be about his liver function? About his vision?

4. When should he take this medication?

# 36 Antihistamines, Decongestants, Antitussives, and Expectorants

**Select the best answer for each question.**

1. The nurse who is providing patient teaching about antihistamine use will include which information? *(Select all that apply.)*
   a. Antihistamines are best tolerated when taken with meals.
   b. The patient can chew gum if he or she experiences dry mouth.
   c. Drowsiness is a frequent side effect of antihistamines.
   d. Over-the-counter medications are generally safe to use with antihistamines.
   e. The patient should avoid drinking alcoholic beverages while on these drugs.

2. A patient asks the nurse about the newer antihistamines. He wants one that does not cause drowsiness. Which drug is appropriate?
   a. Loratadine
   b. Diphenhydramine
   c. Dimenhydrinate
   d. Meclizine

3. Which drugs are considered first-line drugs for the treatment of nasal congestion? *(Select all that apply.)*
   a. Antihistamines such as diphenhydramine
   b. Decongestants such as naphazoline
   c. Antitussives such as dextromethorphan
   d. Expectorants such as guaifenesin
   e. Inhaled corticosteroids such as beclomethasone

4. When giving an antitussive, the nurse remembers that they are used primarily for what reason?
   a. To relieve nasal congestion
   b. To thin secretions to ease removal of excessive secretions
   c. To stop the cough reflex when the cough is nonproductive
   d. To suppress productive and nonproductive coughs

5. The nurse is administering an expectorant and will provide which teaching?
   a. Avoid fluids for 30 to 35 minutes after the dose.
   b. Drink extra fluids, unless contraindicated, to aid in expectoration of sputum.
   c. Avoid driving or operating heavy machinery while taking this medication.
   d. Expect secretions to become thicker.

6. A patient has been self-medicating with diphenhydramine to help her sleep. She calls the clinic nurse to ask, "Why do I feel so tired during the day after I take this pill? I get a good night's sleep!" Which statement by the nurse is correct?
   a. "You are probably getting too much sleep."
   b. "You are taking too much of the drug."
   c. "This drug is not really meant to help people sleep."
   d. "This drug often causes a 'hangover effect' during the day after taking it."

7. A patient is asking about taking an antihistamine for springtime allergies. The nurse assesses for contraindications to antihistamine therapy. Which of these conditions, if present, would be a contraindication? *(Select all that apply.)*
   a. Type 2 diabetes mellitus
   b. Benign prostatic hyperplasia
   c. Hyperthyroidism
   d. Narrow-angle glaucoma
   e. Asthma

8. Which outcome would the nurse recognize as a positive response to guaifenesin?
   a. Decreased wheezing
   b. Increase in respiratory rate
   c. Increase in sputum production
   d. Decreased use of accessory muscles for breathing

9. Which of the following represents the only intranasal anticholinergic drug in use today?
   a. Flunisolide
   b. Fluticasone
   c. Ipratropium.
   d. Ciclesonide

10. Which fact should the nurse provide to the patient with a new prescription for oxymetazoline?
    a. Limit intake of caffeine.
    b. Limit use of the medication to 3 days.
    c. Take the medication with a full glass of water.
    d. The onset of action is immediate.

11. A patient is to receive guaifenesin, 300 mg, via his nasogastric tube. The available medication is syrup, 100 mg/5 mL.
    a. How many milliliters will the nurse administer?

    _____

    b. Mark the medication cup with your answer.

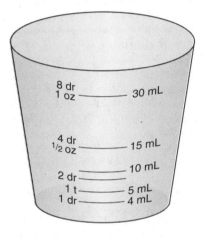

12. A 5-year-old child is to receive a one-time dose of diphenhydramine, 6.25 mg PO. The medication is available in a liquid syrup form with a concentration of 12.5 mg/5 mL. How many milliliters will the nurse administer for this dose?

    _____

### CRITICAL THINKING AND APPLICATION

**Answer the following questions on a separate sheet of paper.**

13. Mrs. L. was seen in the office several days ago with a common cold. She has been on decongestant therapy with naphazoline nasal spray since that time. Today she calls to say, "I thought I was getting over this, but suddenly my nose is more stuffed up than ever." Does Mrs. L. possibly need a stronger dosage of the decongestant? Explain your answer.

14. Keith has been using a topical nasal decongestant for the past few days. He calls the health care provider's office to report that he is feeling nervous and dizzy and that his heart seems to be racing. What might be the cause of Keith's symptoms?

15. How does benzonatate differ from other antitussive drugs in its mechanism of action? In its drug interaction profile?

16. One day the nurse encounters her neighbor Irene as she is returning home from work. Irene is on her way to the drugstore, she tells the nurse, because she has been experiencing a nonproductive cough and wants to get a cough medicine "to loosen things up." The nurse recalls that Irene mentioned a few months ago that she has problems with her thyroid. How should the nurse respond to Irene's comment? Explain your answer.

17. Lisa is a 5-year-old patient who has bronchitis accompanied by a nonproductive cough. The provider has prescribed Robitussin DM for the cough. Lisa's father tells the nurse that his 11-year-old son was prescribed Robitussin A-C several months earlier for a severe cough. He asks whether his son's cough medicine would help Lisa because "there's plenty left in the bottle." What will the nurse tell him?

18. Britney gave birth recently and is breastfeeding her baby. She calls the pediatrician's office because she wants to take an over-the-counter antihistamine for her allergies. "It's okay now that I've given birth, right?" What is the nurse's best answer?

### CASE STUDY

**Read the scenario, and answer the following questions on a separate sheet of paper.**

James, a 35-year-old electrician, is seen in the emergency department with a rash on his arms and hands that appeared after he was working in his yard. You suspect that the physician will prescribe topical diphenhydramine, but during the nursing assessment, James tells you that he has diabetes.

1. How does James's diabetes affect his possible treatment with diphenhydramine?

2. If James does receive a topical diphenhydramine preparation, what other drug might be found in combination with it?

3. The topical medication did not help his rash, and James has been switched to oral diphenhydramine. He tells you that he expects to return to work tomorrow and hopes this medication "does the trick." What cautions, if any, should James be aware of while taking this medication?

4. Are there any concerns with drug interactions?

# 37 Respiratory Drugs

**Select the best answer for each of the following.**

1. The nurse is teaching a group of patients about the use of bronchodilators. It is important to remind them that overuse of bronchodilators may cause which adverse effects? *(Select all that apply.)*
   a. Blurred vision
   b. Increased heart rate
   c. Decreased heart rate
   d. Nausea
   e. Nervousness
   f. Tremors

2. For patients taking a leukotriene receptor antagonist, the nurse should include which information in the patient teaching?
   a. If a dose is missed, the patient may take a double dose to maintain blood levels.
   b. The patient should gargle or rinse the mouth after using the inhaler.
   c. The medication should be taken at the first sign of bronchospasm.
   d. Improvement should be seen within a week of use.

3. Which drug acts by blocking leukotrienes, thus reducing inflammation in the lungs?
   a. Cromolyn
   b. Montelukast
   c. Theophylline
   d. Albuterol

4. A patient is experiencing status asthmaticus. The nurse will prepare to administer which drug first?
   a. Epinephrine
   b. Methylprednisolone
   c. Cromolyn
   d. Montelukast

5. When a patient is taking parenteral xanthine derivatives such as aminophylline, the nurse should monitor for which adverse effect?
   a. Decreased respirations
   b. Hypotension
   c. Tachycardia
   d. Hypoglycemia

6. The nurse would be correct in identifying which of the following levels as representative of a therapeutic level of theophylline?
   a. 0 to 5 mcg/mL
   b. 5 to 15 mcg/mL
   c. 15 to 25 mcg/mL
   d. 25 mcg/mL or greater

7. Which of the following patient factors would most concern the nurse in a patient who is taking theophylline?
   a. The patient has increased fluid intake.
   b. The patient smokes a pack of cigarettes a day.
   c. The patient has bradycardia.
   d. The patient complains of sleepiness.

8. A patient who has asthma may be prescribed which type of inhaled drug for its antiinflammatory effects?
   a. Corticosteroid
   b. Anticholinergic
   c. Xanthine derivative
   d. Beta adrenergic

9. A patient is to receive a new prescription for an ipratropium inhaler. The nurse will assess for which potential contraindications? *(Select all that apply.)*
   a. Allergy to soy lecithin
   b. Allergy to peanuts
   c. Allergy to iodine products
   d. Hypertension
   e. Seizure disorders

10. A patient has a new prescription for an ipratropium bromide/albuterol sulfate metered-dose inhaler. The patient is to take two puffs, four times a day. The inhaler contains 200 "puffs." In how many days should the patient replace the inhaler?

    _____

11. A 6-year-old child is to receive albuterol 0.2 mg/kg PO two times a day. The child weighs 40 lb. How many milligrams will the child receive per dose? *(Record answer using one decimal place.)*

    _____

**Answer the following questions on a separate sheet of paper.**

12. Tom, a 70-year-old retiree who smoked for 40 years, has been diagnosed with chronic obstructive pulmonary disease (COPD); the treatment regimen prescribed includes theophylline. After a few weeks, Tom tells the nurse that he is experiencing nausea and "bad heartburn at night." The laboratory studies show the level of theophylline in his blood to be 30 mcg/mL. What condition might Tom be experiencing, and how can it be corrected?

13. Sylvia has come to the clinic today complaining of nausea, palpitations, and anxiety. She says that her heart feels "as if it's going to fly out of my chest." Physical examination confirms an increased heart rate. Sylvia's records indicate that she has asthma, for which she uses an albuterol inhaler. When asked about the inhaler, she states that she uses it "whenever I feel short of breath." What is causing Sylvia's complaints?

14. Mrs. V., a 65-year-old office manager, has arthritis, glaucoma, and emphysema. The health care provider is planning treatment for her emphysema.
    a. What three types of drugs might be considered for the treatment of COPD?
    b. What factor must the provider keep in mind when determining the best drug for Mrs. V.?

15. Several months ago, the physician prescribed an orally administered corticosteroid for Mr. Z., who has chronic bronchial asthma.
    a. What are the disadvantages of administering the corticosteroids orally? Is there an alternative route?
    b. Today the physician adds beclomethasone dipropionate to Mr. Z.'s drug regimen and reduces the dosage of the oral corticosteroid. Why was the oral corticosteroid not discontinued? Why should Mr. Z. rinse his mouth with water after use?

16. Alice has been treated for asthma for several months and has the following inhalers: albuterol and fluticasone. Which one should she choose if she experiences an asthma attack? Explain your answer.

17. Justin calls the nurse at the office because he experiences "palpitations and a racing heart" every morning after breakfast. He is taking theophylline as part of his treatment for asthma. Upon questioning, he states that he has been drinking an extra cup of coffee in the morning "to get going" because his coughing has kept him from sleeping well. What could be his problem?

## CASE STUDY

**Read the scenario, and answer the following questions on a separate sheet of paper.**

Jennie has been treated for adult-onset asthma for 3 years. She has been doing fairly well with her inhalers, but today she receives a prescription for montelukast one 10-mg tablet daily.

1. How does this medication differ from the corticosteroids that are used to reduce inflammation?

2. Jennie says, "I hope this medicine works better than the other one I took when I had an asthma attack." How will you reply?

3. Jennie takes ibuprofen on occasion for arthritis pain. How do you advise Jennie regarding taking over-the-counter drugs with montelukast?

4. After 3 months, Jennie stops taking the montelukast. She says, "My symptoms are better, and I don't want to take medicine unless I need it." Is this appropriate?

## CRITICAL THINKING CROSSWORD

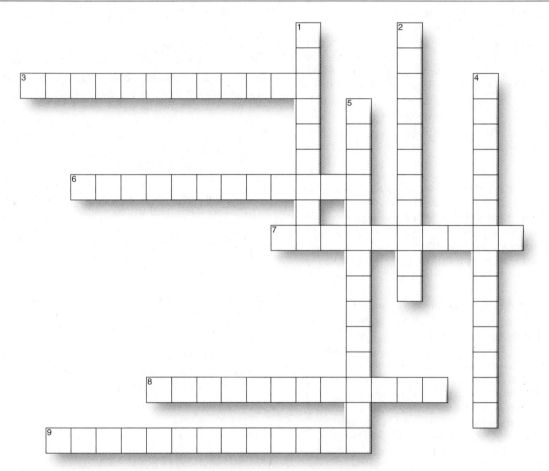

**Across**

3. Antibiotics taken before exposure to an infectious organism in an effort to prevent the development of infection
6. This class of antibiotics may cause tooth discoloration in children younger than age 8 years.
7. Anaphylactic reactions are common with this class of antibiotics.
8. Antibiotics that kill bacteria
9. There is a chance of cross-reactivity between this class of antibiotics and the class in 7 Across.

**Down**

1. The classification for the drug erythromycin
2. This class of antibiotics is commonly used for urinary tract infections.
4. Antibiotics that inhibit the growth of bacteria
5. An infection that occurs during antimicrobial treatment for another infection and involves overgrowth of a nonsusceptible organism

**Select the best answer for each question.**

1. The nurse is reviewing the drugs ordered for a patient. A drug interaction occurs between penicillins and which drugs? *(Select all that apply.)*
   a. Alcohol
   b. Oral contraceptives
   c. Digoxin
   d. Nonsteroidal antiinflammatory drugs
   e. Warfarin
   f. Anticonvulsants

2. Which intervention is the priority for the nurse to perform before beginning antibiotic therapy?
   a. Obtain a specimen for culture and sensitivity.
   b. Give with an antacid to reduce gastrointestinal (GI) upset.
   c. Monitor for adverse effects.
   d. Restrict oral fluids.

3. The nurse will instruct a patient who is receiving a tetracycline antibiotic to take it using which guideline?
   a. It needs to be taken with milk.
   b. It needs to be taken with 8 oz of water.
   c. It needs to be taken 30 minutes before iron preparations are taken.
   d. An antacid should also be taken to decrease GI discomfort.

4. A patient is to receive antibiotic therapy with a cephalosporin. When assessing the patient's drug history, the nurse recognizes that an allergy to which drug class may be a possible contraindication to cephalosporin therapy?
   a. Cardiac glycosides
   b. Thiazide diuretics
   c. Penicillins
   d. Macrolides

5. When asked about drug allergies, a patient says, "I can't take sulfa drugs because I'm allergic to them." Which question will the nurse ask next?
   a. "Do you have any other drug allergies?"
   b. "Who prescribed that drug for you?"
   c. "How long ago did this happen?"
   d. "What happened when you took the sulfa drug?"

6. Which statement accurately describes the action of antiseptics?
   a. They are used to kill organisms on nonliving objects.
   b. They are used to kill organisms on living tissue.
   c. They are used to sterilize equipment.
   d. They are used to inhibit the growth of organisms on living tissue.

7. The nurse knows the use of tetracyclines is limited in children because of the occurrence of which side effect?
   a. Stunting of the growth plate
   b. Threat of sunburn
   c. Discoloration of teeth
   d. Pseudomembranous colitis

8. Which statement accurately describes the method of action of penicillin?
   a. Interruption of bacterial protein synthesis
   b. Inhibition of bacterial cell wall synthesis
   c. Interruption of bacterial DNA replication
   d. Increased bacterial cell wall permeability

9. During a class on health care–associated infections, the nurse shares several facts about these infections. Which statements about health care–associated infections are true? *(Select all that apply.)*
   a. They are contracted in the home or community.
   b. They are contracted in a hospital or institution.
   c. They are more difficult to treat.
   d. The organisms that cause these infections are more virulent.
   e. The infection is incubating at the time of admission.

10. A patient is to receive 2 million units of penicillin G potassium per day, every 6 hours in IV piggyback doses. The medication is available in vials of 1 million units/50 mL, and each dose needs to be mixed in 50 mL of $D_5W$. How many milliliters will the nurse draw up for each IV piggyback dose?

    _____

11. A patient is to receive medication through a feeding tube. The order reads, "Give amoxicillin 250 mg per feeding tube every 8 hours." When reconstituted, the concentration of the medication is 125 mg/5 mL. How many milliliters will the nurse give per dose?

    _____

## CRITICAL THINKING AND APPLICATION

**Answer the following questions on a separate sheet of paper.**

12. A patient is receiving imipenem–cilastatin (Primaxin) and asks the nurse, "Why does that medicine bag have two names listed? Am I receiving two drugs?" What is the best explanation for the patient?

13. Mr. R., a 50-year-old banker, is scheduled for colon surgery tomorrow. The surgeon is planning to administer a prophylactic antibiotic. What drug is frequently used for this purpose? Why?

14. Sean is a 19-year-old college freshman who has been diagnosed with gonorrhea. The provider has prescribed doxycycline therapy. During the nursing assessment, Sean discusses his diet, which includes "lots of meat, milk, and veggies." Sean also tells the nurse that he jogs frequently and is a member of the tennis team.

    a. In addition to instruction about sexually transmitted infections, what patient teaching about the medication does Sean require?

    b. A few days later, Sean calls and complains of an upset stomach and diarrhea. What does the nurse suspect might be wrong with Sean?

15. Sandra has bronchitis and has been taking an antibiotic for 1 week. She calls the nurse and complains of severe genital itching and a whitish discharge in her vaginal area. What has happened, and what caused it?

CASE STUDY

**Read the scenario, and answer the following questions on a separate sheet of paper.**

A 78-year-old patient admitted to the hospital with a stroke 2 days earlier has developed a urinary tract infection. His Foley catheter is draining urine that is cloudy and dark yellowish-orange with a strong odor. He is receiving an intravenous heparin infusion and has a history of type 2 diabetes. The physician orders co-trimoxazole (Bactrim).

1. What will the nurse assess before giving this medication?

2. Are there any potential drug interactions?

3. Why was this particular antibiotic chosen?

4. Is this antibiotic bactericidal or bacteriostatic? Explain.

# 39 Antibiotics Part 2

**Select the best answer for each question.**

1. When patients are receiving aminoglycosides, the nurse must monitor for tinnitus and dizziness, which may indicate which problem?
   a. Cardiotoxicity
   b. Hepatotoxicity
   c. Ototoxicity
   d. Nephrotoxicity

2. A patient is being prepared for colon surgery and will be receiving neomycin tablets during the day before surgery. He asks the nurse why he needs to take this medicine before he even has surgery. What is the nurse's best response?
   a. "This medicine helps clear out your bowels before surgery."
   b. "It helps reduce the number of bacteria in your intestines before surgery."
   c. "It is given to sterilize your bowel before surgery."
   d. "It is given to prevent an infection after surgery."

3. A patient has been admitted to the unit with a stage IV pressure ulcer. After 2 days, the wound culture results come back positive for methicillin-resistant *Staphylococcus aureus* (MRSA). The nurse knows that the drug of choice for the treatment of MRSA infection is which drug?
   a. Vancomycin
   b. Gentamicin
   c. Ciprofloxacin
   d. Colistimethate

4. A patient who is receiving vancomycin therapy needs to notify the nurse immediately if which effects are noted? *(Select all that apply.)*
   a. Ringing in the ears
   b. Dizziness
   c. Hearing loss
   d. Flushing of the face
   e. Nausea

5. Which is a common adverse effect that occurs when vancomycin (Vancocin) is infused too quickly?
   a. Bone marrow suppression
   b. Tubular necrosis
   c. Red man's syndrome
   d. Colitis

6. Which statement accurately describes the method of action of quinolones?
   a. Interruption of bacterial protein synthesis
   b. Inhibition of bacterial cell wall synthesis
   c. Interruption of bacterial DNA replication
   d. Increased bacterial cell wall permeability

7. After an infusion of colistimethate (Coly-Mycin), the nurse will report to the prescriber if the patient complains of which adverse effects? *(Select all that apply.)*
   a. Numbness
   b. Vertigo
   c. Upset stomach
   d. Insomnia
   e. Dizziness

8. The nurse is reviewing the list of medications for a patient who will be starting antibiotic therapy with an aminoglycoside. Which medications, if present, may present a potential interaction with the aminoglycoside? *(Select all that apply.)*
   a. Metoprolol, a beta blocker
   b. Furosemide, a loop diuretic
   c. Warfarin, an oral anticoagulant
   d. Vancomycin, an antibiotic
   e. Levothyroxine, a thyroid hormone

9. Which laboratory test will the nurse monitor in the patient taking daptomycin?
   a. Liver function studies
   b. Red blood cell counts
   c. Platelet levels
   d. Creatinine phosphokinase

**97**

10. A patient will be taking oral neomycin before having bowel surgery. The order reads, "Give 1 g per hour for 4 doses PO." The patient cannot swallow pills, so an oral solution has been ordered. The solution is 125 mg/5 mL. How many milliliters will the nurse

    give for each 1-g dose? _____

11. The order reads, "Give colistimethate 2.5 mg/kg/day IVPB. Infuse over 5 minutes." The patient weighs 165 pounds. How many milligrams will the patient receive per dose? *(Record answer using one decimal*

    *place.)* _____

## CRITICAL THINKING AND APPLICATION

**Answer the following questions on a separate sheet of paper.**

12. Angie has a severe infection and is receiving an aminoglycoside once a day. She says, "They tell me I have a terrible infection. Why am I not getting the antibiotic more than once a day? I don't understand!" What will the nurse tell her?

13. Explain the concept of "trough" levels during aminoglycoside therapy and the way in which renal function is monitored.

14. Greg has been taking amiodarone for a heart rhythm problem. He has developed an infection from an open wound, and the sensitivity report indicates that levofloxacin (Levaquin) is the best choice to fight this infection. Are there any concerns?

15. Nitrofurantoin has been ordered for a patient who has a severe urinary tract infection caused by *Escherichia coli*. Explain why this drug is used for this type of infection.

## CASE STUDY

**Read the scenario, and answer the following questions on a separate sheet of paper.**

Virgil has been admitted to your unit and prescribed aminoglycoside therapy as part of treatment for a urinary tract infection with *Pseudomonas*. He is 65 years old, awake, and alert, but he is anxious about his problem and wants to "hurry up and get better."

1. For which two serious toxicities will you monitor? What are their symptoms, and how can they be prevented?

2. The physician adds penicillin to Virgil's drug regimen. Explain the reason for this.

3. Virgil's "trough" aminoglycoside level is 3.0 mcg/mL, and his serum creatinine level is increased from 2 days earlier. Are these results a concern? What will you do? Explain.

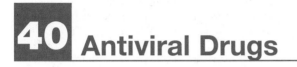

# 40 Antiviral Drugs

## CHAPTER REVIEW AND NCLEX® EXAMINATION PREPARATION

**Select the best answer for each question.**

1. The nurse is administering acyclovir and recalls that it is considered the drug of choice for treatment of which viral infection?
   a. Cytomegalovirus (CMV)
   b. Human immunodeficiency virus (HIV)
   c. Respiratory syncytial virus (RSV)
   d. Varicella-zoster virus (VZV)

2. When administering ganciclovir, the nurse keeps in mind that the main dose-limiting toxicity for this drug is which condition?
   a. Renal failure
   b. Gastrointestinal disturbances
   c. Peripheral neuropathy
   d. Bone marrow suppression

3. When reviewing the health history of a patient who is to receive foscarnet, the nurse knows that which condition would be a contraindication to its use?
   a. Renal failure
   b. CMV retinitis
   c. Asthma
   d. Immunosuppression

4. When reviewing the use of amantadine, the nurse expects that the drug would be used most appropriately in which patient?
   a. A 29-year-old man who tests positive for HIV
   b. A 22-year-old woman who is in her eighth month of pregnancy and tests positive for HIV
   c. A heart transplant patient who has influenza A
   d. Older adult patients who require prophylaxis for influenza B

5. A patient calls the clinic nurse to ask for oseltamivir (Tamiflu) "because I was exposed to the flu over the weekend at a family reunion." The nurse knows that Tamiflu is indicated for which conditions? *(Select all that apply.)*
   a. Prevention of infection after exposure to influenza virus types A and B
   b. Reduction of the duration of influenza in adults
   c. Treatment of topical herpes simplex virus infections
   d. Reduction of the severity of shingles symptoms
   e. Treatment of lower respiratory tract infections caused by respiratory syncytial virus

6. The nurse is preparing to administer the aerosol form of ribavirin. Which condition is a contraindication to the drug?
   a. Asthma
   b. Pregnancy
   c. Hypertension
   d. Type 2 diabetes

7. The method of action of antiviral agents is identified by which statement?
   a. Inhibiting the virus's ability to replicate
   b. Interfering with receptor site activity
   c. Interrupting the viral cell wall membrane
   d. Destroying the nucleus of the cell

8. Which of the following agents would the nurse expect to be used in the treatment of hepatitis C? *(Select all that apply.)*
   a. Sofosbuvir
   b. Daclatasvir
   c. Ribavirin
   d. Oseltamivir
   e. Zanamivir

**99**

9. Viral infections and viruses are more difficult to eradicate than bacteria for which reason?
   a. Viruses replicate at a faster rate.
   b. Viruses grow as an attachment to host cells and must first be removed from the cell wall.
   c. Viruses require folic acid synthesis.
   d. Viruses replicate only inside host cells, so medications must enter the cell.

10. The order reads, "Give acyclovir, 0.25 g IVPB now." The medication comes in a vial that contains 1000 mg. The label reads, "Add 20 mL of diluent for a solution that contains 50 mg/mL." The medication will be added to 100 mL $D_5W$ for IV piggyback infusion. How many milliliters of reconstituted medication will the nurse add to the 100-mL bag for infusion? _____

11. The order for a 1-year-old child reads, "Give amantadine 4.4 mg/kg/day in 2 divided doses." The child weighs 22 lb. How many milligrams will the child receive per dose? _____

## CRITICAL THINKING AND APPLICATION

**Answer the following questions on a separate sheet of paper.**

12. Amy is 12 weeks into her pregnancy when she discovers that she is HIV positive. Amy is very upset and says, "I won't live long enough to have this baby. We're both going to die." Is it possible to treat Amy, the fetus, or both? Explain your answer.

13. Bailey, a 53-year-old teacher, has shingles.
    a. What drug will the nurse expect the physician to prescribe?
    b. Several months later, Bailey calls the office to say that her symptoms have returned. What action will the nurse expect to be taken now?

14. Brenda, age 2 years, has bronchopneumonia caused by respiratory syncytial virus (RSV).
    a. What antiviral drug is used to treat RSV?
    b. Brenda's mother wonders whether the treatment will be completed before Brenda's birthday, which is 2 weeks away. What will the nurse tell her?

15. A 25-year-old man has acquired immunodeficiency syndrome (AIDS). He was treated with zidovudine for several months, but now the physician has switched him to didanosine powder. What frequently is the reason that patients are switched from zidovudine to another anti-HIV drug?

16. The nurse overhears a coworker explaining to a student nurse the procedure for administering acyclovir intravenously. "After the acyclovir is diluted in sterile water," the coworker says, "we'll administer this over at least an hour." Should the nurse intervene? Explain your answer.

17. Stacy has had flu symptoms for 4 days and feels miserable. She calls the nurse practitioner in the clinic to ask for "that medicine, Tamiflu, that is supposed to make the flu symptoms better." Will Stacy receive this medication at this time? Explain your answer.

18. Matt has had an organ transplant. What antiviral drug may be used, even though he does not have a viral infection at this time?

## CASE STUDY

**Read the scenario, and answer the following questions on a separate sheet of paper.**

Mr. C., a 30-year-old stockbroker, has been diagnosed with genital herpes simplex type 2 (HSV-2) infection. The health care provider has prescribed topical acyclovir (Zovirax).

1. What patient teaching do you provide to Mr. C. regarding administration of this drug?

2. Mr. C. asks you how long it will take for the acyclovir to cure his herpes. What is your reply?

3. What else will you discuss with Mr. C., who is sexually active?

4. HSV-2 is closely related to which other viruses?

# 41 Antitubercular Drugs

**Select the best answer for each question.**

1. A patient will be receiving long-term isoniazid (INH) therapy. What laboratory tests are most important for the nurse to monitor during therapy?
   a. Liver enzyme levels
   b. Hematocrit and hemoglobin level
   c. Creatinine level
   d. Platelet count

2. The nurse should include which information in the teaching plan for a patient who is taking isoniazid (INH)?
   a. Urine and saliva may be reddish-orange.
   b. Pyridoxine (vitamin $B_6$) should be added to the regimen.
   c. Injection sites should be rotated daily.
   d. The medication should be taken with an antacid to reduce gastric distress.

3. Which teaching point is the priority when educating the patient beginning antitubercular therapy? *(Select all that apply.)*
   a. Take medications as ordered and at the same time every day.
   b. Take medications on an empty stomach.
   c. Monitor blood glucose daily.
   d. Increase intake of green leafy vegetables.

4. A patient newly diagnosed with tuberculosis asks the nurse how long he will need to take "all this medicine." The nurse replies that drug therapy for active tuberculosis may need to last how long?
   a. 6 months
   b. 12 months
   c. 24 months
   d. A lifetime

5. The nurse is explaining antitubercular therapy to a patient. The patient asks, "Why do I have to take so many different medications?" What is the nurse's best response?
   a. "It helps prevent the tuberculosis from becoming resistant to the drugs."
   b. "It makes sure that the disease is cured."
   c. "These medications will reduce symptoms immediately."
   d. "You will have fewer side effects."

6. The nurse would correctly identify the method of action of ethambutol as which of the following?
   a. Inhibiting protein synthesis
   b. Inhibiting mycobacterial ATP synthase
   c. Altering cell wall synthesis
   d. Unknown method of action

7. The nurse would correctly identify the method of action of isoniazid (INH) as which of the following?
   a. Inhibiting protein synthesis
   b. Inhibiting mycobacterial ATP synthase
   c. Altering cell wall synthesis
   d. Unknown method of action

8. The nurse is reviewing the medication list of a patient who has been newly diagnosed with tuberculosis and will be taking rifampin. Which classes of drugs, if taken with rifampin, may cause increased metabolism? *(Select all that apply.)*
   a. Beta blockers
   b. Proton pump inhibitors
   c. Selective serotonin reuptake inhibitors
   d. Oral anticoagulants
   e. Oral antidiabetic drugs

9. The nurse would be correct in identifying which findings as possible side effects of bedaquiline? *(Select all that apply.)*
   a. Headache
   b. Chest pain
   c. Nausea
   d. QT prolongation
   e. Paresthesias

**101**

10. The patient is to receive isoniazid (INH) 0.3 g daily. The medication is available as 100-mg tablets. How many tablets will the nurse

    administer per dose? _____

11. The patient has new orders for pyrazinamide, 30 mg/kg/day. The patient weighs 132 lb. How many milligrams will the patient receive per day?

    Is this dosage safe? _____

## CRITICAL THINKING AND APPLICATION

**Answer the following questions on a separate sheet of paper.**

12. Diane, a 33-year-old proofreader, has been pre-scribed prophylactic isoniazid (INH) treatment.
    a. What laboratory studies should be performed before the start of therapy? Why?
    b. After Diane has taken isoniazid (INH) for 2 months, the physician significantly reduces her dosage of the drug. Why might that be?

13. Ms. I. is undergoing antitubercular therapy that includes streptomycin and rifampin.
    a. How is streptomycin administered?
    b. Ms. I. takes an oral contraceptive. Is that a concern given Ms. I.'s antitubercular therapy? Explain your answer.

14. Why would an eye examination be performed before instituting antitubercular therapy?

15. Mr. F. is on antitubercular therapy. During his first follow-up visit, he is evasive when the nurse asks him about his compliance with his therapy regimen. He does tell the nurse that he has been very busy lately, entertaining various clients "at everything from cocktail parties to big sit-down dinners."
    a. What issues will the nurse discuss with Mr. F.?
    b. Several weeks later, Mr. F. returns for another follow-up visit. On examination, the nurse sees no apparent signs of tuberculosis. How can Mr. F.'s therapeutic response be confirmed?

16. Frannie is a homeless 68-year-old woman who lives in a shelter some of the time. She was diagnosed with tuberculosis at the community health clinic, and antitubercular therapy has been instituted.
    a. What patient education issues are of particular concern in Frannie's case?
    b. Frannie is staying at the shelter and seems to be handling her medication regimen well, but one day she comes by the clinic to tell the nurse that she is afraid the medication may be bad for her. "Whenever I go to the bathroom, everything is reddish-orange," she says. What do you suspect is going on, and what do you tell Frannie?

## CASE STUDY

**Read the scenario, and answer the following questions on a separate sheet of paper.**

George, a 73-year-old retired plant foreman, has been diagnosed with tuberculosis. Nursing assessment reveals a history of gout and diabetes. He also has a history of heavy drinking.

1. What considerations will the physician keep in mind when deciding on a first-line drug for George?

2. George tells you that he has been told that he has a "liver problem." His medical record mentions that he is a slow acetylator. How does this affect his therapy?

3. How will his history of "heavy drinking" affect his therapy?

4. You instruct George about taking vitamin $B_6$ along with the isoniazid (INH) therapy. When he asks you why this is necessary, what will you tell him?

# 42 Antifungal Drugs

**Match each definition with the corresponding term.**

1. _____ Single-celled fungi that reproduce by budding

2. _____ One of the major chemical groups of antifungal drugs; includes amphotericin B and nystatin

3. _____ A very large, diverse group of eukaryotic, thallus-forming microorganisms that requires an external carbon source

4. _____ Another of the major groups of antifungal drugs; includes ketoconazole

5. _____ A term for fungal infection of the mouth

6. _____ One of the older antifungal drugs that acts by preventing susceptible fungi from reproducing

7. _____ The drug of choice for many severe, systemic fungal infections; also, the oldest antifungal drug

8. _____ An antifungal drug commonly used to treat candidal diaper rash

9. _____ An infection caused by fungi

10. _____ Multicellular fungi characterized by long, branching filaments called *hyphae*, which entwine to form a mycelium

a. Thrush
b. Molds
c. Griseofulvin
d. Mycosis
e. Polyenes
f. Fungi
g. Imidazoles
h. Amphotericin B
i. Nystatin
j. Yeast

**Select the best answer for each question.**

11. An infant has thrush. The nurse expects to administer which drug for the treatment of thrush?
    a. Amphotericin B
    b. Fluconazole
    c. Nystatin
    d. Miconazole

12. During an infusion of amphotericin B, the nurse monitors for which adverse effects? *(Select all that apply.)*
    a. Nausea
    b. Fever
    c. Malaise
    d. Constipation
    e. Chills
    f. Hypertension

13. A patient calls the gynecologic clinic because she has begun to menstruate while taking vaginal cream for a vaginal infection. She asks the nurse, "What should I do about taking this vaginal medicine right now?" Which is the nurse's best response?
    a. "You need to stop the medication until the menstrual flow has stopped."
    b. "Just take the medication at night only."
    c. "You should stop the medication for 3 days and then start it again."
    d. "It's okay to continue to take the medication."

14. A patient will be receiving a one-dose treatment for vaginal candidiasis. The nurse expects to administer which drug?
    a. Ketoconazole
    b. Fluconazole
    c. Griseofulvin
    d. Terbinafine

15. The nurse is administering an antifungal drug to a patient who has a severe systemic fungal infection. Which drug is most appropriate for this patient?
    a. Amphotericin B
    b. Fluconazole
    c. Griseofulvin
    d. Flucytosine

**103**

16. In an effort to prevent the complications associated with intravenous infusion of antifungal drugs such as amphotericin B, the nurse will administer them over which time frame?
    a. 30 minutes
    b. 60 minutes
    c. 1 to 2 hours
    d. 2 to 6 hours

17. The nurse is administering a new order for amphotericin B and reviews the patient's current medications. Which medications, if also ordered, may cause an interaction with the amphotericin B? *(Select all that apply.)*
    a. Digoxin, a cardiac glycoside
    b. Metoprolol, a beta blocker
    c. Warfarin, an oral anticoagulant
    d. Levothyroxine, a hormone replacement
    e. Hydrochlorothiazide, a thiazide diuretic

18. Amphotericin B would be contraindicated in which patients? *(Select all that apply.)*
    a. One with severe bone marrow suppression
    b. One with ulcer disease
    c. One with renal impairment
    d. One with hypertension
    e. One with asthma

19. The order reads, "Give amphotericin B 20 mg in 300 mL $D_5W$ over 6 hours." The nurse will set the infusion pump to what rate? _____

20. A patient is to receive voriconazole as follows: 6 mg/kg q12h × 2 doses, then change to 4 mg/kg q12h. The patient weighs 242 lb. How much will the patient receive for each 6-mg/kg dose? The 4-mg/kg dose? _____

## CRITICAL THINKING AND APPLICATION

**Answer the following questions on a separate sheet of paper.**

21. Mr. K. has cryptococcal meningitis, and the physician has prescribed fluconazole (Diflucan).
    a. Why did the physician choose this drug rather than one of the other -azole antifungals?
    b. The results of Mr. K.'s cerebrospinal fluid culture eventually come back negative. When he hears the good news, he says, "Great! I'm tired of taking this medicine." What will be the nurse's response?

22. The physician is planning intravenous amphotericin B therapy for James.
    a. What guidelines will the nurse follow in administering the drug?
    b. What adverse effects will the nurse expect James to experience?
    c. Should the nurse stop the infusion if those effects occur? Explain your answer.

23. Chrissie has a prescription for nystatin oral troches to treat thrush. After a few days, she calls the nurse practitioner to report that her mouth is not better. "I've been chewing them slowly every time I take one. I don't understand why it's not working!" she says. What is the nurse's response?

24. David has a severe fungal infection, and the physician has prescribed a lipid formulation of amphotericin B (Fungizone). Why was this formulation ordered, and what are the advantages and disadvantages?

## CASE STUDY

**Read the scenario, and answer the following questions on a separate sheet of paper.**

Sally has pneumonia with invasive aspergillosis. She has been treated for 2 weeks without showing much improvement, and the physician is considering starting voriconazole (Vfend) therapy. Sally is also receiving a medication for treatment of a cardiac dysrhythmia.

1. What is the reason for starting voriconazole therapy now rather than earlier?

2. What consideration may arise depending on the cardiac medication she is taking?

3. What needs to be monitored while she is taking voriconazole?

# 43 Antimalarial, Antiprotozoal, and Anthelmintic Drugs

**Select the best answer for each question.**

1. Before beginning antiprotozoal therapy, the nurse will assess for which possible contraindications?
   a. Underlying renal or liver disease and pregnancy
   b. Porphyria and glucose-6-phosphate dehydrogenase (G6PD) deficiency
   c. Glaucoma, cataracts, anemia, and petechiae
   d. Constipation, gastritis, and lactose intolerance

2. An 18-month-old toddler develops an abrupt onset of diarrhea. Results of the stool specimen suggest giardiasis as the cause. The nurse would anticipate the provider to write a prescription for which drug?
   a. Metronidazole
   b. Pentamidine
   c. Atovaquone
   d. Praziquantel

3. The patient being treated with albendazole is experiencing infestations with which helminth?
   a. Flukes
   b. Tapeworms
   c. Nematodes
   d. Flatworms

4. The nurse will warn the patient taking metronidazole about which possible adverse effects? *(Select all that apply.)*
   a. Reddish-orange urine
   b. Anorexia
   c. Cough
   d. Weakness
   e. Headache
   f. A metallic taste in the mouth

5. A patient is taking quinine therapy for malaria. The prescriber has decided to add a sulfonamide or tetracycline drug along with the quinine. When the nurse gives the patient the prescription for this new medication, the patient is upset about having to take "another pill." What is the nurse's best explanation for the second drug?
   a. "The antibiotic treats the bacterial infections that accompany malaria."
   b. "The antibiotic reduces the severe adverse effects of quinine."
   c. "The antibiotic will help the quinine to work more effectively against the malaria."
   d. "The antibiotic therapy is also needed to kill the parasite that causes malaria."

6. Which drugs are used mainly for the management of *Pneumocystis jiroveci* (formerly *Pneumocystis carinii*) pneumonia? *(Select all that apply.)*
   a. Metronidazole
   b. Pentamidine
   c. Ivermectin
   d. Pyrantel
   e. Atovaquone

7. The nurse is reviewing anthelmintic therapy. Which statement is true regarding anthelmintic therapy?
   a. The medication can be stopped after symptoms disappear.
   b. Anthelmintics are more effective in their parenteral forms.
   c. Anthelmintics are broad in their actions and can be substituted easily for one another if a given medication is not well tolerated.
   d. Specific anthelmintic drugs are used to target specific organisms.

8. The nurse is reviewing the medication list of a patient with a new prescription for mefloquine. Which drugs may have an interaction with the mefloquine? *(Select all that apply.)*
   a. Beta blockers
   b. Antidiabetic drugs
   c. Calcium channel blockers
   d. Proton pump inhibitors
   e. Thiazide diuretics

9. A patient with *Pneumocystis jiroveci* pneumonia will be receiving pentamidine intravenously. The order reads, "Give 4 mg/kg/day once daily." The medication comes in a 300-mg vial and is to be reconstituted with 5 mL of sterile water, with a resulting concentration of 60 mg/mL. The dose will then be added to a 100-mL bag of D$_5$W for the infusion. The patient weighs 154 lb. What is the dose for this patient, and how many milliliters of medication will the nurse add to the infusion bag? *(Record answer using one decimal place.)* _____

10. A patient is to receive mefloquine 1250 mg in a single dose for treatment of malaria. The medication is available in 250-mg tablets. How many tablets will the patient receive? _____

## CRITICAL THINKING AND APPLICATION

**Answer the following questions on a separate sheet of paper.**

11. Professor H. has just returned from a research sabbatical in Africa, where she did not adequately protect herself from mosquito exposure; thus she has contracted malaria. What kind of parasite causes malaria? Which drug is recommended if the parasite is in the exoerythrocytic phase of development? What exactly is the exoerythrocytic phase?

12. Professor H.'s nurse practitioner would like to prescribe the drug identified in the answer to Question 11. The patient will be assessed for which contraindications?

13. Professor H.'s husband, who accompanied her on her trip, has even more recently begun to develop signs of malaria. He is given chloroquine, a 4-aminoquinoline derivative. Unlike his wife, however, Mr. H. sees no diminishing of his symptoms. His strain of malaria appears to be chloroquine resistant. What alternative(s) will the nurse practitioner suggest for Mr. H.?

14. The medical clinic has a full waiting room this morning. Patient A is being seen for an intestinal disorder that he acquired after swimming in a local lake. Patient B has acquired immunodeficiency syndrome (AIDS) and is showing early signs of pneumonia. Patient C is being treated and evaluated on a regular basis for a sexually transmitted infection. Here's your challenge: All three patients have something in common in terms of the causes of their disorders. Describe what that could be. Second, based on that commonality, predict what disorder, of those discussed in this chapter, each patient may have. (Hint: One patient has giardiasis.) Third, select the drugs you think the physician is likely to prescribe for each patient.

## CASE STUDY

**Read the scenario, and answer the following questions on a separate sheet of paper.**

Sandra, age 15 years, has been diagnosed with an infestation of intestinal roundworms, specifically ascariasis, after a visit to another country. You are preparing to medicate her with pyrantel.

1. How is this infestation diagnosed?

2. What are the contraindications to therapy with pyrantel?

3. What is the method of action of pyrantel?

4. The recommended dosage for pyrantel is 11 mg/kg, up to a maximum of 1 g, in a one-time dose. If Sandra weighs 57 kg, what dose will she receive?

5. What are the expected adverse effects of this medication?

# 44 Antiinflammatory and Antigout Drugs

**Select the best answer for each question.**

1. When teaching a patient about the common adverse effects of therapy with nonsteroidal antiinflammatory drugs (NSAIDs), the nurse will mention which possible adverse effect?
   a. Dizziness
   b. Heartburn
   c. Palpitations
   d. Diarrhea

2. A 13-year-old patient has the flu, and her mother is concerned about her fever of 103° F (39.4° C). Which of these medications will the prescriber suggest to treat the teen's fever?
   a. Aspirin
   b. Acetaminophen (Tylenol)
   c. Indomethacin (Indocin)
   d. Ketorolac (Toradol)

3. A patient is receiving treatment with allopurinol for an acute flare-up of gout. Which statements will the nurse include during patient teaching? *(Select all that apply.)*
   a. "Be sure to avoid alcohol and caffeine."
   b. "Take the medication with meals to prevent stomach problems."
   c. "You need to take this medication on an empty stomach to improve absorption."
   d. "You need to increase fluid intake to up to 3 liters per day."
   e. "Call your provider immediately if you note any skin rashes or abnormalities."

4. When reviewing the health history of a patient who is to receive NSAID therapy, the nurse keeps in mind that contraindications for the use of these drugs include which condition?
   a. Pericarditis
   b. Osteoarthritis
   c. Bleeding disorders
   d. Juvenile rheumatoid arthritis

5. The nurse is reviewing the use of the COX-2 inhibitor celecoxib (Celebrex). Which conditions are indications for celecoxib? *(Select all that apply.)*
   a. Osteoarthritis
   b. Prevention of thrombotic events
   c. Rheumatoid arthritis
   d. Primary dysmenorrhea
   e. Fever reduction

6. The nurse would be correct in identifying which description as the method of action of febuxostat (Uloric) in the treatment of gout?
   a. Inhibits uric acid production
   b. Increase uric acid secretion
   c. Reduces inflammation
   d. Inhibits deposition of urate crystals

7. The nurse would be correct in identifying which description as the method of action of probenecid in the treatment of gout?
   a. Inhibits uric acid production
   b. Increase uric acid secretion
   c. Reduces inflammation
   d. Inhibits deposition of urate crystals

8. The nurse is reviewing a patient's medications and sees an order for ketorolac. This drug is ordered for which condition?
   a. Fever
   b. Mild pain
   c. Moderate to severe acute pain
   d. Long-term chronic pain conditions

9. Which patient teaching fact is the priority when the nurse is teaching the patient about lesinurad?
   a. Drink at least 2 liters of fluid per day.
   b. Take the medication on an empty stomach.
   c. Add a calcium supplement to the medication regimen.
   d. Use sunscreen or wear long sleeves when outdoors.

10. A child is to receive celecoxib as part of treatment for juvenile rheumatoid arthritis. The dose ordered is 100 mg twice daily PO. The child weighs 33 lb. According to the text, the dosing chart for pediatric administration of celecoxib is as follows:

| Less than 25 kg | 50 mg twice daily PO |
| --- | --- |
| More than 25 kg | 100 mg twice daily PO |

Is the ordered dose appropriate for this child? Explain your answer.

11. The order reads, "Give ketorolac 20 mg IV every 6 hours as needed for pain." The medication is available in a concentration of 15 mg/mL. How much will the nurse draw up for each dose? *(Record answer using one decimal place.)* _____
Mark the syringe to indicate your answer.

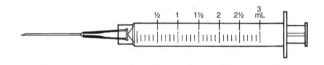

## CRITICAL THINKING AND APPLICATION

**Answer the following questions on a separate sheet of paper.**

12. Ms. B. is brought into the emergency department with severe tinnitus, hearing loss, and some confusion. On examination, the nurse discovers that the patient's blood glucose level is 52 mg/dL. Her husband tells you that she had been experiencing back pain and has been using "a lot of aspirin" over the past few weeks. What do her symptoms and history suggest? Explain your answer.

13. Mr. C. was brought to the emergency department and on arrival states he is experiencing drowsiness, lethargy, and disorientation and reports that he had a seizure while en route to the hospital. His girlfriend tells the nurse that she noticed an empty bottle of ibuprofen by his bed when she found him. What do his symptoms and history suggest? What would the nurse expect if the situation were allowed to progress?

14. Mr. H. has come to the clinic complaining of a severe flare-up of his gout. He tells the nurse that he does not take his medicine on a regular basis because it "kills" his stomach. He also says that he hates to take medicine but hates the gout more. He has a prescription for allopurinol and a follow-up appointment for next month. What patient teaching does Mr. H. need?

15. Eileen has had arthritic joint pain for months, and her current pain management regimen has been less than successful. During a checkup today, she tells the nurse that she has heard of a drug, Toradol, that "works wonders." She wants to try it for "a couple of months" to see if it can help her.
    a. What will the nurse tell her?
    b. What could happen if Eileen takes the ketorolac (Toradol) on a long-term basis?

16. Your neighbor calls you over to "check out this aspirin bottle" that she found in her medicine cabinet. It has a strong vinegary odor. She wants to know if she can still take it for her headaches. What will you tell her?

17. Randy has a history of hypertension and coronary artery disease. Today he is being evaluated for acute gout, and the prescriber is considering febuxostat (Uloric). Are there any concerns, based on Randy's history, if he takes this drug for gout? Explain your answer.

## CASE STUDY

**Read the scenario, and answer the following questions on a separate sheet of paper.**

Sadie has been taking indomethacin (Indocin) as part of therapy for osteoarthritis but lately has noticed that it has been less effective. Her provider has decided to try celecoxib (Celebrex). Sadie has a history of hepatitis (15 years earlier).

1. What advantages might there be to treatment with celecoxib rather than indomethacin?

2. What potential adverse effects will you warn Sadie about before she takes this medication? What should she report?

3. What allergies are important to assess before Sadie takes this medication?

4. She asks you if she can drink her usual glass of wine each evening while taking this medication. What will you tell her?

# 45 Antineoplastic Drugs Part 1: Cancer Overview and Cell Cycle–Specific Drugs

## CRITICAL THINKING CROSSWORD

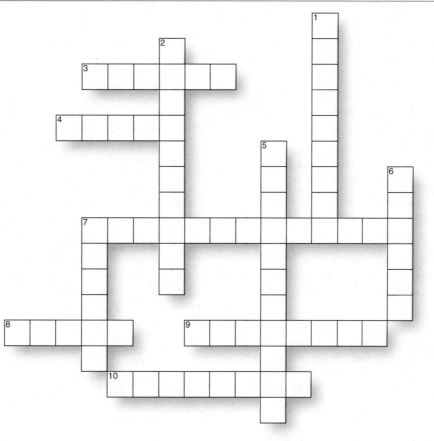

### Across

3. Mr. H. is told that his cancer has metastasized. His physician explains to him that this means it has

   _____ to other areas of his body.

4. Your patient is receiving methotrexate. Your instructor asks for a full description of its mechanism of action, so you explain that it will inhibit dihydro-

   folic reductase from converting _____ acid to a reduced folate and thus ultimately prevent the synthesis of DNA and cell reproduction. The result, you explain, is that the cell will die.

7. Mr. B. has just undergone a series of chemotherapeutic treatments when it is discovered that the antineoplastic drug has leaked into surrounding tissues; in

   other words, _____ of the drug has occurred.

8. Mr. C. is very interested in his chemotherapy process. As you are discussing a drug's action, he hears you use

   the term _____, and he asks you what it means. You explain that this is the point at which the lowest neutrophil count occurs after administration of a chemotherapy agent that causes bone marrow suppression.

9. Ms. F. has been given her first chemotherapy treatment. However, it soon becomes apparent that the adverse effects she is experiencing prevent her from being given dosages that will be high enough to be

   effective. These are dose-_____ adverse effects.

10. Ms. H. has a hematologic malignancy. Her bone marrow is being rapidly replaced with leukemic blasts; she also has abnormal numbers (and forms) of immature white blood cells in her circulation, and even her lymph nodes, spleen, and liver are being infiltrated. Ms. H.'s type of cancer is known as

    _____.

## Down

1. Ms. P. had a biopsy performed on the same day that Ms. L. (6 Down) did. When her biopsy specimen is analyzed, however, the results are the opposite of Ms.

   L.'s; that is, her lump is considered _____.

2. Mr. K. has been treated with methotrexate for its folate-antagonistic properties. Now, however, he seems to be experiencing a toxicity reaction. The

   treatment he will receive will be _____ rescue.

5. Mr. G. is receiving chemotherapy with a drug that is considered cytotoxic during any phase of the cellular growth cycle. This drug is known as cell

   cycle–_____.

6. Ms. L. recently underwent biopsy of a lump near her breast. Several days later, her physician calls and tells her that the lump is noncancerous and therefore is not an immediate threat to life. She is relieved to hear,

   then, that it is _____.

7. Mr. Y.'s physician is not surprised to find that Mr. Y. has nausea and vomiting; the methotrexate therapy is

   displaying a strong _____ potential in this patient.

## CHAPTER REVIEW AND NCLEX® EXAMINATION PREPARATION

**Select the best answer for each question.**

1. When administering antineoplastic drugs, the nurse needs to keep in mind that these drugs include which general adverse effects? *(Select all that apply.)*
   a. Bone marrow suppression
   b. Infertility
   c. Diarrhea
   d. Urinary retention
   e. Nausea and vomiting
   f. Stomatitis

2. A patient will be receiving chemotherapy with paclitaxel. What will the nurse expect to do along with administering this drug?
   a. Administer platelet infusions.
   b. Provide acetaminophen as needed.
   c. Keep the patient on "nothing by mouth" status because of expected nausea and vomiting.
   d. Premedicate with a steroid, an $H_2$ receptor antagonist, and an antihistamine.

3. As the nurse is preparing to give the patient chemotherapy, the patient asks the nurse why more than one drug is used. The nurse will explain that combinations of chemotherapeutic drugs are used to
   a. reduce drug resistance.
   b. reduce the incidence of adverse effects.
   c. decrease the cost of treatment.
   d. reduce treatment time.

4. If extravasation of an antineoplastic drug occurs, what will the nurse do first?
   a. Remove the intravenous catheter immediately.
   b. Stop the drug infusion without removing the intravenous catheter.
   c. Aspirate residual drug or blood from the tube if possible.
   d. Administer the appropriate antidote.

5. During chemotherapy, the nurse will monitor the patient for which symptoms of stomatitis?
   a. Indigestion and heartburn
   b. Severe vomiting and anorexia
   c. Pain or soreness of the mouth
   d. Diarrhea and perianal irritation

6. A patient is receiving leucovorin as part of his chemotherapy regimen. The nurse expects that the patient is receiving which antineoplastic drug?
   a. Cladribine
   b. Fluorouracil
   c. Vincristine
   d. Methotrexate

7. The nursing student asks the pharmacist what it means that an agent is "cell-cycle specific." Which statement is correct?
    a. These drugs are effective in only certain types of cancers.
    b. These drugs are effective throughout all stages of cancer reproduction.
    c. These drugs are effective on slower-growing cells because they target one phase of reproduction.
    d. These drugs are cytotoxic during a specific cycle of cancer cell growth.

8. Which statement is true regarding cancer chemotherapy?
    a. Only selected antineoplastic drugs are effective against all types of cancer.
    b. Most cancer drugs have a high therapeutic index.
    c. A combination of drugs is usually more effective than single-drug therapy.
    d. Side effects can be eliminated with appropriate administration times.

9. The nurse is monitoring a patient who has developed thrombocytopenia after two rounds of chemotherapy. Which signs or symptoms will the nurse look for in this patient? *(Select all that apply.)*
    a. Bruising
    b. Increased fatigue
    c. Ulcerations on mucous membranes inside the mouth
    d. Temperature above 100.5° F (38.1° C)
    e. Increased bleeding from venipunctures

10. A patient will be receiving daily doses of asparaginase. The order is for 200 units/kg/day up to 40,000 units per dose IV. The patient weighs 275 lb. How many units will the patient receive per dose? Is this dose within the safe limit? _____

11. A patient will be receiving chemotherapy with IV cladribine. The order reads, "Give 0.09 mg/kg each day for 7 days." The medication is to be added to 500 mL of normal saline and is available in a 1-mg/mL solution. The patient weighs 200 lb.
    a. How many mg is each daily dose? *(Record answer using one decimal place.)*

    _____

    b. How many milliliters of medication will be added to each infusion? _____

## CASE STUDY

**Read the scenario, and answer the following questions on a separate sheet of paper.**

Allen, a 40-year-old physician, has been diagnosed with acute lymphocytic leukemia and will be receiving chemotherapy with methotrexate. He is scheduled to receive his first treatment today.

1. What is methotrexate's classification, and how does it work?

2. What laboratory test results should be checked before he receives this medication?

3. Allen tells you that he often has problems with ankle pain from an old injury and takes ibuprofen (Motrin) for pain relief. Is this a concern?

4. What other medications may be given along with the methotrexate chemotherapy? Why?

# 46 Antineoplastic Drugs Part 2: Cell Cycle–Nonspecific and Miscellaneous Drugs

## CHAPTER REVIEW AND NCLEX® EXAMINATION PREPARATION

**Select the best answer for each question.**

1. While hanging a new infusion bag of a chemotherapy drug, the nurse accidentally spills a small amount of solution on the floor. What is the nurse's best action?
   a. Let it dry and then mop the floor.
   b. Wipe the area with a paper towel.
   c. Use a spill kit to clean the area.
   d. Ask the housekeeping department to wipe the floor.

2. The nurse is reviewing the medication list for a patient who will be receiving mitotane treatments. A drug from which class would cause the most concern if administered along with the mitotane?
   a. Benzodiazepine
   b. Thyroid replacement hormone
   c. Insulin
   d. Beta blocker

3. A patient receiving chemotherapy for a testicular tumor complains of hearing a "loud ringing sound" in his ears. The nurse expects what to happen next regarding the chemotherapy?
   a. It will continue as ordered.
   b. It will be stopped until the patient's hearing is evaluated.
   c. It will be withheld for a day and then be resumed.
   d. It will be stopped until renal studies are performed.

4. When teaching a patient who is receiving outpatient chemotherapy about potential problems, the nurse needs to mention signs and symptoms of an oncologic emergency, which include which of the following? *(Select all that apply.)*
   a. Swollen tongue
   b. Alopecia
   c. Blood in the urine
   d. Nausea and vomiting
   e. Temperature of 100.5° F (38.1° C) or higher
   f. Chills

5. The nurse monitors very closely for signs of renal toxicity when which of these antineoplastic drugs is given?
   a. Doxorubicin
   b. Cisplatin
   c. Bevacizumab
   d. Mitotane

6. A patient who has cancer is to receive a course of chemotherapy with doxorubicin. Which coexisting condition will require very close monitoring while the patient is taking this drug?
   a. Hypertension
   b. Diabetes mellitus
   c. Gout
   d. Cardiomyopathy

7. The nursing student would correctly identify which description as the method of action of the alkylating agents?
   a. These agents alter the chemical structure of the cells' deoxyribonucleic acid (DNA).
   b. These agents interfere with the ability of the cell to initiate angiogenesis.
   c. These agents enhance the host's autoimmune response.
   d. These agents disrupt cellular cytoplasm, and the cell dies.

8. A patient will be receiving mitotane, and the nurse is reviewing the patient's medication list for potential interactions. Which drugs may interact with mitotane? *(Select all that apply.)*
   a. Digoxin
   b. Warfarin
   c. Phenytoin
   d. Glucophage
   e. Spironolactone

9. The nurse would recognize which symptom as a side effect of cyclophosphamide?
   a. Thrombocytopenia
   b. Vasculitis
   c. Osteopenia
   d. Hemorrhagic cystitis

10. The orders read, "Administer normal saline, 3 L, over 24 hours, beginning 12 hours before the cisplatin chemotherapy begins." The nurse will program the infusion pump to deliver the normal saline at what rate? _____

11. A patient will be receiving cisplatin chemotherapy. The order reads, "Give 100 $mg/m^2$ in 1000 mL $D_5W$ over 22 hours." The nurse will program the infusion pump to deliver the infusion at what rate?

_____

## CRITICAL THINKING AND APPLICATION

**Answer the following questions on a separate sheet of paper.**

12. Describe the concept of cytoprotection, and provide at least two examples of how this may be accomplished during chemotherapy.

13. Mrs. S. has been receiving bleomycin to treat a lung tumor, and lately she has been experiencing increased difficulty breathing. She tells the nurse, "I guess this cancer is getting worse. The medicine is not working." Will the nurse agree, or is there another possible concern?

14. During a busy evening shift, an oncologist tells the nurse that he wants to start Mrs. N.'s chemotherapy immediately. The oncologist asks the nurse to mix the drug as soon as possible and start the infusion. Should the nurse do this? Explain your answer.

15. Mr. G., who had been receiving an infusion of mechlorethamine, has an infiltrated intravenous site. He wants the nurse to pull out the intravenous line immediately because "it hurts so much." What will the nurse do? What will the treatment of extravasation involve?

## CASE STUDY

**Read the scenario, and answer the following questions on a separate sheet of paper.**

Dottie, age 63 years, has been diagnosed with midstage ovarian cancer and will be receiving chemotherapy with cisplatin after surgery. She is understandably anxious about the therapy but says she wants to "beat the cancer."

1. Cisplatin is associated with three main toxicities. Describe each one.

2. Before Dottie receives the therapy, what will be assessed?

3. During therapy, Dottie complains of an "odd tingling" in her toes. Is this a concern? Explain.

4. Dottie tells you that she'd rather "drink nothing" when she is feeling nauseated. Is this a concern? Explain what you need to teach her about fluids.

# 47 Biologic Response–Modifying and Antirheumatic Drugs

**Match each definition with its corresponding term. (Note: Not all terms will be used.)**

1. _____ A type of cytokine that promotes resistance to viral infection in uninfected cells

2. _____ Cytokines that regulate the growth, differentiation, and function of bone marrow stem cells

3. _____ Cytokines that are produced by sensitized T lymphocytes upon contact with antigen particles

4. _____ An immunoglobulin that binds to antigens to form a special complex

5. _____ A substance that is recognized as foreign by the body's immune system

6. _____ Leukocytes of the cell-mediated immune system

7. _____ Leukocytes of the humoral immune system

a. Colony-stimulating factors
b. Antibody
c. B lymphocytes (B cells)
d. T lymphocytes (T cells)
e. Interferons
f. Lymphokine-activated killer cells
g. Lymphokines
h. Antigen
i. Memory cells

**Select the best answer for each question.**

8. The patient reports to the nurse that the medication infliximab prescribed for rheumatoid arthritis is not working. On further questioning, the nurse determines that the patient has been taking the drug for 7 days. Which response by the nurse is most appropriate?
   a. "The medication must be ineffective for you; call the office, and the provider will make a change in drug selection."
   b. "Increase the dosage to two tablets instead of one."
   c. "This medication may take up to 4 to 6 weeks for the full response to occur."
   d. "Are you taking the medication with food?"

9. While teaching a patient about the possible adverse effects of the interferons, the nurse should mention which effects? *(Select all that apply.)*
   a. Myalgia
   b. Fever
   c. Diarrhea
   d. Fatigue
   e. Chills
   f. Dizziness

10. A patient is starting therapy with adalimumab after a course of therapy with methotrexate failed to improve the patient's condition. The nurse recognizes that this patient is being treated for which condition?
    a. Advanced-stage cancer
    b. Multiple sclerosis
    c. Severe rheumatoid arthritis
    d. Systemic lupus erythematosus

11. When administering the drug trastuzumab, the nurse is concerned about the manifestations of any side effect based on which rationale?
    a. The drug has significant drug–drug interactions
    b. The drug is highly protein bound
    c. The drug has a half-life of 10 to 30 days
    d. A central line is required for administration.

12. A patient will be starting therapy with etanercept as part of treatment for severe rheumatoid arthritis. Which conditions, if present, may be a contraindication for this drug? *(Select all that apply.)*
    a. Latex allergy
    b. Active bacterial infection
    c. Diabetes mellitus
    d. Latent tuberculosis
    e. Acute hepatitis B
    f. Peanut allergy

13. The order reads, "Give oprelvekin 50 mcg/kg daily for 14 days subcutaneously. The medication comes in a strength of 5 mg/mL after being reconstituted. The patient weighs 110 lb.

    a. How many milligrams will the patient receive per dose? _____
    b. How many milliliters will the nurse draw up into the syringe for this dose? Mark the syringe with your answer.

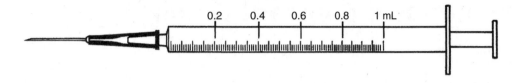

14. A patient is to receive 400 mcg of filgrastim subcut daily for 1 week. The vial contains 480 mcg/1.6 mL. How many

    milliliters will the nurse draw up into the syringe for the dose? _____

## CRITICAL THINKING AND APPLICATION

**Answer the following questions on a separate sheet of paper.**

15. Sonja is to receive interferon therapy as part of the treatment for cancer. Sonja is very athletic and participates in sports activities on a regular basis. The oncologist explains that there is a dose-limiting adverse effect of this type of drug that may have a huge effect on her daily activities. What is this adverse effect, and how will it concern Sonja?

16. Trevor is receiving chemotherapy as part of his treatment for Hodgkin's disease. As he begins therapy, he tells the nurse, "I've seen those commercials about the drugs that increase your white blood cell count. Can't I start taking one of them now to keep my counts from getting so low?" What are the drugs he is referring to, and how will the nurse answer?

17. Brittany has a history of thrombocytopenia, and the results of today's laboratory work have indicated a critically low platelet count. She has received 2 units of platelets, and the oncologist has decided to give her a medication to improve her platelet counts. What drug will be given, how will it be given, and what concerns are there while her platelet count is so low?

18. Dustin will be receiving treatments with methotrexate for severe rheumatoid arthritis. The nurse is reviewing the medication administration record (MAR) and sees the following transcribed order: "Methotrexate, 7.5 mg per day PO." What will be the nurse's next action?

## CASE STUDY

**Read the scenario, and answer the following questions on a separate sheet of paper.**

Donna, a 62-year-old florist, is in the hospital because of severe dehydration after her second round of chemotherapy for ovarian cancer. At this time, the laboratory results revealed a critically low platelet count, and the oncologist has ordered a transfusion of 3 units of platelets. However, Donna states that she cannot accept the platelet transfusion because of her religious convictions. As a result, there are orders to begin therapy with oprelvekin.

1. What is the classification of oprelvekin?

2. What laboratory test results will you monitor while she is taking this medication? Why?

3. Donna says, "I am worried about bleeding. When can this drug be started, and how long will I have to take it?" What will you explain to Donna about how this drug is given?

4. What patient teaching is important while Donna is taking this drug?

Chapter **47 Biologic Response–Modifying and Antirheumatic Drugs**

# 48 Immunosuppressant Drugs

**Select the best answer for each question.**

1. When monitoring patients on immunosuppressant therapy, the nurse must keep in mind that the major adverse effect for patients taking these drugs is which finding?
   a. Severe hypotension with potential renal failure
   b. Increased susceptibility to opportunistic infections
   c. Decreased platelet aggregation
   d. Increased bleeding tendencies

2. A patient is experiencing rejection of a transplanted organ. The nurse expects which drug to be prescribed to manage this?
   a. Azathioprine
   b. Cyclosporine
   c. Muromonab-CD3
   d. Glatiramer acetate

3. The nurse is discussing drug therapy with cyclosporine. Which food product could possibly increase the activity of cyclosporine?
   a. Dairy product
   b. Orange juice
   c. Grapefruit juice
   d. Red wine

4. When teaching patients who are taking oral doses of immunosuppressants, how will the nurse instruct the patient to take the medication?
   a. With food to minimize gastrointestinal upset
   b. On an empty stomach to increase the absorption rate
   c. Only when adverse effects are tolerable
   d. Mixed with water only

5. The nurse providing education for patients taking immunosuppressants will include which information? *(Select all that apply.)*
   a. The mouth and tongue should be inspected carefully for white patches.
   b. Allergic reactions to these drugs are rare.
   c. Patients should avoid crowds to minimize the risk for infection.
   d. Patients should report any fever, sore throat, chills, or joint pain.
   e. Patients should take oral forms with food to avoid gastrointestinal upset.

6. Which statement correctly describes the method of action of the immunosuppressants?
   a. These agents inhibit the antigen–antibody relationship.
   b. These agents suppress the action of T lymphocytes, compromising the immune system.
   c. These agents inhibit prostaglandins, rendering them ineffective in the immune response.
   d. These agents alter the ability of the body to manufacture albumin, and cells lose their integrity and die.

7. Which drugs are indicated for the treatment of multiple sclerosis? *(Select all that apply.)*
   a. Glatiramer acetate
   b. Azathioprine
   c. Basiliximab
   d. Daclizumab
   e. Fingolimod

8. A patient will be taking cyclosporine after transplant surgery. Which of these are potential adverse effects of cyclosporine therapy? *(Select all that apply.)*
   a. Hypertension
   b. Fever
   c. Nephrotoxicity
   d. Fluid retention
   e. Hypotension
   f. Posttransplant diabetes mellitus

9. The order reads, "Give mycophenolate mofetil 1 g PO twice daily." The capsules are available in 250-mg strength. How many capsules will the patient receive per dose? _____

10. A patient is about to undergo transplant surgery and will be receiving a preoperative dose of cyclosporine 8 hours before the surgery. The ordered dose is "cyclosporine, 6 mg/kg/dose, IV, give 8 hours preoperatively." The patient weighs 275 lb. The medication is available as 50 mg/mL.
    a. The dose for this patient is how many milligrams?

    _____

    b. How many milliliters will the nurse administer for this dose? _____

## CRITICAL THINKING AND APPLICATION

**Answer the following questions on a separate sheet of paper.**

11. Mrs. F. is about to undergo kidney transplant surgery. The physician plans for her to start taking sirolimus (Rapamune).
    a. Mrs. F. asks the nurse why she is taking this medication. How will the nurse answer?
    b. Three days before her surgery, an oral antifungal drug is added to Mrs. F.'s regimen. "Why do I have to take this, too?" she asks. How will the nurse answer?

12. A patient on cyclosporine therapy is convinced that the cyclosporine is upsetting his stomach. What can be done to alleviate this problem?

13. A hospitalized patient has asked the nurse to mix the doses of cyclosporine in his disposable Styrofoam cup with milk before he drinks it. What will the nurse do?

14. Tess has had a renal transplant. She is being given muromonab-CD3 intravenously, 5 mg/day in a single bolus. On the second day, she begins to exhibit chest pain, dyspnea, and wheezing. What is happening? What does the nurse need to do at this time? What can be ordered to reduce these problems?

15. John has relapsing-remitting multiple sclerosis and is in the hospital because of an acute exacerbation. The physician talks to him about a "different type" of therapy with an immunosuppressant drug. What drug will be used, and how can it help John?

## CASE STUDY

**Read the scenario, and answer the following questions on a separate sheet of paper.**

Mr. K. had renal transplant surgery 6 months ago and so far has had no problems with organ rejection. He is taking cyclosporine in a maintenance dose. He wants to go back to work and is in for a checkup before approval is given for a return to his job.

1. He asks if he will have to continue the cyclosporine. What is your response?

2. He complains of difficulty swallowing, and as you examine his mouth, you look for signs of oral candidiasis. What findings would indicate that he has this condition?

3. After 2 weeks at work, Mr. K. calls to report that he has the flu. He has a sore throat, chills, and achy joints, and he is very tired. What is your advice?

4. Mr. K. tells you that his job sometimes requires him to travel to remote areas of the world. What concerns are there with vaccinations, if any?

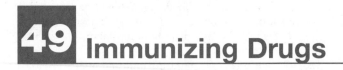

# 49 Immunizing Drugs

1. **Complete the following chart by filling in all missing information.**

| Drug | Active or Passive? | Purpose |
|---|---|---|
| a. | b. | Herpes zoster prevention (over age 60) |
| Hib | c. | d. |
| e. | Active | Hepatitis B prophylaxis |
| f. | g. | Postpartum antibody suppression |
| BCG vaccine | h. | i. |
| DTaP | j. | k. |
| Tetanus immunoglobulin | l. | m. |
| Td | n. | o. |

**Select the best answer for each question.**

2. The immunity that is passed from a mother to her nursing infant through antibodies in breast milk is known as which type of immunity?
   a. Artificially acquired passive immunity
   b. Naturally acquired passive immunity
   c. Active immunity
   d. Genetic immunity

3. Which substance contains microorganisms that trigger the formation of antibodies against specific pathogens?
   a. Antivenin
   b. Serum
   c. Toxoid
   d. Vaccine

4. When reviewing various immunizing drugs, the nurse recalls that one product is purposefully administered to pregnant women. Which is an example of this type of product?
   a. Poliovirus vaccine
   b. Tetanus immune globulin
   c. $Rh_O(D)$ immune globulin
   d. Black widow spider antivenin

5. The nurse is preparing to give a second dose of DTaP vaccine to a 6-month-old infant. The infant's mother tells the nurse that the last time he received this vaccination, the injection site on his leg became warm and slightly reddened. Which is the nurse's best action?
   a. Explain that these effects can be expected and give the medication.
   b. Give half the prescribed dose this week and the other half next week if tolerated well.
   c. Skip the dose and notify the physician.
   d. Wait 6 months and then administer the dose.

6. A nurse has been stuck by a used needle while starting an intravenous line. Which preparation is used as prophylaxis against disease after exposure to blood and body fluids?
   a. Hib vaccine
   b. $Rh_O(D)$ immune globulin
   c. Hepatitis B immune globulin
   d. Hepatitis antitoxin

7. The nurse is providing patient teaching to a 24-year-old woman regarding the human papillomavirus (HPV) vaccine. Which statement by the woman indicates that more teaching is needed? *(Select all that apply.)*
   a. "This vaccine only takes one injection."
   b. "I need to have this vaccine before I turn 26."
   c. "It is safe to get this vaccine if I am pregnant."
   d. "This vaccination prevents the virus that commonly causes genital warts."
   e. "My 13-year-old sister should have this vaccine, too."

8. A student nurse was informed of the need for a "booster" injection for hepatitis B. The student asks the health center nurse why another injection is indicated because the series of three injections was completed. Select the nurse's best response.
   a. "Too much time has elapsed between the second and third injections, and you need a second 'third shot.'"
   b. "With the three injections, your body did not manufacture enough antibodies, and to be therapeutic, you need another injection."
   c. "You have an altered immune response and may never be protected from hepatitis B."
   d. "One of the initial injections you received must have been ineffective."

9. Which of the following statements is true about the zoster vaccine?
   a. It can be safely administered to immunocompromised patients.
   b. It requires three doses over 12 months.
   c. It is indicated for individuals 50 years of age and older.
   d. It is effective against the chickenpox virus and can be administered to children.

10. A newborn will be receiving her first dose of hepatitis B vaccine (inactivated). The dose is 5 mcg IM at birth and then again at 1 month and 6 months. Five mcg is equivalent to how many mg?

_____

11. A 7-month-old infant will be receiving influenza virus vaccine (Fluzone), 0.25 mL IM. Mark the correct dose on the syringe.

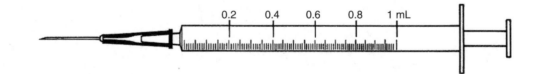

**Answer the following questions on a separate sheet of paper.**

12. Emily, age 25 years, has stepped on a rusty piece of metal and will be receiving a tetanus booster after the wound is cleansed and stitched. Her last tetanus booster, a Td, was 10 years ago. Which booster is she likely to receive today? Explain your answer.

13. Jim, a cabinetmaker, is cut by a woodworking tool and comes to the clinic for stitches. When the nurse asks him about his tetanus vaccination history, he says, "I have no idea when my last tetanus shot was—I thought that once I had all the shots for school, I was set for life! Surely I don't need any more." What will the nurse explain to Jim?

14. Mrs. T., an 82-year-old widow, is in the office for a follow-up appointment to evaluate her emphysema. The physician recommends that she have an influenza virus vaccine. As the nurse prepares the injection, Mrs. T. says, "I had a flu shot last year—why do I need another one this year?" What is the nurse's explanation to her?

15. Mr. S. brings his toddler, Carl, in for a 12-month well-child checkup. Before the nurse gives the measles, mumps, and rubella (MMR) vaccine injection, what adverse effects will she tell Mr. S. to watch for in Carl's response to the immunization? What can be done to relieve these adverse effects?

16. There have been news reports about anthrax threats. Your neighbor is worried and asks you which type of anthrax is the most deadly. What does he mean by "which type," and what is the answer to his question?

17. Paul has received several immunizations in preparation for an overseas trip. He expected to feel some soreness at the injection sites, but the next morning, he wakes up with swelling of the face and tongue, difficulty breathing, shortness of breath, nausea and vomiting, and a fever of 102° F (38.9° C). What is happening, and what should he do?

## CASE STUDY

**Read the scenario, and answer the following questions on a separate sheet of paper.**

You are volunteering at a local animal shelter and helping to care for a sick dog that has just been admitted. During the examination, the dog nips both you and the veterinarian. A little later, the veterinarian tells you that she fears that the dog has rabies and that both of you have been exposed. The veterinarian tells you that she has received a vaccine for rabies but that you will need to be vaccinated immediately.

1. Is rabies a virus or a bacterium?

2. Did the vaccine the veterinarian received previously give her active or passive immunization? Explain.

3. Will the vaccine you receive give you active or passive immunization? Explain why this particular type of vaccine is preferred in your situation.

# 50 Acid-Controlling Drugs

**Match each definition with its corresponding term. (Note: Not all terms will be used; some definitions may have more than one answer; some terms may be used more than once.)**

1. _____ Drugs known as $H_2$ blockers that reduce acid secretion in the stomach

2. _____ Drugs that block all acid secretion in the stomach

3. _____ Generic name for a cytoprotective drug

4. _____ The cells responsible for producing and secreting hydrochloric acid in the stomach

5. _____ A type of antacid that can cause diarrhea

6. _____ Antacids that have constipating effects

7. _____ The cause of many peptic ulcers

8. _____ Drugs used to relieve the painful symptoms associated with gas

9. _____ A type of antacid that may contribute to the development of kidney stones

10. _____ A highly soluble antacid form with a quick onset but short duration of action

a. Aluminum-containing antacids
b. Calcium-containing antacids
c. Magnesium-containing antacids
d. Antiflatulents
e. Proton pump inhibitors
f. *Helicobacter pylori*
g. Sodium bicarbonate
h. Histamine type 2 receptor antagonists
i. Sucralfate
j. Chief cells
k. Parietal cells

**Select the best answer for each question.**

11. A patient with renal failure wants to take an antacid for "sour stomach." The nurse needs to consider that some antacids may be dangerous when taken by patients with renal failure and will recommend which type of antacid?
    a. Activated charcoal
    b. Aluminum-containing antacids
    c. Calcium-containing antacids
    d. Magnesium-containing antacids

12. A patient with peptic ulcer disease will be starting medication therapy. He tells the nurse that he smokes and wonders if that will affect his treatment. Which is the nurse's best response?
    a. "Smoking has no effect on these medications."
    b. "The actions of antacids are less potent when you smoke."
    c. "Smoking has been shown to decrease the effectiveness of $H_2$ blockers."
    d. "Smoking has been shown to increase the adverse effects of $H_2$ blockers."

13. Which drug class would be used as first-line therapy for gastroesophageal reflux disease (GERD) that has not responded to customary medical treatment?
    a. $H_2$ blockers
    b. Antacids
    c. Mucosal protectants
    d. Proton pump inhibitors

14. The nurse is administering a proton pump inhibitor during morning medication rounds. Which statements about proton pump inhibitors are true? *(Select all that apply.)*
    a. They should be taken 1 hour before antacids.
    b. They should be taken 30 to 60 minutes before meals.
    c. They should be taken with meals.
    d. They are part of the treatment of patients with *H. pylori* infections.
    e. There are very few adverse effects with these drugs.

15. A pregnant woman asks the nurse about taking an antacid for indigestion. What is the nurse's best response?
    a. "You won't be allowed to take an antacid while you are pregnant."
    b. "Let's check with your obstetrician to see what is recommended."
    c. "Go ahead and use an aluminum-based antacid."
    d. "Sodium bicarbonate would be the safest choice."

16. Which patient should be advised to limit or avoid the use of sodium bicarbonate as an antacid? *(Select all that apply.)*
    a. A patient who is 6 months pregnant
    b. A patient with hypertension
    c. A patient with heart failure
    d. A patient with gout
    e. A patient with scleroderma

17. When caring for an older adult patient diagnosed with peptic ulcer disease and receiving each of the following medications, the nurse would relate the onset of confusion as a possible side effect of which medication?
    a. Antacids
    b. Carafate
    c. H$_2$ antagonists
    d. Cytotec

18. Which statement correctly describes the benefit of misoprostol in the treatment of ulcer disease?
    a. It reduces the secretion of hydrochloric acid.
    b. It neutralizes stomach acid.
    c. It enhances the production of protective mucus.
    d. It facilitates gastric emptying.

19. A patient is to receive cimetidine, 300 mg IVPB twice a day. The medication is available in a concentration of 150 mg/mL. How many milliliters will the nurse draw up to prepare for the IVPB dose?

_____

20. The patient is to receive pantoprazole 40 mg, mixed in 100 mL of D$_5$W over 30 minutes, IV. The nurse will set the infusion pump to what rate?

_____

## CRITICAL THINKING AND APPLICATION

**Answer the following questions on a separate sheet of paper.**

21. A neighbor, Mr. M., comes over to get advice on antacids. He says he has taken Maalox "for years" for indigestion, but it is no longer helping. He asks the nurse, "Can you recommend another antacid or one of those expensive, fancy pills that the pharmacy sells? Or should I just take baking soda?" How will the nurse respond?

22. Mrs. K. is advised to take omeprazole (Prilosec) capsules to treat her severe case of GERD; nothing else has worked. Develop a patient teaching plan that will instruct Mrs. K. about how to take this medication.

23. Mr. A. has called to ask which antacid he should take. He has been to the store and is confused by the great variety on the shelves. He says he needs something for "occasional heartburn" when he eats something too spicy. He has a history of heart failure and is taking antihypertensive drugs. What type of antacid should he take, and what other instructions will he need?

24. Mr. S. is taking enteric-coated aspirin for mild arthritis symptoms. He tells the nurse that he plans to take the aspirin with his favorite antacid, Maalox, because he does not want any stomach problems. What will the nurse tell him?

25. The nurse is caring for a patient who has been transferred to the step-down unit after spending 1 week in the intensive care unit after a myocardial infarction. The nurse notices that the patient's medication list includes a proton pump inhibitor, but there is no mention of any GI disorders on his chart. What is the reason for this medication?

## CASE STUDY

**Read the scenario, and answer the following questions on a separate sheet of paper.**

Edna, age 78 years, has been self-treating with antacids for "heartburn" for 6 months. After an upper gastrointestinal tract endoscopy, she has been diagnosed with GERD. The decision has been made to start treatment with cimetidine (Tagamet). Edna has been generally healthy except for a history of asthma. She says that she does not smoke but that she enjoys going to a bingo session every Saturday for a few hours, where there is smoking, beer, and pizza.

1. When Edna sees the prescription for cimetidine, she asks, "Why do I need a prescription? I can buy this over the counter!" What will you say in reply?
2. How will the cimetidine help her GERD?
3. What cautions, if any, are associated with the use of cimetidine?
4. Will staying in a smoke-filled room affect her therapy? Explain.

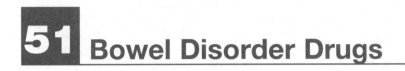

**CRITICAL THINKING CROSSWORD**

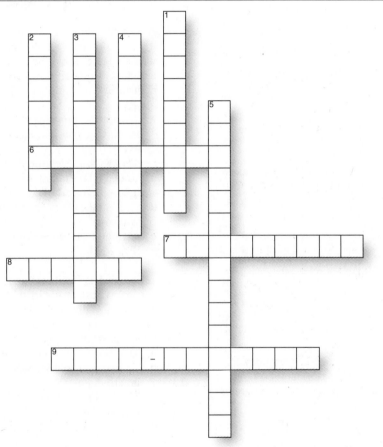

## Across

6. A type of laxative that softens the stool
7. Another word for intestinal flora modifier
8. One type of laxative that increases osmotic pressure in the small intestine, increasing water content and resulting in distention
9. Laxatives that absorb water into the intestine, increasing the volume and distending the bowel (two words)

## Down

1. Antidiarrheal drug that acts by coating the walls of the gastrointestinal tract, and binding to causative bacteria or toxin to allow elimination via the stool
2. Drugs that decrease bowel motility
3. Another type of laxative that increases fecal water content in the large intestine, resulting in distention, increased peristalsis, and evacuation
4. A laxative that stimulates the nerves that supply the intestine, which results in increased peristalsis
5. Antidiarrheal drug that acts by decreasing peristalsis and muscular tone of the intestine, thus slowing the movement of substances through the gastrointestinal tract

**123**

**Select the best answer for each question.**

1. The nurse is reviewing the use of bismuth subsalicylate. This medication would be the most appropriate choice for which patient?
   a. A 7-year-old child who has chickenpox
   b. A 23-year-old woman who has severe abdominal pain
   c. A 45-year-old man who is complaining of constipation
   d. A 58-year-old man who developed diarrhea after traveling out of the country

2. The nurse will teach a patient who is self-treating with bismuth subsalicylate (Pepto-Bismol) to avoid which drug because of the possibility of toxicity?
   a. Aspirin
   b. Acetaminophen
   c. Calcium supplements
   d. Vitamin tablets

3. A patient asks for an over-the-counter medication that will provide rapid relief of constipation. After ruling out possible contraindications, which drug would be most appropriate?
   a. Psyllium
   b. Methylcellulose
   c. Docusate sodium
   d. Magnesium hydroxide

4. A patient who has been taking Pepto-Bismol for diarrhea telephones the nurse and states, "My stools are black, and I think I am bleeding rectally!" Select the nurse's best response.
   a. "Yes, you may be right; go the emergency department immediately."
   b. "Have you been taking any additional vitamins with iron?"
   c. "This is an expected response to the Pepto-Bismol."
   d. "Contact your doctor and ask for a stool evaluation."

5. The patient asks the nurse why increased fiber intake is a solution for constipation. Select the nurse's best response.
   a. "Fiber increases peristaltic waves, increasing fecal movement."
   b. "Fiber lowers the surface tension of GI fluids."
   c. "Fiber increases bulk and distends the bowel to initiate reflex bowel activity."
   d. "Fiber initiates the adrenergic response, increasing the flow of catecholamines into the bowel."

6. A patient has been given PEG-3350 in a solution of polyethylene glycol as preparation for a colonoscopy. He started having diarrhea after about 45 minutes. Two hours later, he tells the nurse that "the diarrhea has not stopped yet." What will the nurse do?
   a. Give the patient an antidiarrheal drug, such as loperamide.
   b. Give the patient another dose of the GoLYTELY to finish cleansing his bowel.
   c. Remind the patient that it may take up to 4 hours to completely evacuate the bowel.
   d. Report this to the physician immediately.

7. A 79-year-old woman visits the clinic today and tells the nurse that her "bowels just aren't right." She wants advice on the best laxative to take so that she can have a bowel movement every day. Which are appropriate responses by the nurse? *(Select all that apply.)*
   a. "A normal bowel pattern does not necessarily mean that you will have a bowel movement every day."
   b. "Try taking Metamucil with sips of water."
   c. "You can try taking Milk of Magnesia every other day—it's a mild laxative."
   d. "Let's talk about increasing fluids and fiber in your diet."
   e. "Mineral oil would be safe for long-term use if needed."

8. A patient has been taking alosetron for 3 weeks as part of treatment for irritable bowel syndrome. Today she calls the clinic to report that she has been experiencing constipation. The nurse will expect which priority action to be taken?
   a. The dose will be increased by 1 mg.
   b. The patient will be told to take a bulk-forming laxative.
   c. The patient will be given Milk of Magnesia to relieve the constipation quickly.
   d. The drug will be discontinued immediately.

9. Which of the following statements is accurate about the selective serotonin 5-HT$_3$ receptor antagonist Alosetron?
   a. It is indicated for women only.
   b. It is indicated for gastric ulcers only.
   c. It can improve constipation.
   d. Its use is limited to hospitalized patients.

10. The order for a child with severe diarrhea reads: "Give diphenoxylate with atropine 0.3 mg/kg/day in 4 divided doses." The medication is available in an oral solution with a concentration of 2.5 mg/5 mL. The child weighs 44 lb.
    a. How many milligrams will the child receive per dose? _____
    b. How many milliliters will the child receive per dose? _____

11. The order for a child reads: "Give lactulose 5 g, PO daily after breakfast." The medication is available as an oral solution in a unit-dose package that contains 10 g/15 mL. How many milliliters will the nurse administer per dose? _____

## CRITICAL THINKING AND APPLICATION

**Answer the following questions on a separate sheet of paper.**

12. Anna has called the health clinic in a panic. She says that she has been taking Pepto-Bismol for diarrhea and noticed this morning that her tongue "is a funny color." She asks, "Have I overdosed on this stuff? What should I do?" What will the nurse tell Anna?

13. Mrs. B. is a 65-year-old retiree with osteoporosis and narrow-angle glaucoma. She has recently developed diarrhea, and the physician is considering antidiarrheal therapy. Mrs. B. tells the nurse that her husband recently "had a bout of diarrhea" for which he took Donnatal. Mrs. B. wonders whether Donnatal would help in her case. What will the nurse tell her?

14. Hillary has come to the physician's office complaining of constipation. During the nurse's assessment, Hillary mentions that she recently started graduate school and has not had time lately to keep up her usual exercise regimen and that her diet "is a disaster." She says that on some days, all she has time to do is grab a milkshake or cheese and crackers at the student center. She also tells the nurse that she has been taking antacids for "heartburn." What might be causing Hillary's constipation?

15. Ira, age 45 years, has chronic constipation.
    a. What are the advantages of bulk-forming laxatives in treating Ira's problem?
    b. The provider prescribes psyllium. What instructions will the nurse give Ira regarding its administration?

16. Drake is a 5-year-old boy with constipation. The family nurse practitioner has suggested the use of glycerin suppositories.
    a. Why is glycerin a good choice for Drake?
    b. The parents will monitor for what adverse effects?

## CASE STUDY

**Read the scenario, and answer the following questions on a separate sheet of paper.**

Charles, age 54 years, recently completed a 2-week course of antibiotic therapy for pneumonia. He is now experiencing severe diarrhea.

1. What is the probable cause of his diarrhea?

2. What antidiarrheal product is indicated for Charles?

3. How does it work?

4. Is it considered a drug or a dietary supplement? Explain.

# 52 Antiemetic and Antinausea Drugs

**Select the best answer for each question.**

1. The nurse is giving medication to reduce nausea. Which antiemetic drug class is known to cause drying of secretions and drowsiness when given? *(Select all that apply.)*
   a. Antihistamines
   b. Antidopaminergic drugs
   c. Serotonin blockers
   d. Tetrahydrocannabinoids
   e. Anticholinergic drugs

2. A nurse is reviewing chemotherapy with a newly-hired nurse on the oncology unit. Which antinausea drug or drug class is indicated for preventing chemotherapy-induced nausea and vomiting? *(Select all that apply.)*
   a. Antihistamines
   b. Antidopaminergic drugs
   c. Serotonin blockers
   d. Phosphorated carbohydrate solution
   e. Tetrahydrocannabinoids

3. When reviewing the drugs used for nausea and vomiting, the nurse recalls that which drug is a synthetic derivative of the major active substance in marijuana?
   a. Ondansetron
   b. Metoclopramide
   c. Prochlorperazine
   d. Dronabinol

4. A patient is undergoing chemotherapy. When giving antiemetics, the nurse will remember that these drugs are most effective against nausea when given at which time?
   a. Before meals
   b. At bedtime
   c. Before the chemotherapy begins
   d. Just after the chemotherapy begins

5. When giving dronabinol to a patient with acquired immunodeficiency syndrome (AIDS), the nurse knows that this drug may also have what therapeutic effect in addition to reducing nausea?
   a. Euphoria
   b. Enhanced appetite
   c. Reduced pain
   d. Enhanced sleep

6. A patient calls the clinic to ask for something for his upset stomach. He admits to "eating a lot of food that's bad for me" the night before and wants something to help him to feel better. The nurse expects that which drug will be most appropriate for this patient?
   a. Metoclopramide
   b. Prochlorperazine
   c. Aprepitant
   d. Phosphorated carbohydrate solution

7. A mother discovers that her child has eaten half a bottle of children's multivitamins. Which is the appropriate first action in this situation?
   a. Give one dose of antacid and repeat in 30 minutes.
   b. Take the child to the pediatric clinic.
   c. Call the national poison control hotline for instructions.
   d. Call 911 for emergency transport to a hospital.

8. Which classification of antiemetics works by blocking dopamine receptors in the chemo trigger zone (CTZ)?
   a. Neurokinin blockers
   b. Serotonin blockers
   c. Prokinetic drugs
   d. Anticholinergic drugs

9. The nurse would recognize that aprepitant is primarily indicated to treat which disorder?
   a. Hyperemesis gravidarum
   b. Achlorhydria
   c. Nausea associated with chemotherapy
   d. Pyloric stenosis

10. The order reads: "Give prochlorperazine 10 mg IM every 4 hours as needed for nausea. Maximum of 4 doses/day." The medication is available in an ampule that contains 5 mg/mL. Mark the syringe with the amount the nurse will administer for each dose.

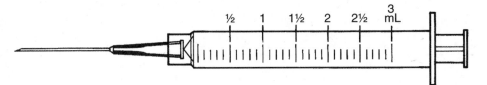

11. A patient is about to receive his first chemotherapy treatment with a drug that is known to cause nausea and vomiting. One of the premedication orders reads, "Give ondansetron PO 24 mg ½ hour before chemotherapy begins." The medication is ordered in a syrup that contains 4 mg/5 mL because the patient does not like to take pills. How many

milliliters of medication will the nurse administer for this dose? _____

## CRITICAL THINKING AND APPLICATION

**Answer the following questions on a separate sheet of paper.**

12. Petra has gastroesophageal reflux disease, and the health care provider has ordered oral metoclopramide (Reglan), four times a day for 2 weeks.
    a. What instructions will the nurse give Petra regarding administration of the medication?
    b. A few days later, Petra calls to say that she thinks the medication is "too strong." She also mentions that her evening routine includes "a couple of glasses of wine." What will the nurse tell Petra?

13. Nellie has been prescribed prochlorperazine (Compazine) via an intramuscular injection. She is on "nothing by mouth" status and has no intravenous access at this time. The nurse is preparing the injection when Nellie says, "I hate shots. Can't I just take it by mouth?" What alternatives are there for this drug, and what will the nurse do?

14. Chuck, age 33 years, is in a later stage of AIDS. He has lost a lot of weight and has no appetite. His physician has prescribed dronabinol (Marinol). When Chuck finds out that this medication is derived from marijuana, he becomes very upset. "Why is the doctor giving me pot?" he asks. What will the nurse explain?

## CASE STUDY

**Read the scenario, and answer the following questions on a separate sheet of paper.**

Mr. O. is preparing for his second course of chemotherapy as part of treatment for leukemia. One of the chemotherapy premedications is ondansetron. His chemotherapy will occur daily for 1 week.

1. What are potential contraindications to the use of ondansetron?

2. Mr. O. tells you that when he is at home, he still has nausea and is puzzled because "I take the medicine for nausea as soon as I feel nauseated." How will you address his comments?

3. One day Mr. O. complains to you that he gets a headache every time ondansetron is administered. What should you do?

# 53 Vitamins and Minerals

**Match each definition with the corresponding term.**

1. _____ A specialized protein that catalyzes bio-chemical reactions

2. _____ A condition that results from a deficiency of cyanocobalamin

3. _____ A nonprotein substance that combines with a protein molecule to form an active enzyme

4. _____ A condition caused by a vitamin D deficiency that is characterized by soft, pliable bones

5. _____ An inorganic substance that, when ingested, attaches to enzymes or other organic molecules

6. _____ An organic compound essential in small quantities for normal physiologic and metabolic functioning of the body

7. _____ A condition resulting from an ascorbic acid deficiency

8. _____ An essential organic compound that can be dissolved and stored in the liver and fatty tissues

9. _____ Biologically active chemicals that make up vitamin E compounds

10. _____ A disease of the peripheral nerves caused by a dietary deficiency of thiamine

11. _____ An essential organic compound that can be dissolved in water but is not stored in the body for long periods of time

12. _____ A disease resulting from a niacin deficiency or a metabolic defect that interferes with the conversion of tryptophan to niacin
   a. Beriberi
   b. Coenzyme
   c. Enzyme
   d. Fat-soluble vitamin
   e. Mineral
   f. Pellagra
   g. Pernicious anemia
   h. Rickets
   i. Scurvy
   j. Tocopherols
   k. Vitamin
   l. Water-soluble vitamin

**Select the best answer for each question.**

13. When giving vitamins, the nurse needs to remember that certain vitamins can be toxic if consumed in excess amounts. These include which vitamins? *(Select all that apply.)*
   a. Vitamin A
   b. Vitamin C
   c. Niacin
   d. Vitamin D
   e. Vitamin K
   f. Folic acid

14. A patient believes that taking megadoses of vitamin C is healthy. What should the nurse tell the patient about megadoses of vitamin C?
   a. They are usually nontoxic because vitamin C is water soluble.
   b. They can produce nausea, vomiting, headache, and abdominal cramps.
   c. Megadoses of vitamin C can lead to scurvy-like symptoms.
   d. They may cause dangerous heart dysrhythmias.

15. The nursing student would correctly identify which site as the storage location for the fat-soluble vitamins?
    a. The pancreas
    b. The bone marrow
    c. The spleen
    d. The liver
16. In addition to its use in maintaining homeostasis, the nurse would recognize a secondary use for vitamin $B_3$ as a treatment for which disorder?
    a. Night blindness
    b. Anemia
    c. Hyperlipidemia
    d. Azotemia

17. A patient has ingested an excessive amount of water-soluble vitamins. The nurse expects what to happen?
    a. The body will store them in muscle and fat tissue until needed.
    b. They are stored in the liver until needed.
    c. They will circulate in the blood, bound to proteins, until needed.
    d. Excess amounts will be excreted in the urine.

18. When reviewing the diet of a patient who has a calcium deficiency, the nurse recalls that efficient absorption of calcium in the diet requires adequate amounts of which substance?
    a. Magnesium
    b. Intrinsic factor
    c. Coenzymes
    d. Vitamin D

19. The nurse would be correct in identifying the major cause of cyanocobalamin deficiency to be which disorder?
    a. Alcoholism
    b. Renal failure
    c. Malabsorption
    d. Drug therapy

20. A patient is to receive 1 L of $D_5W$ with one ampule of multivitamins over the next 10 hours. The nurse will set the infusion pump at what rate for this

    IV infusion? _____

21. The order reads, "Give vitamin K 2 mg subcutaneously now." The patient is a child, age 5 years. The medication is available in an ampule, 1 mg/0.5 mL. How many milliliters will the

    nurse draw up for the injection? _____

## CRITICAL THINKING AND APPLICATION

**Answer the following questions on a separate sheet of paper.**

22. After Mr. W. is treated for colitis with a broad-spectrum antibiotic, he begins to show signs of hypoprothrombinemia caused by vitamin K deficiency. How did this happen, and how will he receive supplements?
23. Mrs. S. has developed vitamin D deficiency as a result of long-term use of lubricant laxatives. She is advised to take supplements for her vitamin D deficiency. However, her health care provider also advises her to get vitamin D through more natural sources. Explain the "natural sources" of vitamin D.

24. Ms. E. has recently undergone an ileal resection and is experiencing some signs of malabsorption. When routine laboratory tests are performed, the nurse discovers that she is mildly anemic.
    a. What type of anemia does the nurse expect?
    b. What about her condition is contributing to this deficiency?
    c. How is this condition treated?

25. Mr. G. is hospitalized with severe hypocalcemia and will be receiving intravenous calcium. What are the safety concerns when giving intravenous calcium?

## CASE STUDY

**Read the scenario, and answer the following questions on a separate sheet of paper.**

A patient with a long history of alcoholism has been admitted to the intensive care unit with an irregular cardiac rhythm and increased confusion. His magnesium level was noted to be 1.2 mg/dL, so he was placed on an intravenous magnesium infusion.

1. What is the normal serum magnesium level?

2. What is your priority when assessing the patient during intravenous magnesium infusion?

3. Twelve hours later, you note that the patient's respirations are 10 breaths/minute, and his Achilles tendon reflexes are diminished. What will you do next?

4. What is the antidote to magnesium toxicity?

# 54 Anemia Drugs

**Select the best answer for each question.**

1. Three days after beginning therapy with oral iron tablets, a patient calls the office, saying, "I'm very worried because my bowel movements are black!" What will the nurse do?
   a. Instruct the patient to stop the iron tablets for a week.
   b. Instruct the patient to take the tablets every other day instead of daily.
   c. Ask the patient to come into the office for a checkup.
   d. Explain to the patient that this is an expected effect of the medication.

2. A patient will be taking an oral iron preparation. Which of these are possible adverse effects? *(Select all that apply.)*
   a. Dizziness
   b. Nausea
   c. Vomiting
   d. Drowsiness
   e. Orthostatic hypotension
   f. Stomach cramps

3. The nurse is preparing to administer folic acid. What occurs if folic acid is given to treat anemia without determining the underlying cause of the anemia?
   a. Erythropoiesis is inhibited.
   b. Excessive levels of folic acid may accumulate, causing toxicity.
   c. The symptoms of pernicious anemia may be masked, delaying treatment.
   d. Intestinal intrinsic factor is destroyed.

4. A patient is about to receive folic acid supplementation. The nurse knows that indications for folic acid supplementation include which of the following? *(Select all that apply.)*
   a. Iron-deficiency anemia
   b. Tropical sprue
   c. Prevention of fetal neural tube defects
   d. Pernicious anemia
   e. Hemolytic anemia

5. When teaching a patient about oral iron preparations, the nurse will include which instructions? *(Select all that apply.)*
   a. Mix the liquid iron preparations with antacids to reduce gastrointestinal distress.
   b. Take the iron with meals if gastrointestinal distress occurs.
   c. Liquid forms should be taken through a straw to avoid discoloration of tooth enamel.
   d. Oral forms should be taken with juice or water, not milk.
   e. Iron products will turn the stools black.

6. A patient will be receiving darbepoetin as part of treatment for post chemotherapy bone marrow suppression. Which finding is a contraindication to darbepoetin therapy?
   a. Pulse rate of 100 beats/min
   b. Blood pressure of 128/79 mm Hg
   c. Hemoglobin level of 11 g/dL
   d. White blood cell count of 7000/mm$^3$

7. The nurse is preparing to give iron sucrose (Venofer) to a 58-year-old patient and will monitor for which common adverse effect?
   a. Hypotension
   b. Dyspnea
   c. Itching
   d. Cramps

8. Which laboratory finding would indicate to the nurse that the patient is responding favorably to epoetin alfa?
   a. An increase in reticulocytes
   b. A decrease in clotting time
   c. An increase in platelets
   d. A decrease in leukocytes

9. The nurse would be correct in identifying that iron sucrose would be appropriate in the treatment of anemia secondary to which disorder?
   a. Emphysema
   b. Chronic renal disease
   c. Hemorrhage from trauma
   d. Hypoalbuminemia

**130**

10. A patient will be receiving epoetin alfa 150 units/kg, subcutaneously, three times a week. The patient weighs 110 lb. The medication is available in a concentration of 10,000 units/mL. How many milliliters will the nurse administer for each dose? *(Record answer using two decimal places.)* _____ Mark the syringe with your answer.

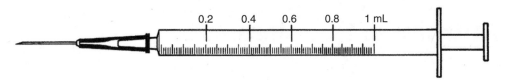

11. A 5-year-old child who is receiving hemodialysis is to receive eight doses of sodium ferric gluconate (Ferrlecit), 1.5 mg/kg IV, with future dialysis sessions. The child weighs 38 lb. How many milligrams is each dose?

    *(Record answer using a whole number.)* _____

## CRITICAL THINKING AND APPLICATION

**Answer the following questions on a separate sheet of paper.**

12. Mr. P. is prescribed intramuscular iron dextran. However, before the nurse can give him his first injection, the pharmacist suggests that she give him a smaller dose of 25 mg first. Why does the pharmacist suggest this? How should intramuscular iron dextran be administered?

13. Mrs. S. will be taking iron for treatment of anemia, and her provider instructed her to take it with orange juice. She asks the nurse for an explanation of this. What will the nurse tell her?

14. What are the advantages of receiving ferric gluconate or iron sucrose injections instead of iron dextran?

15. Connie, age 58 years, is in the hospital because of extreme weakness. She has a history of chronic renal failure, and there is a new order for epoetin alfa. What laboratory results are monitored during epoetin therapy? Why?

## CASE STUDY

**Read the scenario, and answer the following questions on a separate sheet of paper.**

Maureen has been given ferrous fumarate capsules with instructions to take two capsules twice a day as part of her treatment for iron-deficiency anemia.

1. She asks you if she can take this drug with meals. What is your answer?

2. What else will you warn her to expect with this medication?

3. After 1 week, Maureen calls you because she does not like to swallow capsules. She says that her mother has iron tablets that are labeled ferrous sulfate. She wants to know if she can take those tablets instead. What do you tell her?

4. Because Maureen does not like the capsules, her iron preparation has been switched to an oral liquid suspension. While you are teaching her how to give herself the correct dosage, what else is important for you to tell her about liquid iron preparations?

# 55 Nutritional Supplements

## CRITICAL THINKING CROSSWORD

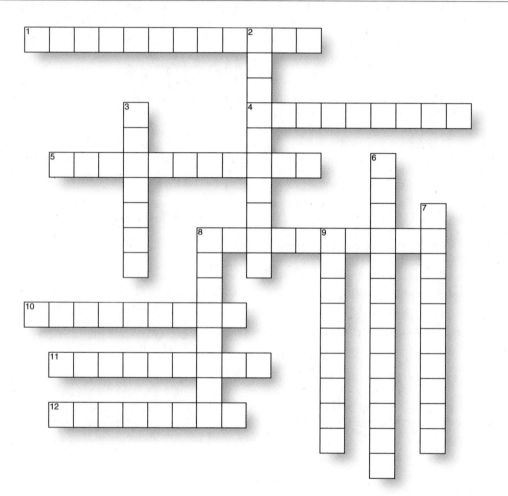

**Across**

1. Mr. G. is receiving an oral antibiotic when it is determined that he is going to need nutritional supplementation as well. However, you are concerned that the nutritional supplement will decrease the absorption of this drug because of high gastric acid content or prolonged emptying time. What is the generic name of this antibiotic?

4. Ms. C. needs amino acids in nutritional supplements. The main use, or primary role, of amino acids is

    protein synthesis or _____.

5. Mr. H. is about to receive a(n) _____, in which a feeding tube will be surgically inserted directly into his stomach.

8. Mrs. P. is worried about her husband, who has post-surgical nausea. She sees that his roommate is receiving total parenteral nutrition (TPN) and asks, "Can't you do that for my husband, just while he's so nauseated?" TPN, you explain, is to be used only when enteral support is impossible or when the

gastrointestinal tract's _____ or functional capacity is insufficient.

10. Ms. D. comes to the clinic when a cut on her hand "just won't heal up." She also says that as long as she is here, she would like to report symptoms of hair loss and a scaly rash on her skin. She wants a prescription for her skin problem, but the provider says, "There's something more going on here." After performing some laboratory work, it is found that Ms. D. also has a decreased platelet level and some evidence of possible fatty liver. The provider states

that Ms. D. has essential _____ (two words) deficiency.

11. Mr. J. is having trouble eating, which has resulted in an inadequate intake of dietary amino acids. His provider explains that he needs nutritional supplementation through enteral nutrition to ensure that he gets enough of these amino acids because they cannot be produced by his own body. Mr. J.

has a deficiency of _____ amino acids.

12. Mr. C., a college sophomore, takes a great deal of interest in the supplementary nutritional product he is receiving and asks to read the label. He says, "There are some amino acids missing from this. Why aren't you giving me all of them?" You explain that some amino acids, all but eight, are manufactured

in the body, using _____ sources.

**Down**

2. When Ms. C. (from 4 Across) asks why she needs amino acid supplemental feedings, you explain that amino acids promote growth and help with wound healing. One of the principal ways they do so is by reducing or slowing the breakdown of proteins, or

_____.

3. Mr. and Mrs. R. drink Ensure to meet a few extra nutritional needs they have experienced with aging. Their nephew recently had surgery, and while recovering, he received nasogastric delivery of a modular formulation to supplement a polymeric feeding formulation he needed. When their grandson was an infant, his parents supplemented his breastfeeding with an infant nutritional formulation. Each member of the family discussed here has

received some form of _____ nutrition.

6. The amino acids in 8 Down are _____ amino acids.

7. You are explaining to Mrs. N.'s family that the parenteral nutritional supplementation you are about to start will help her by bypassing the entire gastrointestinal system, eliminating the need for absorption,

_____, and excretion.

8. The nursing student is reviewing amino acids and is trying to recall the two amino acids that are not produced in large enough quantities during infancy and childhood. One of these is histidine; the other

one is _____.

9. Mr. K. has been receiving peripheral parenteral nutrition. During an assessment, you note that his vein becomes inflamed. What problem is this?

**Select the best answer for each question.**

1. The nurse is assessing a patient who is receiving a peripheral parenteral nutrition (PPN) infusion. The maximum concentration of dextrose in PPN infusions is which percentage?
   a. 10%
   b. 20%
   c. 50%
   d. 100%

2. A patient has a need for a nutritional supplement that contains complex nutrients derived from proteins, carbohydrates, and fat. However, this patient is lactose intolerant. The nurse knows that which product would be most suitable for this patient?
   a. Casec
   b. Polycose
   c. Ensure
   d. Vivonex

3. When monitoring a patient who is receiving TPN through a central line, the nurse will observe for which complications? *(Select all that apply.)*
   a. Pneumothorax
   b. Aspiration
   c. Hyperglycemia
   d. Infection
   e. Air embolus

4. A patient who is just starting to take enteral nutritional supplements will be taught by the nurse to expect which most common adverse effect?
   a. Anorexia
   b. Constipation
   c. Diarrhea
   d. Flatulence

5. When reviewing a patient's need for nutritional supplementation, the nurse remembers that PPN is most appropriate for which type of patient?
   a. Patients who will receive parenteral nutrition for less than 2 weeks
   b. Patients who will receive parenteral nutrition for more than 2 weeks
   c. Patients with severe nutritional problems
   d. Patients who wish to reduce their weight

6. A patient with type 1 diabetes mellitus will be receiving enteral nutrition for 4 months after surgery. Which of these nutritional solutions is most appropriate for this patient?
   a. Jevity
   b. Polycose
   c. Ensure
   d. Glucerna

7. Which prescription for lipid emulsion calorie replacement would most concern the nurse?
   a. The emulsion provides 20% of total daily calories.
   b. The emulsion provides 30% of total daily calories.
   c. The emulsion provides 40% of total daily calories.
   d. The emulsion provides 60% of total daily calories.

8. What is the nurse's priority assessment before administering any enteral feeding?
   a. Heart rate
   b. Bowel sounds
   c. Urine specific gravity
   d. Electrolyte and albumin levels

9. A patient will be receiving TPN. The first bag is to infuse at 50 mL/hr for 4 hours, then at 75 mL/hr for 4 hours, then at 100 mL/hr thereafter. What is the intravenous intake for the TPN over the first

   12 hours of the infusion? _____

10. A patient is receiving a PEG tube feeding of Glucerna at 70 mL/hour via a feeding pump. What will be the PEG tube intake over a 24-hour period?

    _____

## CRITICAL THINKING AND APPLICATION

**Answer the following questions on a separate sheet of paper.**

11. Ms. S. is receiving an enteral feeding through a PEG tube.
    a. What symptoms would she develop if she were lactose intolerant?
    b. Her tube feeding rate is 50 mL/hr. After 24 hours, you note that the residual amount is 120 mL. What is the nurse's priority action?

12. Mr. R., who is on TPN therapy, has a weak pulse, hypertension, tachycardia, and decreased urine output. He seems somewhat confused, and the nurse finds that he now has pitting edema in his ankles. What is happening, and what are the priority actions of the nurse?

**Read the scenario, and answer the following questions on a separate sheet of paper.**

You are caring for Mrs. T., who is receiving peripheral parenteral nutrition (PPN) through an intravenous (IV) line in her right forearm. Your assessment shows that bag No. 3 is infusing at 100 mL/hr via an infusion pump, and the bag has about 300 mL remaining. The site is intact, without redness or swelling.

1. Two hours later, Mrs. T. calls you because she accidentally pulled the IV line out of her arm. The remaining 100 mL of PPN has spilled on the floor. You have tried to reinsert the IV line but have not yet had success. What could occur if you cannot restart the infusion?

2. At last, the IV line has been reinserted, but you then discover that bag No. 4 has not yet been ordered from the pharmacy. What will you hang until PPN bag No. 4 is ready?

3. What else will you monitor while Mrs. T. is receiving PPN?

# 56 Dermatologic Drugs

**Select the best answer for each question.**

1. Which statement accurately describes antifungal therapy for topical infections?
   a. The length of treatment required to eradicate the organism may be from several weeks to as long as 1 year.
   b. Antifungal therapy works best when the affected area is exposed to sunlight.
   c. Oral drugs are the preferred drugs for treating topical fungal infections.
   d. Antifungal therapy is palliative only; fungi are rarely eradicated from topical areas.

2. When instructing a patient on how to use miconazole vaginal cream for vaginal yeast infections, the nurse will keep in mind that this medication will be given in which manner?
   a. Insert once every other day at bedtime for 1 week.
   b. Insert once daily at bedtime for 7 consecutive days.
   c. A one-time dose is administered in the morning.
   d. Insert every night at bedtime until symptoms stop.

3. When instructing a patient about the actions and uses of benzoyl peroxide, the patient asks when positive results from the medication can be expected. Which statement indicates the nurse's best response?
   a. 7 days
   b. 2 to 3 weeks
   c. 3 to 4 weeks
   d. 4 to 6 weeks

4. A patient has a painful sunburn that covers a large area of her body and has asked the nurse for "something to make it feel better." The nurse keeps in mind that which formulation of topical medication will be easiest to use to cover this large area?
   a. Aerosol spray
   b. Gel
   c. Oil
   d. Cream

5. A patient needs a medication that has excellent emollient properties. Because she works as a swimming coach, the medication prescribed should not wash off when it comes in contact with water. If each has the same healing properties, which formulation would be the best for this patient?
   a. Aerosol spray
   b. Oil
   c. Gel
   d. Cream

6. The nurse is administering topical antiviral drugs. Which statements about these drugs are true? *(Select all that apply.)*
   a. Common adverse effects include stinging, itching, and rash.
   b. Topically applied acyclovir does not cure viral skin infections but does seem to decrease the healing time and pain.
   c. Topically applied acyclovir can cure viral skin infections if applied as soon as symptoms appear.
   d. Antiviral drugs are applied topically for the treatment of both initial and recurrent herpes simplex infections.
   e. Topical antiviral drugs are used more often than systemic antiviral drugs for the treatment of viral skin conditions.

7. A 22-year-old woman is taking isotretinoin as part of the treatment for severe cystic acne. Which statement about isotretinoin therapy is true?
   a. This drug reduces acne by causing skin peeling.
   b. Its use is contraindicated if she is allergic to erythromycin.
   c. She will need to apply it twice a day to her face after washing her face thoroughly.
   d. She will need to use two forms of birth control while taking this medication.

8. Before using povidone-iodine solution to prepare skin for surgery, the nurse will ask the patient about allergies to which substance?
   a. Shellfish
   b. Penicillin
   c. Mercury
   d. Milk

9. A patient will be receiving fluorouracil cream as part of treatment for basal cell carcinoma of the skin on her nose. The nurse will instruct the patient about which possible adverse effects? *(Select all that apply.)*
   a. Swelling
   b. Scaling
   c. Pallor
   d. Burning
   e. Tenderness

10. The nurse notes the patient has an order for silver sulfadiazine. The nurse would anticipate the patient is experiencing which diagnosis?
    a. Impetigo
    b. Folliculitis
    c. Burns
    d. Cellulitis

11. The order for a patient who has a severely infected skin wound reads, "Administer clindamycin (Cleocin) 300 mg diluted in 50 mL 0.9% NS IVPB every 6 hours. Infuse over 30 minutes." When calculating the rate for this IVPB, the nurse will set the infusion pump to what rate? _____

12. A patient will be receiving intravenous amphotericin B (Fungizone) for a severe fungal infection that has not responded to other medications. The order reads, "75 mg in 1000 mL $D_5W$ to infuse over 6 hours." The nurse will set the infusion pump to what rate?

   _____

## CRITICAL THINKING AND APPLICATION

**Answer the following questions on a separate sheet of paper.**

13. Mr. M. has a topical skin infection. He is prescribed clindamycin (Cleocin T). He has never used this drug before. What assessments are important before the nurse administers this drug?

14. The nurse is getting ready to apply topical erythromycin to a patient's skin rash. The affected area of the skin is not oozing or even moist, but the nurse wears gloves. Why?

15. Mr. L.'s two children brought "something" home from school, and within 1 day, he had "it," too. He tells the nurse that he has applied lindane (Kwell) to everyone's scalp, but he has come to the clinic to have his children and himself checked because he is not confident that he has "taken care of things properly." For what are Mr. L. and his children being treated? Describe for him the basic steps in using lindane. What other measures does he need to take?

16. A newly admitted patient has a stage III pressure ulcer that shows areas of exudate along with areas of healed granulation tissue. The orders for wound care include application of cadexomer iodine (Iodosorb). Explain what needs to be assessed before applying this medication and its purpose in wound care.

17. A patient with an infected pressure ulcer that contains an area of eschar needs to have the area surgically débrided, but instead the physician orders collagenase (Santyl) treatment of the wound. What could be the reason for this order instead of surgery, and what is the purpose of this medication?

## CASE STUDY

**Read the scenario, and answer the following questions on a separate sheet of paper.**

Judy is in the clinic today because she burned her arm last evening while frying chicken. She has a second-degree burn over a 5-inch area of her forearm. She did not apply anything to it overnight, and the wound is reddened and peeling.

1. The physician instructs you to apply silver sulfadiazine (Silvadene) cream to the site. What needs to be done before the cream is applied?

2. You instruct Judy that the area will need to be kept covered. Why is this necessary?

3. Do you need to wear gloves when applying this cream? Explain.

4. Are there any adverse effects associated with this medication?

# 57 Ophthalmic Drugs

**Match each definition with the corresponding term. (Note: Not all terms will be used.)**

1. _____ Adjustment of the lens of the eye for variations in distance

2. _____ Inflammation of the eyelids

3. _____ The clear, watery fluid that circulates in the anterior and posterior chambers of the eye

4. _____ An abnormal condition of the lens of the eye, characterized by loss of transparency

5. _____ Paralysis of the ciliary muscles, which prevents accommodation of the lens for variations in distance

6. _____ Excessive intraocular pressure caused by obstruction of the outflow of aqueous humor

7. _____ The mucous membrane that lines the eyelids and the exposed anterior surface of the eye

8. _____ Drugs that constrict the pupil

9. _____ The vascular middle layer of the eye, containing the iris, ciliary body, and choroid

10. _____ Drugs that dilate the pupil

a. Cycloplegia
b. Conjunctiva
c. Accommodation
d. Glaucoma
e. Mydriatics
f. Miotics
g. Uvea
h. Blepharitis
i. Vitreous humor
j. Aqueous humor
k. Cataract

**Select the best answer for each question.**

11. When reviewing the medical record of a patient with a new order for a carbonic anhydrase inhibitor, the nurse knows that which condition would be a potential problem for a patient taking this drug?
    a. Glaucoma
    b. Ocular hypertension
    c. Allergy to sulfa drugs
    d. Allergy to penicillin

12. During an ophthalmic procedure, the patient receives ophthalmic acetylcholine. The nurse is aware that which effect is the purpose of administering this drug?
    a. To produce mydriasis for ophthalmic examination
    b. To produce immediate miosis during ophthalmic surgery
    c. To cause cycloplegia to allow for measurement of intraocular pressure
    d. To provide topical anesthesia during ophthalmic surgery

13. The nurse identifies which description as the method of action of pilocarpine in treating glaucoma?
    a. Producing miosis, increasing outflow of aqueous humor
    b. Decreasing the production and formation of aqueous humor
    c. Vasoconstriction, thereby inhibiting the flow of aqueous humor
    d. Producing cycloplegia, decreasing pupillary response

14. When giving latanoprost eyedrops, the nurse will advise the patient of which possible adverse effects?
    a. Temporary eye color changes, from light eye colors to brown
    b. Permanent eye color changes, from light eye colors to brown
    c. Photosensitivity
    d. Bradycardia and hypotension

15. A patient has come to the emergency department with an eye injury. After fluorescein (AK-Fluor) is applied, the physician sees an area with a green halo. This indicates which condition?
    a. A corneal defect
    b. A conjunctival lesion
    c. The presence of a hard contact lens
    d. A foreign object

16. When applying ophthalmic drugs, the nurse will follow which instructions? *(Select all that apply.)*
    a. Apply drops directly onto the cornea.
    b. Apply drops into the conjunctival sac.
    c. Apply pressure to the inner canthus for 1 minute after medication administration.
    d. Apply ointments in a thin layer.
    e. Avoid touching the eye with the tip of the medication dropper.

17. A newborn infant is about to receive medication that prevents gonorrheal eye infection. The nurse will prepare to administer which drug?
    a. Dexamethasone ointment
    b. Gentamicin solution
    c. Erythromycin ointment
    d. Sulfacetamide solution

18. The nurse identifies which description as the method of action of betaxolol in treating glaucoma?
    a. Producing miosis, increasing outflow of aqueous humor
    b. Decreasing the production and formation of aqueous humor
    c. Vasodilation, increasing blood flow to the optic nerve
    d. Producing cycloplegia, decreasing pupillary response

19. A patient will be receiving acetazolamide, 250 mg PO four times a day, as part of treatment for glaucoma. The tablets are available in 125-mg strength. How many tablets will the patient receive

    per dose? _____

20. A patient has an order for an IV to infuse at 75 mL/hr. The IV will infuse by gravity drip; the administration set delivers 15 gtt/mL. What is the gtt/min that the nurse will need to use for this infusion?

    _____

## CRITICAL THINKING AND APPLICATION

**Answer the following questions on a separate sheet of paper.**

21. Jonathan has blue eyes; Julie has brown eyes. Why would the drug effects of the miotics on the iris be less pronounced in Julie?

22. Mrs. N., a 60-year-old librarian, has open-angle glaucoma. The ophthalmologist prescribes dipivefrin (Propine).
    a. Why might the physician have chosen that drug over epinephrine?
    b. What effects will the nurse tell Mrs. N. to expect when first taking dipivefrin?
    c. Will the nurse expect any serious reactions to the drug? Explain your answer.

23. The ophthalmologist prescribes a beta-adrenergic blocker for Ned, who has ocular hypertension. Ned experiences what he calls "an allergic reaction" to the drug, and the physician changes Ned's medication to another beta-blocking drug, timolol (Timoptic). Because both of these drugs are beta-adrenergic blockers and Ned had a reaction to the first drug, why would the physician simply switch Ned to another drug in the same category?

24. The nurse is preparing to administer sulfacetamide to Tony, a patient with an eye infection.
    a. Why will the nurse cleanse Tony's eye before administering the medication?
    b. Before using the sulfacetamide, the nurse examines it and then throws the solution away and orders another container of sulfacetamide. Why did the nurse do this?

25. Louisa has an inflammatory disorder of the eye for which the nurse practitioner has prescribed a topical ophthalmic nonsteroidal antiinflammatory drug (NSAID). Why was an NSAID chosen over a corticosteroid?

26. Ms. L. has been prescribed ophthalmic corticosteroid drops for an inflammation of her eye. The next day she calls the clinic and tells the nurse, "These drops sting so much when I use them that I can't even put in my contacts." What is the priority when the nurse responds to her statement?

27. The nurse is administering medications to a patient. The patient will receive both latanoprost (Xalatan) eyedrops and pilocarpine (Pilocar) eye gel at the same time. Which drug needs to be given first? Explain your answer.

**Read the scenario, and answer the following questions on a separate sheet of paper.**

Mr. W., age 72 years, has developed a bacterial ocular infection and has a prescription for erythromycin ocular ointment. You are teaching him how to self-administer the medication.

1. How will this drug be administered?

2. You will educate Mr. W. about what safety precautions to take after he receives a dose of this medication?

3. After receiving the first dose, Mr. W. complains that the medication "burns and stings." What will you say to Mr. W. about this?

4. Mr. W. tells you, "I have some eyedrops from a few months ago when I had some allergy problems. I am sure they will help me now. Can I take them with this ointment?" What is your best response?

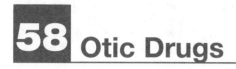
# 58 Otic Drugs

**Select the best answer for each question.**

1. When assessing for otitis media, the nurse remembers that common symptoms of this condition include which of the following? *(Select all that apply.)*
   a. Pain
   b. Malaise
   c. Ear drainage
   d. Hearing loss
   e. Fever

2. A patient with a severe middle ear infection will generally require treatment with which type of drug?
   a. Topical steroids
   b. Systemic steroids
   c. Topical antibiotics
   d. Systemic antibiotics

3. The patient with external otitis asks the nurse why the physician placed a small piece of cotton in the patient's ear and told the patient to leave it in place. How should the nurse respond?
   a. "The physician made an error; I will remove the cotton."
   b. "The cotton traps the medication and doesn't allow it to exit the ear."
   c. "The cotton is designed to gradually reabsorb over the next 24 hours."
   d. "The cotton is called a wick and enables the medication to get to the infected area more effectively."

4. An older adult patient has a buildup of cerumen in his left ear. The nurse expects that this patient will receive which type of drug for this problem?
   a. Antifungal
   b. Wax emulsifier
   c. Steroid
   d. Local analgesic

5. Before giving eardrops, the nurse checks for potential contraindications to the use of otic preparations, such as which of these conditions?
   a. Eardrum perforation
   b. Infection
   c. Presence of cerumen
   d. Mastoiditis

6. A child has a case of otitis media. The nurse knows that otitis media in children is usually preceded by
   a. participation on a swim team.
   b. injury with a foreign object.
   c. upper respiratory tract infection.
   d. mastoiditis.

7. The nurse is preparing to administer Cortic and Acetasol HC. The nurse would anticipate the patient is experiencing which disorder?
   a. Viral otitis externa
   b. Bacterial otitis media
   c. Fungal otitis media
   d. Bacterial otitis externa

8. A child with an ear infection will be receiving amoxicillin suspension PO. The order reads: "Give 125 mg (5 mL) three times a day PO." The child weighs 11 kg.
   a. How many milligrams of medication will this child receive in 24 hours? _____
   b. The safe dosage range of the medication is 20 to 40 mg/kg/day. What is the safe range (in milligrams) for this child? _____
   c. Is the ordered dose within the safe range? _____
   d. Mark on the medication cup how many milliliters the patient will receive for this dose.

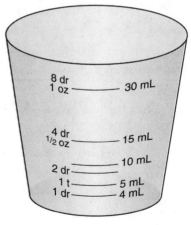

**Answer the following questions on a separate sheet of paper.**

9. A patient calls the clinic complaining of severe pain in, and drainage from, his left ear. He also says he "had a little mishap" on his motorcycle yesterday. What will the nurse tell him?

10. Why are antiinfective otic drugs frequently combined with steroids?

11. André, a 30-year-old teacher, has an ear infection and a new prescription for eardrops.
    a. What might be done before he takes the eardrops?
    b. What safety measures are important to inform André about regarding self-administration of the eardrops?

12. Mrs. F., a 52-year-old office manager, has come to the clinic today complaining of a painful, "itchy" left ear. The physician's assistant diagnoses an infection of the external auditory canal and prescribes eardrop medication that contains a combination of polymyxin B and hydrocortisone.
    a. What is the advantage of using a product containing hydrocortisone?
    b. What would be a contraindication to Mrs. F.'s use of these eardrops?

13. Why do so many otic combination products contain local anesthetic drugs?

14. Ben, a 2-year-old toddler, attends day care, and his brother Drew is a 6-year-old kindergartener. They both require otic drugs for ear infections.
    a. What instructions will the nurse give the boys' parents regarding instillation of the drops?
    b. A few days after they are first seen, the boys' mother brings them back for a follow-up visit. Ben and Drew do not seem to be in pain, and there is no redness or swelling in either child's ears. What does this mean?

15. During a home visit, the nurse observes Esther's husband preparing her eardrops. He puts a glass of water in the microwave, saying that he will soak the bottle of eardrops in hot water to warm them up.
    a. Why is this a concern?
    b. Immediately after her husband instills the drops, Esther sits up and asks whether they are now doing everything right. What will the nurse tell her?

16. A 4-year-old child will be receiving oral amoxicillin suspension for treatment for otitis media. The nurse gives the prescription to the child's mother and asks her if she has any questions. The mother states, "Just to make sure, I will pour this liquid into his ears, correct? And I can stop it when his symptoms go away, right?" What is the priority when answering her questions?

## CASE STUDY

**Read the scenario, and answer the following questions on a separate sheet of paper.**

Mark, who is 45 years old, comes to the office complaining of a "heavy" feeling in his left ear, with slight pain and decreased hearing. When you walk into the examination room, you find Mark inserting a cotton-tipped applicator into his ear "to scratch it."

1. What is a possible reason for his symptoms?

2. What can be done to address this problem?

3. You give Mark a container of carbamide peroxide drops. Before you continue, he asks you how many times a day he needs to take this medication and whether he can take it with meals. How is this medication given?

4. Why is there a combination of carbamide peroxide and glycerin in the Debrox?

# Overview of Dosage Calculations

There are many important aspects to consider when performing dosage calculations, but probably the most important one is common sense. If a drug dose calculation does not seem right, then most likely it is not. The administration of drugs to patients is a shared responsibility among the patient, prescriber, pharmacist, and nurse. All those involved have a moral, ethical, and legal responsibility to ensure that the administration takes place in a safe and effective way. There are many checks and balances in the system to guarantee that this happens. The necessary basic calculations involved in the safe and accurate administration of medications to patients are described in this section.

Calculating drug doses is one small part of the overall process of pharmacologic therapy. Before you actually calculate a drug dose, you must follow many steps. The nurse will evaluate the patient and the prescribed medication for the following "rights": right patient, right drug, right dose, right time, and right route. In addition, the nurse must document correctly after the drug is given. Other principles to follow to decrease the likelihood of mistakes are to calculate doses systematically and to perform calculations consistently time after time so that the process becomes easier with each calculation.[1]

It also helps to have a peer check your calculations, especially if the dose seems unusual or the math is very difficult. Make use of a calculator to help you with the arithmetic. Remember that common sense should prevail. If a calculation shows that you are to give 25 mg of digoxin and the strongest strength is 0.25 mg, common sense tells you that the patient should not be given 100 pills, especially because drug dosage forms are usually manufactured with the most commonly prescribed dosages in mind.

You must have basic arithmetic skills before beginning. The following basic principles may need to be reviewed:

- Basic multiplication
- Basic division
- Roman numerals
- Fractions (reducing to lowest terms, addition, subtraction, multiplication, division, mixed numbers)
- Decimals (addition, subtraction, multiplication, division)
- Ratios and percentages (changing a fraction to a percentage, changing a ratio to a percentage)
- Solving for $x$ in a simple equation

## RULES TO REMEMBER

- Before calculating a drug dose for a particular patient, you must first convert all units of measure to a SINGLE unit of measure if this has not already been done. For example, do NOT attempt to guess a dosage if the drug is ordered in grains but the drug label is in milligrams. The best approach is to convert to the units of measure used on the drug label. You may have to convert the patient's weight from pounds to kilograms if the medication is ordered to be given per kilogram of weight.
- **Rounding.** Always round your answers to the nearest dose that is measurable after verifying that the dose is correct for that patient.
  - If a tablet is scored, you may round to the nearest half tablet.
    **Examples:**   1.8 tablets: give 2 tablets
                   1.2 tablets: give 1 tablet
  - If a tablet is unscored, call the pharmacy. It is very difficult to cut an unscored tablet accurately. Remember that enteric-coated, sustained-release, or extended-release formulations cannot be cut or crushed!
  - Recheck your calculations if the dose is more than one or two tablets.

---

[1]Disclaimer: Please note that the drugs and dosages within this chapter are examples for educational purposes only; please refer to appropriate drug resources for dosage information.

- To round liquids, look at the equipment you plan to use. Some syringes are marked in tenths or hundredths of a milliliter. Larger syringes are marked in 0.2-mL increments. Tuberculin syringes are marked in hundredths. For liquid medications, NEVER round up to the nearest WHOLE number. If the answer is 1.8 mL, DO NOT round up to 2 mL. Rounding up in these situations may lead to overdosing. However, if you are using an electronic infusion pump, you will probably need to round to the nearest whole number.
- To round to the nearest tenth, look at the hundredths column. If it is 0.5 or more, round UP to the next tenth (using one decimal place).

  **Example:** To round to the nearest tenth (using one decimal place):

    1.78 or 1.75: round to 1.8

    1.32 or 1.34: round to 1.3
- A syringe calibrated in hundredths permits more exact measurement of small doses. To round to the nearest hundredth, look at the thousandth column. If it is 0.005 or more, round UP to the next hundredth (using two decimal places).

  **Example:** To round to the nearest hundredth (using two decimal places):

    1.847: round to 1.85

    1.653: round to 1.65
- NOTE: Never round liquid medications to the nearest whole number. If the answer is 1.6 mL, DO NOT round up to 2 mL! Such increases may lead to overdoses.
- PEDIATRIC DOSES are rounded to the TENTHS place, not whole numbers. Rounding to whole numbers may lead to overdoses.

■ **Leading Zeros.** Always insert a zero (0) in front of decimals when the number is less than a whole number. This draws attention to the decimal and avoids potential errors.

  **Example:** 0.05 is CORRECT.

    .05 is NOT correct.

■ **Trailing Zeros.** Never place a lone zero after a decimal point. If the decimal is not noticed, a dangerous dosage error may occur.

  **Example:** 3 is CORRECT.

    3.0 is NOT correct and may be mistaken for 30.

■ **Labeling.** Always label your answers with the appropriate unit. If the problem asks for the number of tablets, write "tablets." If you are to give an injection, use "mL." Heparin and insulin, however, use "units" instead of "mg" or "mcg." Problems using an intravenous (IV) infusion pump are always asking for mL/hr. THINK about what the question is asking, and then label your answer appropriately.

■ **Common Sense.** Use common sense! Drug companies typically formulate medications that are close to the usual doses and medications that can provide the ordered dose with one or two tablets. If your answer indicates that you need to give 60 mL intramuscularly, CHECK IT AGAIN! Remember, you can only give 2 to 3 mL intramuscularly, depending on institution policies, so a dosage of 60 mL would be inappropriate.

## INTERPRETING MEDICATION LABELS

Medication labels contain a great amount of information—much of it in small print. The drug manufacturer prints some labels; others are prepared by pharmacy technicians or pharmacists for institutional use. The most important information follows:

■ Generic name—The first letter is usually lowercase; this is the name used by all companies that produce the drug.

■ Trade, brand, or proprietary name—The first letter is usually capitalized; this name is used only by the manufacturer of the drug and may be followed by the "®" symbol.

■ Unit dose per milliliter, per tablet, per capsule, and so on

■ Total amount in the container

- Route(s)
- Directions for preparation, if needed
- Directions for storage
- Expiration date

Other information, such as a specification for adult or pediatric use, may be noted on the label.

**Example:**

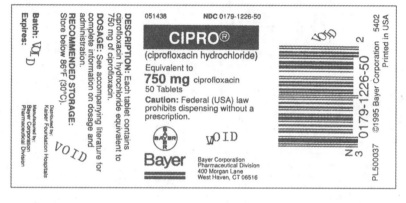

Generic name:        ciprofloxacin hydrochloride
Trade name:        Cipro
Unit dose:        750 mg per tablet
Total amount in container:        50 tablets
Route:        (It is assumed that tablets are oral route.)

**For the following labels, identify the information requested:**

1.

Generic name: _____

Trade name: _____

Unit dose: _____

Total amount in container: _____

Route: _____

**2.**

AMOXIL®
125mg/5mL

125mg/5mL
NDC 0029-6008-23

**AMOXIL®**
AMOXICILLIN
FOR ORAL
SUSPENSION

**Directions for mixing:** Tap bottle
until all powder flows freely. Add
approximately 1/3 total amount of
water for reconstitution (total=78 mL);
shake vigorously to wet powder.
Add remaining water; again shake
vigorously. Each 5 mL (1 teaspoonful)
will contain amoxicillin trihydrate
equivalent to 125 mg amoxicillin.
**Usual Adult Dosage:** 250 to
500 mg every 8 hours.
**Usual Child Dosage:** 20 to
40 mg/kg/day in divided doses every
8 hours, depending on age, weight and
infection severity. See accompanying
prescribing information.

**Keep tightly closed.**
**Shake well before using.**
**Refrigeration preferable but not required.**
**Discard suspension after 14 days.**

100mL
(when reconstituted)

SB SmithKline Beecham

NSN 6505-01-153-3862
**Net contents:** Equivalent to 2.5 grams amoxicillin.
Store dry powder at room temperature.
SmithKline Beecham Pharmaceuticals
Philadelphia, PA 19101

Rx only

3 0029-6008-23 1

LOT
EXP.
9405793-F

Generic name: _____

Trade name: _____

Unit dose: _____

Total amount in container: _____

Route: _____

**3.**

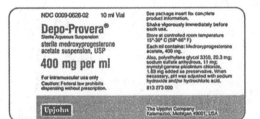

NDC 0009-0626-02    10 ml Vial

**Depo-Provera®**
Sterile Aqueous Suspension
sterile medroxyprogesterone
acetate suspension, USP

**400 mg per ml**

For intramuscular use only
Caution: Federal law prohibits
dispensing without prescription.

Upjohn

See package insert for complete
product information.
Shake vigorously immediately before
each use.
Store at controlled room temperature
15°–30° C (59°–86° F)
Each ml contains: Medroxyprogesterone
acetate, 400 mg.
Also, polyethylene glycol 3350, 20.3 mg;
sodium sulfate anhydrous, 11 mg;
myristyl-gamma picolinium chloride,
1.69 mg added as preservative. When
necessary, pH was adjusted with sodium
hydroxide and/or hydrochloric acid.
813 273 000

The Upjohn Company
Kalamazoo, Michigan 49001, USA

Generic name: _____

Trade name: _____

Unit dose: _____

Total amount in container: _____

Route: _____

**4.**

Single-Dose Vial      For IV or IM use
Contains Benzyl Alcohol as a Preservative
See package insert for complete
product information.
Per 2 mL (when mixed):
* hydrocortisone sodium succinate equiv.
to hydrocortisone, 250 mg. Protect
solution from light. Discard after 3 days.

814 070 205   Reconstituted ..........
The Upjohn Company
Kalamazoo, MI 49001, USA

2 mL Act-O-Vial®      NDC 0009-0909-08

**Solu-Cortef®** Sterile Powder
hydrocortisone sodium succinate
for injection, USP

**250 mg***

Generic name: _____

Trade name: _____

Unit dose: _____

Total amount in container: _____

Route: _____

There is more than one way to calculate dosages; the examples in this guide use the principles of ratio and proportion to calculate how much medication to give. A proportion is a way of stating a relationship of equality between two ratios. Ratio and proportion problems can be used to calculate ONE of the numbers in the equation if it is not known. The simple rule to use is this:

*The product of the outside terms equals the product of the inside terms.*

If one of the terms is not known, it is designated as $x$. The problem is then set up to solve for $x$.

**Example:**
The problem "1 : 100 :: 4 : $x$" actually means:
"The relationship of 1 to 100 is the same as the relationship of 4 to $x$." The $x$ is unknown.

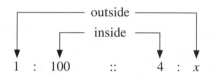

1 and $x$ are the "outsides"; 100 and 4 are the "insides." To solve for $x$, multiply the "outsides" ($1 \times x$) together, multiply the "insides" ($100 \times 4$) together, and form an equation:

$(1 \times x) = (100 \times 4)$
$1x = 400$
$x = 400$

**Proof:** You may prove your equation as follows: Insert the answer for $x$ in the original equation; then solve.

$1 \times 400 = 400$ (outsides)
$100 \times 4 = 400$ (insides)
$400 = 400$; the answer for $x$ is correct.

**Example:**
$5 : 25 :: 15 : x$

Multiply the "outsides" and the "insides" and form an equation; then solve for $x$.
$(5 \times x) = (25 \times 15)$
$5x = 375$
$x = 375/5$
$x = 75$

**Proof:**
$5 \times 75 = 375$
$25 \times 15 = 375$
$375 = 375$

The following chart provides a few common equivalents used in pharmacology. These equivalents are then used in ratio and proportion problems to calculate appropriate dosages.

| Metric Equivalents | Other Equivalents |
|---|---|
| **Weight** <br> 1 mg (milligram) = 1000 mcg (micrograms) <br> 1 g (gram) = 1000 mg (milligrams) <br> 1 kg (kilogram) = 1000 g (grams) | **Weight** <br> 1 g (gram) = 1000 mg <br> 1 kg (kilogram) = 2.2 lb (pounds) |
| **Volume** <br> 1000 mL (milliliters) = 1 L (liter) | **Volume** <br> 1 oz (ounce) = 30 mL (milliliters) <br> 1 tsp (teaspoon) = 5 mL <br> 1 tbsp (tablespoon) = 15 mL <br> 2 tbsp = 30 mL |

To find basic equivalents from one unit of measure to another, use the ratio and proportion approach.

**Example 1:** The drug dosage is 500 mg. You have scored tablets on hand that are 1 g each. How many tablets will you give?

You have *grams* on hand. You need to change the *milligrams* needed to the equivalent grams on hand.

Find the proper equivalents:
Equivalent: 1 g = 1000 mg
Next, set up the ratio and proportion equation.
On the LEFT side, put the ratio that you know: 1 g is 1000 mg.
On the RIGHT side, put the ratio that you want to know: How many g ($x$) is 500 mg?

*Know*         *Want to Know*
1 g : 1000 mg :: $x$ g : 500 mg

Solve for $x$: $(1 \times 500) = (1000 \times x)$; $500 = 1000x$; $x = 500/1000$; $x = 0.5$
You will give 0.5 (half) of the 1-g tablet, which equals 500 mg.

To double-check your answer, substitute your answer for the $x$ and solve. The "outsides" should equal the "insides."
$1 \times 500 = 500$; $1000 \times 0.5 = 500$; $500 = 500$

**Example 2:** Cough syrup, 45 mL, is ordered. The cough syrup comes in a 2-oz bottle. How many ounces do you give?
You have 2 oz on hand. You need to give 45 mL.
Equivalent: 1 oz = 30 mL

*Know:* 1 oz is 30 mL; *Want to Know:* How many ounces is 45 mL?

*Know*         *Want to Know*
1 oz : 30 mL :: $x$ oz : 45 mL

$(1 \times 45) = (30 \times x)$; $45 = 30x$; $x = 45/30 = 1.5$ oz = 45 mL
**Proof:** $1 \times 45 = 45$; $30 \times 1.5 = 45$; $45 = 45$

**Example 3:** Mabel weighs 122 lb. How many kilograms does she weigh?
Equivalent: 1 kg = 2.2 lb

*Know*         *Want to Know*
1 kg : 2.2 lb :: $x$ kg : 122 lb

$(1 \times 122) = (2.2 \times x)$; $122 = 2.2x$; $122/2.2 = x$; $x = 55.45$ kg; round off to tenths: 55.5 kg
**Proof:** $1 \times 122 = 122$; $2.2 \times 55.45 = 121.99$ (rounds to 122)

**Example 4:** You have an injectable solution that is 50-mg strength. How many mcg are in 50 mg?
Equivalent: 1 mg = 1000 mcg

*Know*          *Want to Know*
1 mg : 1000 mcg :: 50 mg : $x$ mcg

$(1 \times x) = (1000 \times 50)$; $1x = 50,000$; $x = 50,000$; therefore 50 mg = 50,000 mcg
**Proof:** $1 \times 50,000 = 50,000$; $1000 \times 50 = 50,000$

**Example 5:** Elixir is ordered as follows: "Give 2 tsp PO now." How many milliliters will you give?
Equivalent: 1 tsp = 5 mL

*Know*          *Want to Know*
1 tsp : 5 mL :: 2 tsp : $x$ mL

$(1 \times x) = (5 \times 2)$; $1x = 10$; $x = 10$ mL
**Proof:** $1 \times 10 = 10$; $5 \times 2 = 10$; $10 = 10$
So, give 10 mL to equal 2 tsp.

**Example 6:** You have an injection that delivers 75 mcg. How many milligrams does it deliver?
Equivalent: 1 mg = 1000 mcg

*Know*          *Want to Know*
1 mg : 1000 mcg :: $x$ mg : 75 mcg

$(1 \times 75) = (1000 \times x)$; $75 = 1000x$; $x = 75/1000$; $x = 0.075$
So, 75 mcg = 0.075 mg. (Don't forget the leading zero!)
**Proof:** $1 \times 75 = 75$; $1000 \times 0.075 = 75$; $75 = 75$

---

### PRACTICE PROBLEMS

**Calculate the following conversions.**

| | | |
|---|---|---|
| 1. 600 mg | = | _____ mcg |
| 2. 1500 mg | = | _____ mcg |
| 3. 5000 mcg | = | _____ mg |
| 4. 5 g | = | _____ mg |
| 5. 2.5 g | = | _____ mg |
| 6. 900 mg | = | _____ g |
| 7. 8 kg | = | _____ g |
| 8. 750 mL | = | _____ L |
| 9. 975 L | = | _____ mL |
| 10. 500 mL | = | _____ L |

| | | |
|---|---|---|
| 11. gr xvi 0.5 g | = | _____ mg |
| 12. 90 mg | = | _____ gr |
| 13. 4 tsp | = | _____ mL |
| 14. 60 mL | = | _____ tsp |
| 15. 90 mL | = | _____ tbsp |
| 16. 3 oz | = | _____ mL |
| 17. 6 mL | = | _____ oz |
| 18. 90 kg | = | _____ lb |
| 19. 150 lb | = | _____ kg |
| 20. 11 kg | = | _____ lb |

To calculate oral dosages of medications, use the same ratio and proportion procedures described in Section I. Label all terms, and check your answers by proving them.

The first step in doing medication dosage calculation problems is examining the order and the medication on hand. The units for both the order and the medication on hand MUST be the same units (e.g., milligrams, milliliters). If they are not the same, then a conversion must first be done to change the ordered dose to the same units as the medication on hand.

Remember these rules:

- NEVER substitute one form of a medication for another even if the dosage amount is the same. Parenteral forms of oral drugs are not equivalent, and the resulting drug effects might be dangerous.
- Do not forget to place a zero in front of a decimal point (e.g., 0.75 mg). It reminds you that the number is a decimal, not a whole number.
- Convert the drug ordered to the units of the drug on hand.
- Place what you have on hand (what you know)—information from the label—on the LEFT side of the equation.
- Place what is ordered (what you want to know) on the RIGHT side of the equation.
- Solve the equation as described in Section I.
- ALWAYS label the units of your answer (e.g., tablets, capsules, mL).
- Consult the pharmacist before splitting a tablet. Enteric-coated tablets and most capsules must not be broken.

**Example 1:** The prescription reads, "Give 500 mg PO." The unit dose is 250 mg/tablet. How many tablets will you give?

**Ordered:** 500 mg          **Unit dose:** 250 mg/tablet
**NOTE:** Units match (mg).

*Know*                *Want to Know*
250 mg : 1 tablet :: 500 mg : $x$ tablet

$(250 \times x) = (1 \times 500)$; $250x = 500$; $x = 500/250 = 2$
**Answer:** Give 2 tablets.
**Proof:** $250 \times 2 = 500$; $1 \times 500 = 500$; $500 = 500$

**Example 2:** The order is to give 175 mg. The tablets on hand are 350-mg scored tablets. How many tablets will you give?

**Ordered:** 175 mg          **Unit dose:** 350 mg/tablet
**NOTE:** Units match (mg).

*Know*                *Want to Know*
350 mg : 1 tablet :: 175 mg : $x$ tablet

$(350 \times x) = (1 \times 175)$; $350x = 175$; $x = 175/350 = 0.5$
**Answer:** Give 0.5 tablet (half of the scored tablet).
**Proof:** $350 \times 0.5 = 175$; $1 \times 175 = 175$; $175 = 175$

**Example 3:** You are asked to administer 100 mg of a drug. You have 0.05-g tablets on hand. How many tablets will you give?

**Ordered:** 100 mg          **Unit dose:** 0.05 g/tablet
**NOTE:** Units do not match (mg and g).
**First:** Calculate: 100 mg = $x$ g (equivalent: 1 g = 1000 mg)

*Know*      *Want to Know*

1 g : 1000 mg :: *x* g : 100 mg

$(1 \times 100) = (1000 \times x)$; $100 = 1000x$; $x = 100/1000 = 0.1$

100 mg = 0.1 g

Now that you have the ordered dose and the dose on hand in the same units, you can complete the problem.

**Ordered:** 0.1 g (100 mg)          **Unit dose:** 0.05 g/tablet

*Know*         *Want to Know*

0.05 g : 1 tablet :: 0.1 g : *x* tablet

$(0.05 \times x) = (1 \times 0.1)$; $0.05 x = 0.1$; $x \times 0.1/0.05 = 2$

**Answer:** Give 2 tablets.

**Proof:** $0.05 \times 2 = 0.1$; $1 \times 0.1 = 0.1$; $0.1 = 0.1$

**Example 4:** You are instructed to give 0.5 g of a drug. You have 250-mg tablets on hand. How many tablets will you give?

**Ordered:** 0.5 g      **Unit dose:** 250 mg/tablet

**NOTE:** Units do not match (g and mg).

**First:** Calculate: 0.5 g = *x* mg (equivalent: 1 g = 1000 mg)

*Know*         *Want to Know*

1 g : 1000 mg :: 0.5 g : *x* mg

$(1 \times x) = (1000 \times 0.5)$; $1x = 500$; $x = 500$

0.5 g = 500 mg

Now that you have the ordered dose and the dose on hand in the same units, you can complete the problem.

**Ordered:** 500 mg (0.5 g)          **Unit dose:** 250 mg/tablet

*Know*         *Want to Know*

250 mg : 1 tablet :: 500 mg : *x* tablet

$(250 \times x) = (1 \times 500)$; $250x = 500$; $x = 500/250 = 2$

**Answer:** Give 2 tablets.

**Proof:** $250 \times 2 = 500$; $1 \times 500 = 500$; $500 = 500$

**Example 5:** You are to administer 200 mg of guaifenesin (Robitussin) syrup. You have a bottle labeled 100 mg/5 mL. How many milliliters will you give?

**Ordered:** 200 mg         **Unit dose:** 100 mg/5 mL

**NOTE:** Units match (mg).

*Know*         *Want to Know*

100 mg : 5 mL :: 200 mg : *x* mL

$(100 \times x) = (5 \times 200)$; $100x = 1000$; $x = 1000/100 = 10$

**Answer:** Give 10 mL.

**Proof:** $100 \times 10 = 1000$; $5 \times 200 = 1000$; $1000 = 1000$

**Perform the following calculations.**

1. Dose ordered: ascorbic acid 0.5 g PO
   Dose on hand: 500-mg tablets
   How many tablets will you give? _____

2. Dose ordered: digoxin (Lanoxin) 0.5 mg PO
   Dose on hand: 250-mcg tablets
   How many tablets will you give? _____

3. Dose ordered: 0.15 g PO
   Dose on hand: 300-mg tablets
   How many tablets will you give? _____

4. Dose ordered: diphenhydramine (Benadryl)
   syrup 50 mg PO
   Dose on hand: syrup 12.5 mg/5 mL
   How many milliliters will you give? _____

5. Dose ordered: 600 mg PO
   Dose on hand: gr v tablets
   How many tablets will you give? _____

6. Dose ordered: cefaclor (Ceclor) 0.1 g PO
   Dose on hand: oral suspension 125 mg/5 mL
   How many milliliters will you give? _____

7. Dose ordered: zidovudine (Retrovir) 0.3 g PO
   Dose on hand: 100-mg capsules
   How many capsules will you give? _____

8. Dose ordered: potassium chloride liquid 30 mEq PO
   Dose on hand: 20 mEq/15 mL
   How many milliliters will you give? _____

9. Dose ordered: 0.15 g PO
   Dose on hand: 50-mg capsules
   How many capsules will you give? _____

10. Dose ordered: 2 g PO
    Dose on hand: 500-mg tablets
    How many tablets will you give? _____

## SECTION III: RECONSTITUTING MEDICATIONS

Many parenteral medications come in powder or crystal form and must be reconstituted by the addition of a diluent to create a liquid form before administration. Instructions for dissolving medications can be found in the literature that accompanies the medication or on the medication label. In most facilities the pharmacy department has taken over the task of reconstituting medications. However, there are still instances when you may be required to reconstitute a drug and then draw up the proper dose for parenteral use. Medications for intravenous (IV) use that need to be reconstituted are sent with delivery systems that match 50- or 100-mL IV bags, and reconstitution occurs as the nurse prepares the medication for use. Some medications for intramuscular (IM) administration also need to be reconstituted before use. Following are examples of instances in which nurses will be reconstituting medications before use.

As an example, the instructions may read:

*Add 1.2 mL normal saline to make 2 mL of reconstituted solution that yields 100 mg/mL.*

This tells the nurse that the medication takes up 0.8 mL of space: 1.2 mL + 0.8 mL = 2 mL of medication solution. The label of the medication container will tell the nurse how many units, grams, milligrams, or micrograms are in each milliliter of the reconstituted drug. In this example, the dose on hand, after reconstitution, is 100 mg/mL.

Remember these concepts:

- Read all instructions for reconstitution before doing anything! Be sure to ask the pharmacist if you have any questions.
- When reconstituting medications, be certain to use the exact type of diluent indicated and add the exact amount of diluent as directed. Substitutions or inaccurate amounts of diluent can inactivate the medication or alter the concentration, thus altering the dose received by the patient.
- If the container is a multiple-dose vial, the nurse who reconstitutes the medication must put the date, time, amount of diluent used, and his or her initials on the label. Follow the facility's policy for multiple-dose vials.
- Many solutions are unstable after being reconstituted. Be sure to follow the directions on the label for proper storage of reconstituted medications. Follow the facility's policy for labeling the reconstituted solution.
- Make note of the time limit or expiration date for the reconstituted medication. Do not use the medication after it has expired.
- Ratio solutions indicate the number of grams of the medication per total milliliters of solution. For example, a medication that is designated 1:1000 has 1 g of medication per 1000 mL of solution.

**To avoid overdosing, it is essential that the nurse choose the correct ratio solution!**

- Percentage (%) solutions indicate the number of grams of the medication per 100 mL of solution. For example, a medication that is designated 10% has 10 g of drug per 100 mL of solution.
- COMPARE:           "1:1000" indicates 1 g per 1000 mL

                    "10%" indicates 10 g per 100 mL

**As you calculate parenteral dosages:**

- If the amount is greater than 1 mL, round $x$ (the amount to be given) to tenths and use a 3-mL syringe to measure it.
- Small (less than 0.5 mL, or pediatric) dosages are rounded to hundredths and measured in a tuberculin syringe. Tuberculin syringes are calibrated in 0.01-mL increments.
- THINK! For adults, the maximum volume of an IM injection is usually 3 mL. (Facility policies regarding the maximum volume of an IM injection may vary.) Sometimes the dose might have to be given in two divided doses; for example, a dose of 4 mL IM would usually be divided into two 2-mL doses. However, if your calculations yield an unusual number, such as 10 mL IM, look over your calculation and repeat your math! Double-check your calculations with a peer.

**Always remember to note the route ordered. IM doses and IV doses are NOT always the same amount, and the drug formulations may differ. Confusing the route may have fatal results.**

**Example 1:** You receive an order for morphine 12 mg IM. The medication vial reads: "10 mg/mL." How much morphine would you give?
Does this medication require reconstitution?
Would you use a 3-mL or a tuberculin syringe to measure this drug?

**Ordered:** 12 mg         **Unit dose:** 10 mg/mL

*Know*         *Want to Know*
10 mg : 1 mL :: 12 mg : $x$ mL

$(10 \times x) = (1 \times 12); 10x = 12; x = 12/10 = 1.2$
**Answer:** 1.2 mL measured in a 3-mL syringe. This medication does not require reconstitution.
**Proof:** $10 \times 1.2 = 12; 1 \times 12 = 12$

**Example 2:** The ordered dose is 2.5 mg IV.

How much medication would you give?
Does this medication require reconstitution?
Would you use a 3-mL or a tuberculin syringe to measure this drug?

**Ordered:** 2.5 mg         **Unit dose:** 10 mg/1 mL

*Know*         *Want to Know*
10 mg : 1 mL :: 2.5 mg : $x$ mL

$(10 \times x) = (1 \times 2.5); 10x = 2.5; x = 2.5/10 = 0.25$
**Answer:** 0.25 mL measured in a tuberculin syringe. Reconstitution is not needed.
**Proof:** $10 \times 0.25 = 2.5; 1 \times 2.5 = 2.5; 2.5 = 2.5$

**153**

**Example 3:** You receive an order for penicillin G potassium 400,000 units IM.

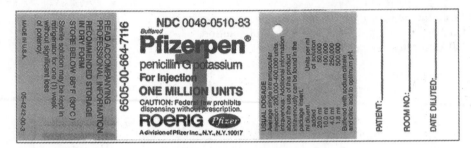

Which dilution would you choose for the ordered dose?
How much penicillin G potassium would you give?
Would you use a 3-mL or a tuberculin syringe to measure this drug?

**Ordered:** 400,000 units      **Unit dose:** Choosing the 1.8 mL diluent amount, the unit dose is 500,000 units/mL.

*Know*            *Want to Know*
500,000 units : 1 mL :: 400,000 : $x$ mL

$(500,000 \times x) = (1 \times 400,000)$; $500,000x = 400,000$; $x = 400,000/500,000 = 0.8$
**Answer:** 0.8 mL measured in either a 3-mL or tuberculin syringe
**Proof:** $500,000 \times 0.8 = 400,000$; $1 \times 400,000 = 400,000$; $400,000 = 400,000$

**NOTE:** Choose the concentration that is close to the ordered dose. Choosing the 1.8-mL diluent amount allows for the injection amount to be small yet easily measured. If you had chosen the 10-mL diluent amount, the injection would have been 4 mL; choosing the 20-mL diluent would have made the injection amount 8 mL. Because of the volume limits for IM injections, both would have required at least two separate injections!

**Example 4:** You receive an order for epinephrine 0.6 mg subcutaneously (subcut). The medication label reads:

> 1-mL ampule
> Epinephrine 1:1000
> For subcut or IM use

What is the dose on hand?
How much epinephrine would you give?
Would you use a 3-mL or a tuberculin syringe to measure the drug?

**First:** Figure the dose on hand.
1:1000 = 1 g in 1000 mL = 1000 mg in 1000 mL = 1 mg in 1 mL
Then complete the problem:

**Ordered:** 0.6 mg            **Unit dose:** 1 mg/mL

*Know*            *Want to Know*
1 mg : 1 mL :: 0.6 mg : $x$ mL

$(1 \times x) = (1 \times 0.6)$; $1x = 0.6$; $x = 0.6$
**Answer:** 0.6 mL measured in either a 3-mL or tuberculin syringe.
**Proof:** $1 \times 0.6 = 0.6$; $1 \times 0.6 = 0.6$; $0.6 = 0.6$

**Example 5:** Calcium gluconate 5 g IV push over 5 minutes.

What is the dose on hand?
How much calcium gluconate would you give?
**First:** Figure the dose on hand.
10% = 10 g in 100 mL = 0.1 g per 1 mL
Then complete the problem:

**Ordered:** 5 g          **Unit dose:** 0.1 g/mL

*Know*            *Want to Know*
0.1 g : 1 mL :: 5 g : $x$ mL

$(0.1 \times x) = (1 \times 5); 0.1x = 5; x = 5/0.1; x = 50$
**Answer:** 50 mL
**Proof:** $0.1 \times 50 = 5; 1 \times 5 = 5; 5 = 5$

## PRACTICE PROBLEMS

**Perform the following calculations.**

1. Dose ordered: thiamine 200 mg IV
   On hand: 10-mL vial, 100 mg/mL

   How much will you give? _____

2. Dose ordered: gentamicin (Garamycin) 60 mg IM
   On hand: 40 mg/mL

   How much will you give? _____

3. Dose ordered: heparin 8000 units subcut
   On hand: 1-mL vial, 10,000 units/mL

   How much will you give? _____

4. Dose ordered: medication 750 mg IV
   On hand: 1-g vial
   Instructions for reconstitution: Add 1.5 mL of sterile water. Reconstituted solution will contain approximately 500 mg of medication solution per milliliter.

   How much will you give? _____

5. Dose ordered: ampicillin 500 mg IV
   On hand: 1-g vial powder for injection
   The reconstituted solution contains 125 mg/5 mL.

   How much will you give? _____

6. Dose ordered: penicillin G potassium 300,000 units IM
   On hand: 1,000,000-unit vial
   Instructions for reconstitution: Using only sterile water, add 9.6 mL to provide 100,000 units/mL, or 4.6 mL to provide 200,000 units/mL. Which concentration would you choose for

   this dose? _____

   How much will you give? _____

7. Dose ordered: epinephrine 750 mcg subcut
   On hand: 1:1000

   How much will you give? _____

8. Dose ordered: medication 0.2 mg IV piggyback (IVPB)
   On hand: 1:5000

   How much will you give? _____

9. Dose ordered: calcium chloride 900 mg IVPB
   On hand: calcium chloride 10% vial. How much

   will you give? _____

10. Dose ordered: magnesium sulfate 4 g IVPB
    On hand: magnesium sulfate 50% vial

    How much will you give? _____

**Overview of Dosage Calculations**

Doses used in pediatric patients must differ from those used in adults. The most common method for calculating doses for pediatric patients is weight based (i.e., milligrams per kilogram). In some cases, dosages may be calculated using body surface area (BSA) calculations.

### Body Surface Area Calculations

The BSA is a common method used to calculate pediatric therapeutic dosages. It requires the use of a chart called a *West nomogram* (see Fig. 3-1 in your text) that converts weight to square meters ($m^2$) of BSA. The average adult is assumed to weigh 140 lb and have a BSA of 1.73 $m^2$. The BSA may be used to calculate the pediatric dose of certain medications.

- For a child of normal height and weight, find the square meters for that weight on the shaded area of the nomogram chart.
  **Example:** Using Figure 3-1 in your text, find the BSA for a child who weighs 40 lb and is 38 inches tall (normal height for her weight). According to the nomogram, the BSA for 40 lb is 0.74 $m^2$.
- For a child who is underweight or overweight, the BSA is indicated at the point where a straight line connecting the height and weight intersects the unshaded surface area (SA) column.
  **Example:** Using Figure 3-1, find the BSA for a child who weighs 25 lb and has a height of 30 inches (underweight). According to the nomogram, the BSA for this child is 0.51 $m^2$.

There are two types of BSA problems.

1. The first type involves medications for which the literature provides recommended dosages in square meters.

**Step 1:** Check the order, and look up the recommended dose.
The order is for 15 mg PO.
The literature states that 40 mg/$m^2$ is safe for children.

**Step 2:** Determine child's height and weight. Then consult the appropriate nomogram to obtain the BSA in square meters. This child weighs 22 lb and has a normal height of 70 cm. The BSA is approximately 0.46 $m^2$.

**Step 3:** Calculate the recommended square meters (mg/$m^2$) dose (from the literature) using ratio and proportion. Then, for a safety check, compare it with the dose ordered.

For this calculation, what you know is the literature's recommendation (40 mg/$m^2$). What you want to know is the milligrams per the child's BSA (which is 0.46 $m^2$).

*Know*          *Want to Know*
40 mg : 1 $m^2$ :: $x$ mg : 0.46 $m^2$

$(40 \times 0.46) = (1 \times x)$; $18.4 = 1x$; $x = 18.4$ (Pediatric doses are rounded to tenths place; do not round to whole numbers.)
**Answer:** 18.4 mg is the safe dose limit.
**Decision:** The order for 15 mg is safe.

**Practice:**
The medication ordered is 100 mg.

**Step 1:** The literature recommends 50 mg/$m^2$ for children.

**Step 2:** The child weighs 10 lb and is a normal height for his weight. The BSA is 0.27 $m^2$.

**Step 3:** Calculate the dose for this child's BSA:

*Know*          *Want to Know*
50 mg : 1 $m^2$ :: $x$ mg : 0.27 $m^2$
$(50 \times 0.27) = (1 \times x)$; $13.5 = 1x$; $x = 13.5$ (Pediatric doses are rounded to tenths place; do not round to whole numbers.)
**Answer:** 13.5 mg is the safe dose limit.
**Decision:** The order for 15 mg exceeds the safe dose limit and therefore is NOT safe. Notify the physician.

2. The second type of BSA involves situations when a recommended dose is cited in the literature for adults but not for children.

**Step 1:** Determine the BSA (in square meters) of the child by dividing the adult dose by 1.73 m² (the average adult's BSA).

**Step 2:** Multiply the result by the average adult dose.

$$\frac{\text{Child's BSA (m}^2)}{\text{Average adult's BSA}} \times \text{Average adult dose of drug} = \text{Estimated child's dose}$$

**Example:** A 6-lb child has a BSA of 0.20 m², and the average adult dose of a drug is 300 mg. What would be the estimated safe dose for a child?

$$\frac{0.20\,\text{m}^2}{1.73\,\text{m}^2} \times 300\,\text{mg} = 34.68\,\text{mg}$$

**Answer:** 34.7 mg is the estimated safe dose for this child. (Round to tenths place for pediatric doses.)

**Practice:**
The average adult dose for a medication is 20 mg. The child has a BSA of 0.6 m². What would be the estimated safe dose for a child?

$$\frac{0.60\,\text{m}^2}{1.73\,\text{m}^2} \times 20\,\text{mg} = 6.94\,\text{mg}$$

**Answer:** 6.9 mg is the estimated safe dose for this child. (Round to tenths place for pediatric doses.)

### Weight-Based Calculations

When calculating the proper dose according to weight, **step 1** involves changing the weight from pounds to kilograms (if necessary).

- Be careful when converting ounces and pounds to kilograms. First, ounces must be converted to part of a pound (by dividing the ounces by 16). Remember, 16 ounces = 1 pound. Therefore 8 oz does not convert to 0.8 lb! Convert 8 oz to pounds by dividing by 16: 8/16 = 0.5; 8 oz = 0.5 lb.
- After you have converted ounces to pounds, then add the ounces to the pounds. For example, 10 lb, 8 oz would equal 10.5 lb. You are now ready to convert pounds to kilograms.
- Remember: 1 kg = 2.2 lb. To convert 10.5 lb to kilograms, divide the pounds by 2.2.
- 1 kg : 2.2 lb :: $x$ kg : 10.5 lb; (1 × 10.5) = (2.2 × $x$); 10.5 = 2.2$x$; $x$ = 10.5/2.2 = 4.8 kg (rounded to tenths)
- DO NOT round pediatric weights to whole numbers!
- After you have converted the child's weight to kilograms, you are ready for step 2.

**Step 2** involves calculating the therapeutic dosage ranges for a child based on his or her weight. The nurse uses the child's weight (in kilograms) to calculate the low and high acceptable doses for that medication. This will give a range of dosage that this child could receive for this medication.

**Step 3** involves THINKING and comparing the ordered dose with the therapeutic dosage range that was calculated for that child. If the ordered dose is under or over the calculated therapeutic dosage range, then do not give the medication and notify the physician.

- **Step 1:** Convert the child's weight from pounds to kilograms.
- **Step 2:** Calculate therapeutic dose range (low and high).
- **Step 3:** (1) Is the ordered dose safe (does not exceed the dosage range)?
  (2) Is the ordered dose therapeutic (falling within the recommended dosage range, not too low)?

**Example 1:** The ordered dose is 50 mg of acetaminophen (Tylenol). The infant weighs 15 lb. The therapeutic dosage range for acetaminophen is 10 to 15 mg/kg/dose.

**Step 1:** Convert pounds to kilograms by dividing 15 by 2.2.
15/2.2 = 6.82; 15 lb = 6.8 kg (Round pediatric weights to tenths, not to whole numbers.)

**Step 2:** Calculate the therapeutic dosage range for this infant based on his weight.
Low dose: 10 mg/kg/dose × 6.8 kg = 68 mg/dose (note that the kilograms cancel out).
High dose: 15 mg/kg/dose × 6.8 kg = 102 mg/dose (note that the kilograms cancel out).
The therapeutic dosage range for this infant is 68 to 102 mg/dose for acetaminophen.

**Step 3:** Compare the ordered dose with the therapeutic dosage range calculated in step 2.
**Answer:** The ordered dose of 50 mg is not therapeutic because it falls under the low recommended dose.

**Question:** If the doctor orders 110 mg of acetaminophen for this infant, would that be a safe and therapeutic dose?
**Answer:** No, it would neither be safe nor therapeutic because it is higher than 102 mg.

**Example 2:** The ordered dose is amoxicillin (Amoxil) 275 mg q 8 hr orally (PO). The patient weighs 35 lb. The therapeutic dosage range for amoxicillin is 20 to 40 mg/kg/24 hr in divided doses.

**Step 1:** Convert pounds to kilograms by dividing 35 by 2.2.
35/2.2 = 15.9; 35 lb = 15.9 kg

**Step 2:** Calculate the therapeutic dosage range for this child based on his weight.
Low dose: 20 mg/kg/24 hr × 15.9 kg = 318 mg/24 hr
High dose: 40 mg/kg/24 hr × 15.9 kg = 636 mg/24 hr

**Note:** These ranges are for 24 hours! The dosage is every 8 hours, so dividing 24 hours by 8 tells us that there will be 3 doses within 24 hours. To figure out the single dosage for the low and high ranges, divide each 24-hour dose by 3:

318 mg/24 hr divided by 3 doses = 106 mg/dose
636 mg/24 hr divided by 3 doses = 212 mg/dose

**Answer:** The safe range for a single dose of amoxicillin for this child is 106 to 212 mg/dose. (An alternate way to determine a single dose is to calculate the amount of medication the ordered dose would provide in 24 hours. In this example, knowing there are three doses given every 8 hours in a 24-hour period, multiplying the dose ordered by 3 would yield the ordered dose for 24 hours: 275 mg × 3 doses = 825 mg/24 hr.)

**Step 3:** Is the ordered dose of 275 mg therapeutic for this child?
**Answer:** No, the ordered dose of 275 mg exceeds the therapeutic dosage range for this patient. Consult the physician. (Note also that the calculated 24-hour dose of 825 mg/24 hr exceeds the high range of 636 mg/24 hr calculated for this child.)

Many pediatric medications come in several concentrations. It is ESSENTIAL to use the correct concentration of medication to ensure accurate dosage and prevent accidental underdosage or overdosage.

**Example:** Acetaminophen comes in many forms, including:
Elixir, 160 mg/5 mL
Liquid suspension, 160 mg/5 mL, 500 mg/5 mL, 500 mg/15 mL
Chewable tablet, 80 mg/tablet
Tablet, 325 or 500 mg/tablet
Orally disintegrating tablet, 80 or 160 mg/tablet
Suppository, 120, 325, or 650 mg
(Note: The infant drops concentration of 80 mg/0.8 mL has been removed from the market.)

A 4-month-old infant weighs 13 lb and has a fever of 101.5° F (38.6° C). What would be the therapeutic dosage range of acetaminophen this infant could receive? The recommended range is 10 to 15 mg/kg/dose.

**Step 1:** 13 lb = 5.9 kg

**Step 2:** Low dose: 10 mg/kg/dose × 5.9 = 59 mg/dose
High dose: 15 mg/kg/dose × 5.9 = 88.5 mg/dose
**Answer:** The therapeutic dosage range for this infant is 59 to 88.5 mg/dose.
Referring to the forms of acetaminophen listed previously, which form would you choose if this infant was to receive a 60-mg dose?
**Answer:** Choose the elixir, 160 mg/5 mL, and administer 1.9 mL with a calibrated oral syringe or dropper (160 mg : 5 mL :: 60 mg : $x$; $x$ = 1.875, which rounds to 1.9 mL).

**Step 3:** Is the ordered dose of 60 mg therapeutic for this infant?
**Answer:** Yes, the 60-mg dose falls within the recommended range of 59 to 88.5 mg/dose for this infant.

Choose the medication form that is manufactured for infants and children. The infant cannot take tablets; suppositories are not the first choice unless the infant cannot take oral medications. Rectal doses may be a little higher than oral doses, and cutting suppositories in half is not recommended because the medication may not be distributed evenly within the suppository. Note: Most liquid medication packages for infants and children have specific instructions for dosing and include the specific dropper to use for measuring liquids.

## PRACTICE PROBLEMS

**Perform the following calculations.**

1. Your 6-year-old patient weighs 40 lb. Morphine sulfate via continuous infusion is ordered at 1 mg/hr. The therapeutic dosage range for continuous IV infusion is 0.025 to 2.6 mg/kg/hr.
   a. What are the low and high doses for this child?

   _____

   b. Is the ordered dose within a safe and therapeutic

   range? _____

2. A 5-year-old child weighs 33 lb. Ibuprofen is ordered at 120 mg PO q 8 hr. The therapeutic dosage range is 5 to 10 mg/kg/dose q 6 hr to q 8 hr, and the maximum dose is 40 mg/kg/24 hr.
   a. What are the low and high doses for this child?

   _____

   b. What is the maximum amount this child can receive

   in 24 hours? _____
   c. Is the ordered dose within a safe and therapeutic

   range? _____

3. A 10-year-old patient weighs 70 lb. Ceftazidime is ordered at 1.7 g q 8 hr IV. The therapeutic dosage range is 100 to 150 mg/kg/24 hr (divided q 8 hr IV).
   a. What are the low and high doses for this child in

   24 hours? _____
   b. What are the low and high doses for this child per

   individual dose? _____
   c. Is the ordered dose within a safe and therapeutic

   range? _____

4. Your patient weighs 15 lb. The medication ordered is 150 mcg bid. The therapeutic dosage range of the medication is 0.02 to 0.05 mg/kg/day.
   a. What are the low and high doses for this child in

   24 hours? _____
   b. What are the low and high doses for this child per

   individual dose? _____
   c. Is the ordered dose within a safe and therapeutic

   range? _____

5. A child weighs 34 lb. The medication ordered is 30 mg IM preoperatively. The therapeutic dosage range is 1 to 2.2 mg/kg.
   a. What are the low and high doses for this child per

   individual dose? _____
   b. Is the ordered dose within a safe and therapeutic

   range? _____

6. For a child weighing 50 lb, medication is ordered at 0.2 mg daily IV. The therapeutic dosage range is 4 to 5 mcg/kg/day.
   a. What are the low and high doses for this child per

   individual dose? _____
   b. Is the ordered dose within a safe and therapeutic

   range? _____

Intravenous (IV) fluids and medications are given over a designated period of time. For instance, the order may read:

*Give 1000 mL normal saline over 8 hours IV.*

For IV lines that infuse with an infusion pump, the milliliters per hour (mL/hr) is calculated.

For IV lines that infuse by gravity, the rate at which an IV medication is given is measured in terms of drops per minute (gtt/min).

To calculate milliliters per hour (mL/hr) and drops per minute (gtt/min), we need to consider what the order contains and what equipment is used. To calculate drops per minute, we need to know the drop factor of the IV tubing. The size of the drops delivered per milliliter can vary with different types of tubing. The drop factor of a certain tubing set is printed on the packaging label.

Adding to the previous order:

*The drop factor for the IV tubing is 15 gtt/mL.*

The order now reads:

*Give 1000 mL normal saline over 8 hours IV. The drop factor is 15 gtt/mL.*

**Step 1:** Calculate milliliters per hour.
We know that 1000 mL is to infuse over 8 hours. We want to know how much is to infuse over 1 hour. Set up the equation:

***Know***          ***Want to Know***
1000 mL : 8 hr :: $x$ mL : 1 hr

$(1000 \times 1) = (8 \times x)$; $1000 = 8x$; $x = 8/1000$; $x = 125$ mL/hr
**Rate:** To give 1000 mL normal saline over 8 hours, give 125 mL/hr for 8 hours.
*A quick way to determine the hourly rate is to divide the total volume by the total time (if the time is in hours): 1000 mL ×*
*8 hr = 125 mL/hr.*

**Step 2:** Calculate the gtt/min.
To set up a gravity IV drip, further calculations are needed. To ensure the proper rate, one must count the drops per minute (gtt/min).

We know the rate is 125 mL/hr and the drop factor is 15 gtt/mL. Because we need to change from hours to minutes, another equivalent we will need is 60 min = 1 hr.

When milliliters per hour is known, the formula for calculating drops per minute is as follows:

$$\frac{\text{Drop factor (gtt/mL)}}{\text{Time (min)}} \times \text{Hourly rate (mL/hr)}$$

Plugging in what we know:

$$\frac{15\,\text{gtt/mL}^*}{60\,\text{min/hr}} \times 125/\text{hr} = x\,\text{gtt/min}$$

*To make it easier to calculate, reduce the 15/60 fraction to 1/4 before multiplying by 125.
1/4 × 125 = 125/4 = 31.25 (round mL/hr to whole numbers)
**Answer:** 31 gtt/min for a gravity drip

**Points to remember:**

■ The drop factor varies per IV tubing set manufacturer. It can range from 10 to 60 gtt/mL.
■ Infusion sets that deliver 60 gtt/mL are called *microdrips*.
**Step 1:** To calculate milliliters per hour, divide the total volume by the total time (in hours).
**Step 2:** To calculate drops per minute when the hourly rate is known, use the formula:

$$\frac{\text{Drop factor (gtt/mL)}}{\text{Time (min)}} \times \text{Hourly rate (mL/hr)}$$

■ THINK! If you are using an infusion pump, you need to calculate milliliters per hour.
■ THINK! Round off your answer to the nearest whole number. You cannot count a partial drop! Also, electronic infusion pumps will usually use the nearest whole number in milliliters. (Exceptions to this may occur in critical care or pediatric settings.)

**Example 1:** The order reads "200 mL to be infused for 1 hr." If the drop factor is 15 gtt/mL, how many drops per minute will be given?
*Start at Step 1 or Step 2?*
Start at Step 1. You need to know the hourly rate in milliliters per hour.

**Step 1:** Calculate milliliters per hour. Divide total volume by the total time (in hours).
200 mL over 1 hr = 200 mL/hr.

**Step 2:** Calculate drops per minute using the formula:

$$\frac{\text{Drop factor}}{\text{Time (min)}} \times \text{Hourly rate} = 15/60 \times 200 = 1/4 \times 200 = 50$$

**Answer:** 50 gtt/min

**Example 2:** The order is for 1000 mL to infuse at 150 mL/hr. The drop factor is 20 gtt/mL. How many drops per minute will be given?
*Start at Step 1 or Step 2?*
Start at Step 2. The hourly rate, 150 mL/hr, has been given.

**Step 2:** Calculate drops per minute using the formula:

$$\frac{\text{Drop factor}}{\text{Time (min)}} \times \text{Hourly rate} = 20/60 \times 150 = 1/3 \times 150 = 50$$

**Answer:** 50 gtt/min

**Example 3:** You receive an order for 200 mL to be infused for 90 minutes. You have a microdrip set (60 gtt/mL). How many drops per minute will be given?
*Start at Step 1 or Step 2?*
Start at Step 1. Calculate the hourly rate. Remember, 60 min = 1 hr.

**Step 1:** Calculate milliliters per hour.

*Know*          *Want to Know*
200 mL : 90 min :: $x$ mL : 60 min

$(200 \times 60) = (90 \times x)$; $12{,}000 = 90x$; $x = 12{,}000/90$ $x = 133.33$
**Rate:** 133 mL/hr (Round to nearest whole number.)

**Step 2:** Calculate drops per minute using the formula:

$$\frac{\text{Drop factor}}{\text{Time (min)}} \times \text{Hourly rate} = 60/60 \times 133 = 133$$

**Answer:** 133 gtt/min
Shortcut: For microdrips, when the drip factor is 60 and the time is 60 minutes, the "60s" cancel out to 1, and the result is that the ordered milliliters per hour = the drops per minute.

**Overview of Dosage Calculations**

# PRACTICE PROBLEMS

**Calculate the following, and prove your answers.**

1. Give 1000 mL of lactated Ringer's solution over 6 hours. The drop factor is 15 gtt/mL.
   *Start at Step 1 or Step 2?*

   a. mL/hr: _____

   b. gtt/min: _____

2. Infuse 600 mL of blood over 3 hours. The blood administration set has a drop factor of 10 gtt/mL.
   *Start at Step 1 or Step 2?*

   a. mL/hr: _____

   b. gtt/min: _____

3. Infuse 1000 mL of normal saline over 12 hours using tubing with a drop factor of 15 gtt/mL.
   *Start at Step 1 or Step 2?*

   a. mL/hr: _____

   b. gtt/min: _____

4. Infuse 200 mL of D$_5$NS over 2 hours using a microdrip set.
   *Start at Step 1 or Step 2?*

   a. mL/hr: _____

   b. gtt/min: _____

   c. What is the drop factor? _____

5. Infuse D$_5$W at 75 mL/hr. The drop factor is 10 gtt/mL.
   *Start at Step 1 or Step 2?*

   gtt/min: _____

6. Infuse D$_5$W at 75 mL/hr. The drop factor is 15 gtt/mL.
   *Start at Step 1 or Step 2?*

   gtt/min: _____

7. Infuse D$_5$W at 75 mL/hr. The drop factor is 20 gtt/mL.
   *Start at Step 1 or Step 2?*

   gtt/min: _____

8. After looking at your answers for Questions 5, 6, and 7, what observation can you make about the relationship between the drop factor and the resulting drops per minute?

9. Give 50 mL of an antibiotic over 30 minutes. You will be using an infusion pump.
   *Start at Step 1 or Step 2?*

   a. mL/hr: _____

   b. gtt/min: _____

   c. Do you need to calculate both milliliters per hour and drops per minute for this situation?

   _____

10. Infuse 500 mL of normal saline over 4 hours using tubing with a drop factor of 60 gtt/mL.
    *Start at Step 1 or Step 2?*

    a. mL/hr: _____

    b. gtt/min: _____

## PRACTICE QUIZ

### Convert the following.

1. 750 mcg   =   _____ mg

2. 8 g        =   _____ mg

3. 250 lb    =   _____ kg

4. 75 kg     =   _____ lb

5. 3 tsp     =   _____ mL

6. gr x 0.6 g  =   _____ mg

### Calculate the following, and prove your answers.

7. Dose ordered: indomethacin (Indocin) (oral suspension) 50 mg qid
   Dose on hand: Oral suspension 25 mg/5 mL
   How much would you give per dose?

   _____

8. Dose ordered: procainamide (Pronestyl) 0.5 g q 4 hr PO
   Dose on hand: 500-mg tablets
   How much would you give per dose?

   _____

9. Dose ordered: phenytoin (Dilantin) 100 mg IV now
   Dose on hand: 5-mL ampule labeled "50 mg/mL"
   How much would you give per dose?

   _____

10. Dose ordered: lidocaine (Xylocaine) 50 mg IV now
    Dose on hand: lidocaine 1% in a 5-mL ampule

    How much would you give? _____

11. Dose ordered: epinephrine 0.25 mg subcut now
    Dose on hand: epinephrine 1:1000 ampule

    How much would you give? _____

12. Dose ordered: heparin 15,000 units IV bolus
    Dose on hand: heparin 10,000 units/mL (5-mL vial)

    How much would you give? _____

13. Dose ordered: furosemide (Lasix) 50 mg PO daily
    Dose on hand: furosemide oral solution, 10 mg/mL
    Child's weight: 22 lb
    Therapeutic dosage range: 1 to 6 mg/kg/day in doses divided every 12 hours
    a. What is the safe and therapeutic range for this child (specify both per day and per dose)?

    _____

    b. Is the ordered dose safe and therapeutic?

    _____

14. Ordered: Infuse normal saline 500 mL over 8 hours. The tubing drop factor is 15.

    a. What is the rate of the IV? _____

    b. What is the drops per minute? _____

15. Ordered: D₅1/2NS to infuse at 50 mL/hr via an infusion pump.
    a. How will this be administered—milliliters per hour or drops per minute? _____

    b. What is the rate? _____

16. Ordered: 1000 mL D₅W to infuse over 24 hours. The tubing drop factor is 60.

    a. What is the rate of the IV? _____

    b. What is the drops per minute? _____

17. Ordered: ticarcillin 500 mg IM q 6 hr
    Dose on hand: Medication powder for injection (See label.)

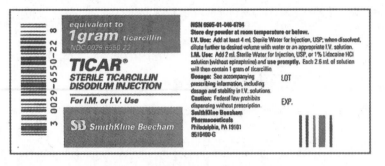

a. How much does this vial contain? _____

b. How much will you give for each dose? _____

18. Ordered: penicillin G 500,000 units IV q 6 hr

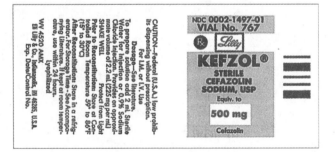

a. What concentration should you choose? _____

b. How much diluent should you add to the vial to obtain this concentration? _____

c. How much medication will you give? _____

d. How do you label the vial? _____

19. A child weighs 31 lb.
    Dose ordered: cefazolin 225 mg IVPB q 6 hr
    Dose on hand: See label.
    Maximum safe dose: 25 to 100 mg/kg/day, divided every 6 hours

a. How much would you give for this dose? _____

b. What is the maximum safe dose for this child in 24 hours? Per dose? _____

c. How much total medication will this child receive in 24 hours? _____

d. Is the ordered dose within a safe and therapeutic range? _____

20. Dose ordered: digoxin (Lanoxin) 125 mcg/day
Dose on hand: pediatric elixir 0.05 mg/mL

How much would you give? _____

21.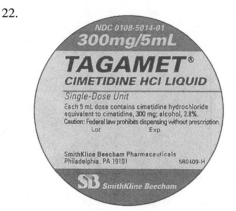

Dose ordered: octreotide acetate (Sandostatin) 0.025 mg IV bolus now
Dose on hand: See label.

How much would you give for this dose? _____

22.

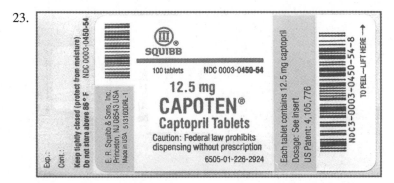

Dose ordered: cimetidine (Tagamet) 800 mg PO at bedtime
Dose on hand: See label.

How much would you give for this dose? _____

23.

Dose ordered: captopril (Capoten) 6.25 mg PO three times/day
Dose on hand: See label.

How much would you give for each dose? _____

24.

N 0469-1155-15    915501

**HEPARIN SODIUM**

*INJECTION, USP*

20,000 USP Units/mL

(Derived from Porcine
Intestinal Mucosa)
For IV or SC Use
1 mL Multiple Dose Vial
Usual Dosage: See Insert.

Fujisawa USA, Inc.
Deerfield, IL 60015-2548

40212F

LOT

EXP

Dose ordered: heparin 15,000 IV push now
Dose on hand: See label.

How much would you give for this dose? _____

25.

NDC 0186-0648-16          5 mL

**Atropine Sulfate**
**Injection, USP**
**0.5 mg** (0.1 mg/mL)
**For IV, IM or SC Use.**          072073R00

**ASTRA®** Astra USA, Inc.
Westborough, MA 01581

4    3    2    1    0 mL

Dose ordered: atropine 0.4 mg IM now
Dose on hand: See label.

How much would you give for this dose? _____

# Answer Key

## CHAPTER 1

**The Nursing Process and Drug Therapy**

**Chapter Review and NCLEX® Examination
Preparation/Critical Thinking and Application**
1. a
2. d
3. c
4. b
5. a, d, e
6. b
7. c
8. 0.25 mg (See Overview of Dosage Calculations, Section I.)
9. 125 mcg (See Overview of Dosage Calculations, Section I.)
10. 1 = d; 2 = e; 3 = b; 4 = a; 5 = c
11. a
12. b
13. S, O, O, O, S, S
14. Answers may vary slightly for each one but should include the following:
    - *Right drug:* Compare drug orders and medication labels. Consider whether the drug is appropriate for that patient. Obtain information about the patient's medical history and a thorough, updated medication history, including over-the-counter medications taken.
    - *Right dose:* Check the order and the label on the medication, and check the "rights" at least three times before administering the medication. Recheck the math calculations for dosages, and contact the physician when clarification is needed. Check the dose and confirm that it is appropriate for the patient's age and size, and check the prescribed dose against the available drug stocks and against the normal dosage range.
    - *Right time:* Assess for a conflict between the pharmacokinetic and pharmacodynamic properties of the drugs prescribed and the patient's lifestyle and likelihood of compliance.
    - *Right route and form:* Never assume the route of administration or change it; always check with the physician or prescriber. Additionally, it is critical to patient safety to be aware of the right form of medication. For example, there are various dosage forms of acetaminophen, a commonly used medication. It is available in oral suspension, tablet, capsule, gelcap, pediatric drops, and rectal suppository dosage forms. Nurses need to give the right drug via the right route with use of the correct dosage form.
    - *Right patient:* Check the patient's identity before administering a medication. Ask for the patient's name, and check the identification band or bracelet to confirm the patient's name, identification number, and allergies. The Joint Commission requires the use of two patient identifiers, such as name and birthday, Social Security number, or medical record number.
    - *Right documentation:* Record the date and time of medication administration, name of medication, dose, route, and site of administration. Don't forget to document the patient's response to the medication.
    - *Right reason and response:*
        - Right reason refers to the appropriateness of the use of the medication for the patient. Confirm the rationale for use through researching the patient's history while also asking the patient the reason he or she is taking the drug. Always revisit the rationale for long-term medication use.
        - Right response refers to the drug and its desired response. Continually assess and evaluate the achievement of the desired response and any undesired response.
15. a. assessment
    b. objective
    c. subjective
    d. analyze
    e. outcomes
    f. outcome criteria
    g. implementation
    h. evaluation
16. The nurse must be sure to question the patient for any allergies, especially drug allergies, before giving the medication. If an allergy is present, question the patient about the type of reaction that occurred, and do not give the medication until the order is clarified with the prescriber.

17. The nurse's role is to always be alert for the Nine Rights. The information obtained from implementing the Nine Rights can lead to early identification of patient problems. The focus of nursing care is on patient safety. The Quality and Safety Education for Nurses (QSEN) project was initiated in 2005. QSEN attempts to address the continued challenge of preparing future nurses with the knowledge, skills, and attitudes (called KSAs) needed to continuously improve the quality and safety of patient care within the health care system. These KSAs that flow out of the QSEN initiatives and are being integrated into nursing education curricula and clinical outcomes. The six major initiatives are patient-centered care, teamwork and collaboration, evidence-based practice, quality improvement, safety, and informatics.

## Case Study

1. See the discussion in Chapter 1 of the textbook under Assessment. Important points include the following:
   - Use of prescription and over-the-counter medications
   - Use of home remedies, herbal treatments, and vitamins
   - Intake of alcohol, tobacco, and caffeine
   - Current or prior use of street drugs
   - Health history
   - Family history
   - Allergies
2. Answers will vary but may include the following:
   - Activity intolerance
   - Acute pain
   - Deficient knowledge
   - Fatigue
   - Ineffective breathing pattern
   - Ineffective health maintenance
   - Ineffective therapeutic regimen management
   - Nausea
   - Risk for aspiration
   - Risk for impaired liver function
   - Risk for injury
   - Risk for falls

   Prioritization will depend on the nursing diagnoses chosen, which are developed with the patient's input. Often, actual diagnoses are prioritized before risk diagnoses.
3. The medication order is missing the route of delivery and the dose amount. Contact the physician to clarify the incomplete order.
4. Again, contact the physician, and never change the medication route without an order.
5. After administering any drug, evaluate the patient's response to the drug therapy. In this case, monitoring intake and output, monitoring vital signs, and watching for orthostatic blood pressure changes are important.

## CHAPTER 2

### Pharmacologic Principles

### Chapter Review and NCLEX® Examination Preparation/Critical Thinking and Application

1. 1 = e; 2 = c; 3 = d; 4 = a; 5 = b
2. c
3. b
4. d
5. a, e
6. c
7. b
8. d
9. 1600
10. a
11. c
12. c
13. b
14. g
15. h
16. e
17. f
18. a
19. d
20. c
21. Because muscles have a greater blood supply than the skin, drugs injected intramuscularly are typically absorbed faster than those injected subcutaneously. Absorption can be increased by applying heat to the injection site or by massaging the injection site, which increases the blood flow to the area and thus enhances absorption.
22. This is an example of supplemental therapy—drug therapy that supplies the body with a substance needed to maintain normal function.
23. Extended-release oral dosage forms must not be crushed because this could cause accelerated release of the drug from the dosage form and possible toxicity. Enteric-coated tablets also are not recommended for crushing. This would cause disruption of the tablet coating designed to protect the stomach lining from the local effects of the drug or protect the drug from being prematurely disrupted by stomach acid.
24. For the pharmaceutical company, the testing has been performed, and for the patient, the cost is reduced.

## Case Study

1. Half-life is the time it takes for half of the original amount of a drug in the body to be eliminated and is a measure of the rate at which drugs are excreted by the body. If the half-life is 2 hours, then in this example, the drug levels would be as follows:
   1600 = 200 mg/L
   1800 = 100 mg/L
   2000 = 50 mg/L
   2200 = 25 mg/L

2. a. He has nausea and vomiting and cannot take medications by mouth. His medications will need to be given parenterally.
   b. Because of his decreased serum albumin level, a smaller amount of drugs that are usually protein bound will be bound to protein, and as a result, more free drug will be circulating, and the duration of drug action may be increased. In addition, his heart failure may result in decreased cardiac output and thus decreased distribution.
   c. His liver failure will result in decreased metabolism of drugs, which increases the chance for drug toxicities if the drugs accumulate in his body.
   d. Because his liver may not be able to effectively metabolize drugs and convert them to water-soluble compounds, excretion through the kidneys may be decreased. This would also contribute to drug accumulation.
3. This situation illustrates prophylactic therapy to *prevent* illness or other undesirable outcomes. Prophylactic intravenous antibiotic therapy may be used to prevent infection during a high-risk surgery or procedure, such as placement of the peripherally inserted central catheter.
4. The therapeutic index is the ratio between the toxic and therapeutic concentrations of a drug. A low therapeutic index means that the difference between a therapeutically active dose and a toxic dose is small. As a result, the drug has a greater likelihood of causing an adverse reaction. The nurse should monitor the patient's response carefully when a drug has a low therapeutic index by looking for signs and symptoms of toxicity and ensuring that drug levels are checked periodically.

## CHAPTER 3

### Lifespan Considerations

### Chapter Review and NCLEX® Examination Preparation/Critical Thinking and Application
1. c
2. a
3. d
4. b
5. a, b, c
6. a
7. 320 mg (See Overview of Dosage Calculations, Section IV.)
8. 0.021 mg (23 lb = 10.5 kg; 2 mcg × 10.5 kg = 21 mcg = 0.021 mg)
9. 0.21 mL

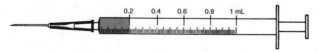

10. a
11. d
12. b
13. e
14. a
15. c
16. Keep in mind that older patients take a greater proportion of both prescription and over-the-counter (OTC) medications, and they commonly take multiple medications on a daily basis. In addition, older adults also have more chronic diseases than younger people. They may see several different specialists, each of whom may prescribe a different set of medications. In addition, some patients self-administer OTC products to ease the discomfort of even more ailments. This use of multiple medications is called *polypharmacy*.
17. Drawing on the information in Table 3-3: Physiologic Changes in the Elderly Patient, a variety of physiologic changes affecting the cardiovascular, gastrointestinal, hepatic, and renal systems may be described.
18. It would be important to prepare her in advance for the teaching session. Let her know what to expect and include her parent, if possible, in the teaching session. It is also important to allow her time to express her feelings about this new diagnosis and the need to test her own blood glucose levels. Allow her to make choices when appropriate (i.e., choosing a glucometer with a special color). After demonstrating the procedure, encourage her participation and allow for return demonstration.
19. From the beginning to the end of life, the human body changes in many ways. These changes have a dramatic effect on the four phases of pharmacokinetics—drug absorption, distribution, metabolism, and excretion. Newborn, pediatric, and older adult patients each have special needs. Drug therapy at both spectrums of life is more likely to result in adverse effects and toxicity. Examples of these differences include decreased first-pass effect and increased intramuscular absorption in neonates and younger pediatric patients and decreased protein binding and increased metabolism in older children. Similar absorption and metabolism changes are seen in older adults as their organs decline in function.

## Case Study
1. Children and teenagers should not take aspirin to treat chickenpox or flulike symptoms because Reye's syndrome—a rare but serious illness—has been associated with aspirin use at these ages. It is important to check for precautions when giving any medication to children.

2. If the toddler does not like taking pills or cannot take pills, have the parent ask the pharmacist for a liquid form of the medication, which may be flavored and better accepted by the child than a pill. Some pediatric medications also come in quick-dissolving oral tablets or films.

3. Most OTC preparations for children have dosages based on the child's weight. The most common dosage calculation method for children is the milligrams-per-kilogram formula. However, for OTC preparations, the manufacturer will convert kilograms to pounds to make dosing by the parents easier.

4. The 5-year-old child received 240 mg (at 160 mg/tsp, 1.5 tsp = 240 mg).

5. The parents should monitor the children's fevers—the expected response is that the fevers will go down. In addition, because the medication also has analgesic effects, signs of discomfort may decrease. The parents should also monitor for any adverse effects of the medication or worsening of the children's illnesses.

## CHAPTER 4

### Cultural, Legal, and Ethical Considerations

### Chapter Review and NCLEX® Examination Preparation/Critical Thinking and Application

1. b
2. a
3. d
4. c
5. b
6. d
7. b, c
8. 6 mL
9.

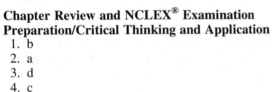
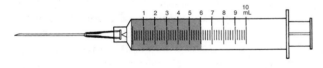

10. a
11. b
12. d
13. a
14. c
15. b
16. a
17. c
18. d
19. b
20. The nurse also has the right to refuse to participate in any treatment or aspect of a patient's care that violates his or her personal ethical principles. However, this must be done without deserting the patient, and in some facilities, the nurse may be transferred to another patient care assignment only if the nurse manager or nurse supervisor approves the transfer. The nurse needs to discuss the situation with the immediate supervisor, and hopefully another solution can be reached. The nurse must always remember, however, that the American Nurses Association's *Code of Ethics* and professional responsibility and accountability require the nurse to provide nonjudgmental nursing care from the start of the patient's treatment until the time of the patient's discharge.

21. Answers will vary depending on the group identified.
    a. Barriers may include language, poverty, access, pride, and beliefs regarding medical practices.
    b. Attitudes will vary depending on the group identified.
    c. Questions may include the following topics: health beliefs and practices, past use of medicine, folk remedies, home remedies, use of over-the-counter drugs and treatments, usual responses to illness, responsiveness to medical treatments, religious practices and beliefs, and dietary habits.

## Case Study

1. You should not give the drugs until it is established that the study has been reviewed by an institutional review board and that the patient has given informed consent. As a professional, the nurse has the responsibility to provide safe nursing care, and it is within the nurse's realm of practice to provide information and assist the patient facing decisions regarding health care. The nurse also has the right to refuse to participate in any treatment or aspect of a patient's care that violates personal ethical principles.

2. Principles include the following:
    1. Autonomy—the patient's right to self-determination. The nurse supports this by ensuring informed consent.
    2. Beneficence—the duty to do good. Will the patient be best served by this course of action?
    3. Nonmaleficence—the duty to do no harm
    4. Veracity—the duty to tell the truth, especially with regard to investigational drugs and informed consent

3. Some patients believe strongly in using home remedies instead of medications. Sometimes these remedies can be integrated into HIV treatment. You should assess and consider health beliefs and practices at the beginning of the therapeutic relationship. Because the patient believes drugs are not needed, the nurse has a duty to provide education so that the patient has the knowledge needed to make a sound judgment.

4. The issue of confidentiality should be discussed. The researchers have a duty to respect privileged information about a patient. Measures that the researchers will use to ensure the confidentiality of participants should be discussed.

## CHAPTER 5

## Medication Errors: Preventing and Responding

**Chapter Review and NCLEX® Examination Preparation/Critical Thinking and Application**
1. adverse drug event
2. adverse drug reaction
3. allergic reaction
4. idiosyncratic
5. False. High-alert medications are not necessarily involved in more errors than other drugs. However, the potential for patient harm is higher with these medications.
6. True, many medications carry expected side effects or allergic responses because they occur frequently and may be identifiable based on the patient. For example, penicillin and cephalosporins carry similar properties, and an allergic response to one may indicate a similar response to the other.
7. The actions include the following: (1) Multiple systems of checks and balances must be in place to prevent medication errors. (2) Prescribers must write legible orders that contain correct information, or orders must be entered electronically, if available. (3) Authoritative resources must be consulted if there is any area of concern or lack of clarity, beginning with the medication order and continuing throughout the entire medication administration process. Do not use faculty members, nursing staff, or fellow nursing students as your authoritative source regarding medications and the safe practice of using appropriate resources. (4) Nurses always need to check the medication order three times before giving the drug and consult with authoritative resources (see earlier in the chapter) if any questions or concerns exist. (5) The Nine Rights of medication administration should be used consistently; their use has been shown to substantially reduce the likelihood of a medication error.
8. The four categories are (1) no error, although circumstances or events occurred that could have led to an error; (2) medication error that causes no harm; (3) medication error that causes harm; and (4) medication error that results in death.
9. Refer to Box 5-1: Examples of High-Alert Medications.
10. Medication reconciliation involves three steps:
    Verification—Collection of the patient's medication information with a focus on medications currently used (including prescription drugs, over-the-counter medications, and supplements)
    Clarification—Professional review of this information to ensure that medications and dosages are appropriate for the patient
    Reconciliation—Further investigation of any discrepancies and changes in medication orders
11. Digoxin 125 mcg PO now
    Lasix 40 mg IV daily (every day)
    Discontinue all meds
    NPH insulin 12 units subcut every morning before breakfast
    Floxin Otic 1 drop right ear bid
    Lactulose 30 mL PO every other day
12. a. One-half of a 50-mg tablet (See Overview of Dosage Calculations, Section II.)
    b. A 50-mg dose, which is a double dose
    c. Because this medication can have an effect on the patient's blood pressure and heart rate, the nurse will immediately check and record the patient's vital signs and caution the patient about not getting out of bed without help. The patient's physician will be notified, and the patient must be monitored frequently throughout the day. In addition to telling the patient about the double dose, the nurse will need to follow facility protocol for reporting a medication error, which would include completing a U.S. Pharmacopeia Medication Errors Reporting Program (USPMERP) report for the national database.
13. b
14. 5 mL
15.

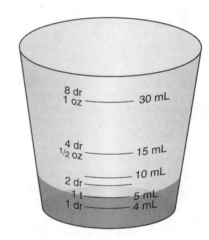

16. c

## Case Study

1. The nursing student needs to inform her instructor of the error immediately. Then together they need to monitor the patient's response and follow the institution's procedure for reporting a medication error. Reporting medication errors is a professional and ethical responsibility.
2. The student could have prevented this error by checking the six rights before giving this medication. In this situation, she missed the right dose. In addition, if the student had understood the rationale for the medication (i.e., the low dose needed for antiplatelet therapy), then she may have avoided this error. One must be knowledgeable about medications and the rationale for their use in a particular patient before administering them.

**171**

3. According to Chapter 5, the recommendation is that the patient should be told of the error both as ethical practice and because of the legal implications.
4. Yes. A medication error is defined as "any preventable adverse drug event involving inappropriate medication use by a patient or health care professional." It may or may not cause harm to the patient.
5. The USPMERP exists to gather and disseminate safety information regarding medications. By reporting this error, the student contributes to the USPMERP database of medication errors and their causes. This service is confidential.

## CHAPTER 6

### Patient Education and Drug Therapy

### Chapter Review and NCLEX® Examination Preparation/Critical Thinking and Application
1. c
2. d
3. a
4. a, b
5. a
6. a
7. 10 mL per dose (See Overview of Dosage Calculations, Section II.)
8.

9. Refer to the information in Chapter 22 for specific information about antihypertensive drug therapy. In addition, Table 6-1 provides information relevant to the development of teaching strategies for the 78-year-old patient.
10. Refer to Box 6-1. Ideally, a health care professional who speaks the mother's language should do the teaching. It is essential that an interpreter be found so that questions from the mother can be answered adequately. Other strategies include using pictures and illustrations and demonstrating by example. In addition, the patient needs to be provided with detailed written instructions in her native language.
11. a. Answers will vary, but the nursing diagnosis addresses deficient knowledge.
    b. Answers will vary, but the nursing diagnosis addresses noncompliance or ineffective health maintenance.
12. Answers will vary, but an example is as follows:
    Outcome criteria: Patient applies patch to a clean, nonhairy area of the skin and rotates application sites.
    Measurement criteria: Patient demonstrates all of the steps in order and with zero errors.

13. Teaching plans will vary somewhat in format, but each should contain the following information:
    a. Some of the assessment items listed in the text in the section Assessment of Learning Needs Related to Drug Therapy
    b. Deficient knowledge
    c. A measurable goal with outcome criteria related to the nursing diagnosis
    d. Specific educational strategies for providing the information needed
    e. Specific questions designed to validate whether learning has occurred

### Case Study
1. Both "deficient knowledge" and "noncompliance" are possible answers. In this case, "deficient knowledge" is probably the most correct because this nursing diagnosis exists when the patient has a lack of or limited understanding about his or her medications. For example, as you will read in Overview of Dosage Calculations, nitroglycerin tablets should not be stored in one's pants pockets because the body heat may destroy the active compounds in the tablets. In addition, the patient was not aware of the importance of not missing doses of antihypertensive medication. Noncompliance exists when the patient does not take the medication as directed or at all, and the data collected indicate that the patient's condition has recurred or has not resolved. In this case, his blood pressure has improved from previous readings despite what he has said about taking his medications.
2. Answers may vary. A goal for the nursing diagnosis of "deficient knowledge" in this case may be the following: "The patient self-administers his prescribed medications on schedule without missing doses." Outcome criteria may include the following: "The patient is able to describe the schedule of medications ordered." "The patient is able to state the rationale for consistent dosing of antihypertensive medications." "The patient is able to state the proper storage and administration of sublingual nitroglycerin tablets." "The patient is able to identify potential side effects of the prescribed medications and knows when to report them."
3. Again, answers may vary. Refer to Box 6-1. Suggestions include the following:
   • A teaching session regarding medication administration needs to be held with both the patient and his wife in attendance. If necessary, find out whether they have any children or neighbors nearby who may be able to assist with medications as needed.
   • Assist the patient in developing a daily time calendar for taking the medications prescribed.
   • Suggest the use of a daily or weekly pill container that can assist in reminding when doses are due. If necessary, a neighbor or the patient's son or daughter can come over periodically to fill this container.

- Discuss and provide written literature on the purposes and side effects of each medication ordered and on other important issues regarding these medications.
4. Confirm whether learning has occurred by asking the patient and his wife questions related to the teaching session. Assess their understanding of the time calendar and the concept of using pill containers. Follow-up can be accomplished via telephone as needed, and a return visit to review medications can be scheduled. In addition, the patient must keep return appointments to the office so that the therapeutic outcomes of the drug therapy (i.e., blood pressure readings) can be measured.

## CHAPTER 7

### Over-the-Counter Drugs and Herbal and Dietary Supplements

### Critical Thinking Crossword
*Across*
2. Ginger
5. Flax
6. Saw palmetto
8. Kava
*Down*
1. Echinacea
2. Ginkgo
3. Ginseng
4. Aloe
6. Soy

### Chapter Review and NCLEX® Examination Preparation/Critical Thinking and Application
1. a, b, d, f
2. d
3. d
4. a, b, c, d
5. c
6. 6000 mg total per day
7. Yes, there is a concern! Acetaminophen doses must not exceed a total of 3 g/day, and hepatic toxicity may occur with excessive doses.
8. c
9. b, e
10. d
11. d
12. Garlic, ginger, ginkgo, ginseng, flax, and valerian
13. Older adults, children, patients with single or multiple acute and chronic illnesses, patients who are frail or in poor health, patients who are debilitated and nutritionally deficient, and those with suppressed immune systems may have more frequent adverse reactions to OTC drugs. In addition, those who have a history of renal, hepatic, cardiac, or vascular disorders may have problems with OTC medications.

14. Normally, OTC medications are used only for short-term treatment of common minor illnesses. Having diarrhea for 3 weeks puts the patient at risk for dehydration. In addition, delaying an evaluation of the cause of the diarrhea also delays the opportunity to treat what could be a serious illness or disease.
15. Answers will vary.

### Case Study
1. The aspirin and garlic tablets may interfere with platelet and clotting functions. If the wine is taken with the kava or valerian, central nervous system depression may occur.
2. The Food and Drug Administration (FDA) has issued a warning about the use of kava and possible liver toxicity. Also, tolerance may develop in patients who use echinacea for longer than 8 weeks.
3. Because she is trying to conceive, she needs to consider the fact that the herbal drugs have not been tested or proved safe for use in pregnancy. Also, aspirin use is contraindicated in pregnancy because of its anti-platelet effects.
4. Herbal products are not required by the FDA to be proven safe or effective. They are classified as dietary supplements and are not subject to the same rules as are drugs. Therefore the patient must receive adequate information about the herbal products, including his or her risks, side effects, and possible benefits.
5. Many patients believe that if a product is "natural," then it is safe. Discuss each product with the patient, and instruct the patient about possible contraindications, safe use, frequency of dosing, specifics about how to take the product, and the way to monitor for both therapeutic effects and complications or toxic effects.

## CHAPTER 8

### Gene Therapy and Pharmacogenomics

### Chapter Review and NCLEX® Examination Preparation/Critical Thinking and Application
1. a
2. f
3. b
4. c
5. d
6. a, c, d
7. a
8. a
9. A major ethical issue related to gene therapy is that of *eugenics*. *Eugenics* is the intentional selection before birth of genotypes that are considered more desirable than others. For similar reasons, the prospect of being able to manipulate genes in human *germ cells* (sperm and eggs), at a preembryonic stage, is also a potential ethical hazard of gene therapy. Theoretically, even

cosmetic modifications could be attempted by using such techniques as a part of routine family planning. Because of ethical concerns such as these, U.S. gene therapy research is limited to somatic cells only. Gene therapy in *germ-line* (reproductive) cells is currently not approved for funding by the National Institutes of Health.

10. Recombinant DNA is DNA that has been artificially synthesized or modified in a laboratory setting. This technology is used to make recombinant forms of drugs such as hormones, vaccines, and antitoxins. An example of this technology is the alteration of the *Escherichia coli* genome so that these bacteria manufacture a recombinant form of human insulin.

11. The general goal of gene therapy is to transfer to the patient exogenous genes that will either provide a temporary substitute for or initiate permanent changes in the patient's own genetic functioning to treat a given disease. Although hundreds of gene therapy clinical trials have been approved by the U.S. Food and Drug Administration (FDA), no gene therapy to date has been approved for routine treatment of disease. Gene therapy techniques are being studied for the treatment of acquired illnesses such as cancer, heart disease, and diabetes.

12. This patient's comment is a clue to a potential genetic issue. An unusual or other-than-expected reaction to a drug in family members might point to a difference in the patient's ability to metabolize certain drugs. It is essential that the nurse investigate this comment further and obtain details about what has happened with the family members, how they reacted to the surgery, and the outcomes. This information will need to be communicated to the patient's surgeon and anesthesiologist. The nurse will tell the patient that although there is no way to predict how he will respond to medication, measures will be taken to ensure his safety.

13. Maintaining privacy and confidentiality is of utmost importance during genetic testing and counseling. The patient is the one who decides whether to include or exclude any family members from the discussion and from knowledge of the results of genetic testing. Nurses must protect against improper disclosure of information to other family members, friends of the family, other health care providers, and insurance providers. The nurse will tell the patient's sister that only the patient is able to share that information.

## Case Study

1. This information about Dale's cousin may be significant! An unusual or other-than-expected reaction to a drug in family members may point to a difference in the patient's ability to metabolize certain drugs. Genetic factors may alter a patient's metabolism of a particular drug, resulting in either increased or decreased drug action.

2. The nurse will ask about the type of medication Dale's cousin received and the type of surgery and will obtain details about the reaction that occurred and the treatment. The nurse will also ask if any other family members have had unusual reactions to drugs and whether Dale himself has had any problems.

3. The family history needs to cover at least three generations and include the current and past health status of each family member.

4. The surgeon and anesthesiologist will work to adjust the planned drug therapy for Dale's surgery according to the genetic variation that has been identified. In addition, during surgery, the patient will be monitored closely for any unusual responses.

### CHAPTER 9

**Photo Atlas of Drug Administration**

## Chapter Review and NCLEX® Examination Preparation/Critical Thinking and Application

1. c
2. a
3. b
4. c
5. c
6. b
7. a
8. c
9. a
10. c
11. a
12. b
13. d
14. b
15. a
16. a, b, d
17. 14 units

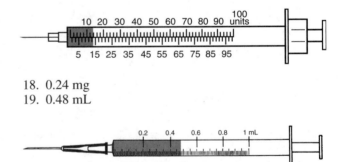

18. 0.24 mg
19. 0.48 mL

20. a. Palpate sites for masses or tenderness and assess the amount of subcutaneous tissue.
    b. Note the integrity and size of the muscle and palpate for tenderness.
    c. Note any lesions or discoloration of the forearm.
21. See the descriptions under textbook Figure 9-38 for each type of injection.

22. Remove the needle and ensure that the site is not bleeding. Discard the medication and syringe, draw up new medication, and repeat the procedure in a different location.
23. Rather than pouring it into a medication cup, draw small volumes of liquid medications into a calibrated oral syringe.
24. 100 divided by 4 (4 puffs/day) = 25 days

## Case Study

1. For an adult, the ventrogluteal site is the preferred injection site; however, immunizations are often given in the deltoid muscle because of the small volume size. If the adult is of average size, choose a needle that is 1 1/2 inches long and 21 to 25 gauge, and insert the needle at a 90-degree angle. For an infant, the preferred site is the vastus lateralis muscle. The needle must be of the correct length to ensure that it reaches muscle tissue, not the subcutaneous layer.
2. For an infant or child younger than 3 years of age, pull the pinna of the ear down and back before the drops are administered. Direct the drops along the sides of the ear rather than directly onto the eardrum. Take the drops out of refrigeration about 1 hour before administering them. The mother needs to stay with her child and ensure that the child lies on her side for 5 to 10 minutes. Gentle massage of the tragus area of the ear with her finger will help distribute the medication down the ear canal.
3. Liquid medication doses under 5 mL must be drawn up in a calibrated oral syringe. A medicine cup does not provide accurate measurements for small doses under 5 mL.
4. Liquids are usually ordered because infants cannot swallow pills or capsules. Do not add the medication to a bottle of formula. The infant may refuse the feeding or may not drink all of the bottle and, as a result, would not get the entire dosage of medication. A plastic disposable oral dosing syringe is recommended for measuring small doses of liquid medications. Position the infant so that the head is slightly elevated. Place the plastic dropper or syringe inside the infant's mouth, beside the tongue, and administer the liquid in small amounts while allowing the infant to swallow each time. Take great care to prevent aspiration. A crying infant can easily aspirate medication.

## CHAPTER 10

### Analgesic Drugs

### Critical Thinking Crossword
*Across*
3. Agonist
5. Acute
11. Superficial
13. Visceral

*Down*
1. Antagonist
2. Adjuvant
4. Tolerance
6. Threshold
7. Somatic
8. Chronic
9. Opioid
10. Opiate
12. Partial

### Chapter Review and NCLEX® Examination Preparation
1. b
2. d
3. c
4. d
5. b, c, e
6. c
7. b, d, e
8. Based on the patient's statements, he was taking a total of 5300 mg of acetaminophen per day! (Two Percocets twice a day equals 1300 mg; two extra-strength acetaminophen tablets four times a day equal 4000 mg.) Yes, this is a concern because the standard maximum daily dose for acetaminophen is 3000 mg/day. He is at risk for liver damage.
9. 3 mL (See Overview of Dosage Calculations, Section II.)
10. 1.2 mL (See Overview of Dosage Calculations, Section II.)
11.

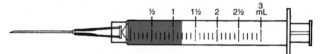

12. f
13. e
14. h
15. g
16. c
17. a
18. i
19. b
20. d

## Case Study
1. Superficial pain, which originates from the skin or mucous membranes
2. All opioids cause some histamine release. It is thought that this histamine release is responsible for many of the unwanted side effects, such as itching.
3. The most serious side effect of opioids is central nervous system depression, which may lead to respiratory depression. Naloxone (Narcan), an opioid reversal drug, may have to be administered to reverse severe respiratory depression.

**175**

4. The use of a nonopioid analgesic with an opioid is known as *adjuvant analgesic therapy*. This allows the use of smaller doses of opioids, which accomplishes two important functions. First, it diminishes some of the side effects that are seen with higher doses of opioids, such as respiratory depression, constipation, and urinary retention. Second, it approaches the pain stimulus by another mechanism of action and has a resulting synergistic beneficial effect in reducing the pain.

## CHAPTER 11

**General and Local Anesthetics**

**Chapter Review and NCLEX® Examination Preparation/Critical Thinking and Application**

1. f
2. g
3. j
4. e
5. d
6. a
7. i
8. c
9. b
10. h
11. a, c, e
12. b
13. a
14. b
15. b, c, e
16. c
17. d
18. b
19. b
20. a
21. 1 = c; 2 = a; 3 = b
22. 0.4 mL (See Overview of Dosage Calculations, Section III.)
23. 0.05 mL (See Overview of Dosage Calculations, Section III.)
24. Pediatric patients are more susceptible to problems such as central nervous system depression, toxicity, atelectasis, pneumonia, and cardiac abnormalities because their hepatic, cardiac, respiratory, and renal systems are not fully developed or fully functional.
25. These drugs cause paralysis of the respiratory muscles. The nurse will need to monitor the mechanical ventilation closely because if the ventilator does not work, the patient will not be able to breathe on his own. Emergency resuscitation equipment must be kept nearby. In addition, these drugs do not cause sedation, and the patient is still able to hear and feel. Most facilities have protocols for sedation during the use of these drugs. However, it is important to remain professional at all times and to take the time to reassure the patient and orient him to his

surroundings, what noises mean, and what procedures are going to be done to him. Remind the family that he is still able to hear what is said.
26. She will be given a combination of intravenous medications that will produce analgesia and amnesia of the procedure, but she will still be alert enough to breathe on her own and follow verbal directions as needed. In some cases, local anesthesia will be used to enhance patient comfort. This type of sedation is called *moderate* (or *procedural*, or *conscious*) *sedation*; it is associated with fewer complications and a shorter recovery time than general anesthesia.
27. Yes, there is a difference. Lidocaine with epinephrine is used when the vasoconstriction effects of epinephrine are needed. The vasoconstriction confines the anesthetic (lidocaine) to the local area of injection and acts to reduce bleeding. The two types of lidocaine are not interchangeable.

## Case Study

1. In balanced anesthesia, minimal doses of a combination of anesthetic drugs (both intravenous and inhaled) are given to achieve the desired level of anesthesia for the surgical procedure. Adjunctive drugs may also be used and commonly include sedative-hypnotics, narcotics, and neuromuscular blocking drugs (NMBDs; depolarizing drugs such as succinylcholine and the nondepolarizing or competitive drugs such as pancuronium or d-tubocurarine). Combining several different drugs makes it possible for general anesthesia to be accomplished with smaller amounts of anesthetic gases and thereby reduces the side effects.
2. The main therapeutic use of the NMBD succinylcholine is to maintain controlled ventilation during surgical procedures. When respiratory muscles are paralyzed by NMBDs, mechanical ventilation is easier because the body's drive to control respirations is eliminated by the drug; this allows the ventilator to have total control of the respirations.
3. Multiple medical conditions (listed in Box 11-4) can predispose an individual to toxicity. These conditions increase the sensitivity of an individual to NMBDs and prolong their effects. Because the patient's temperature has decreased, hypothermia may lead to an increased sensitivity to the medication. In addition, the history of paraplegia is another condition that may predispose this patient to toxicity.
4. Anticholinesterase drugs such as neostigmine, pyridostigmine, and edrophonium are antidotes and are used to reverse muscle paralysis.
5. Local anesthesia is most commonly used in settings in which loss of consciousness, whole-body relaxation, and loss of responsiveness are either unnecessary or unwanted. A lower incidence of toxic effects is associated with the use of local anesthetics because very little of these drugs is absorbed systemically.

6. Regardless of the type of anesthesia a patient is receiving, one of the most important nursing considerations during this time is close and frequent observation of the patient and all body systems, with specific attention to the ABCs of care (airway, breathing, and circulation) and vital signs. Resuscitative equipment and any drug antidote should be kept nearby in case of cardiorespiratory distress or arrest. Other nursing actions include monitoring all aspects of body functions, instituting safety measures, and implementing the physician's orders.

## CHAPTER 12

### Central Nervous System Depressants and Muscle Relaxants

### Chapter Review and NCLEX® Examination Preparation/Critical Thinking and Application
1. a
2. b
3. a
4. d
5. c
6. b
7. b
8. b
9. a, c, d, e
10. a. 7.5 mg
    b. 3.75 mL (See Overview of Dosage Calculations, Section IV.)
11. 10 mL
12.

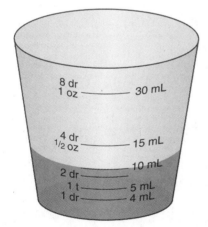

13. An overdose of barbiturates produces central nervous system (CNS) depression ranging from sleep to profound coma and death. Respiratory depression progresses to Cheyne-Stokes respirations, hypoventilation, and cyanosis. Patients often have cold, clammy skin or are hypothermic, and later they can exhibit fever, areflexia, tachycardia, and hypotension. The priority of care would be to maintain the ABCs (airway, breathing, and circulation),

especially respirations because respiratory depression is likely. There is no antidote for barbiturate overdose.

14. These drugs can be taken for insomnia only if their use is limited to the short term (less than 2 to 4 weeks). With long-term use, rebound insomnia and severe withdrawal can develop. If Jackie needs to take something to help her sleep while she is on her trip, the nonbenzodiazepine hypnotics may be an option, and of course, you could provide patient teaching on nonpharmacologic methods to aid sleep.

15. Benzodiazepines can create a significant fall hazard in older adults, and the lowest effective dose must be used in this patient population.

16. a. Ask about allergies, CNS disorders, sleep disorders, diabetes, addictive disorders, personality disorders, thyroid conditions, and renal and liver function.
    b. Alcohol and CNS depressants but also all prescribed or over-the-counter medications and herbal products used
    c. The patient's age matters because these drugs have increased effects in older persons and small children.

17. a. Patient teaching should include information about potential side effects and potential drug interactions. In addition, safety measures to prevent injury stemming from decreased sensorium must be emphasized.
    b. These medications are most effective when used in conjunction with rest and physical therapy.

## Case Study

1. Barbiturates are considered controlled substances because of the potential for misuse and the severe effects that result if they are not used appropriately. Other hypnotic drugs are now used because they have fewer side effects and are safer than the older barbiturates. Barbiturates are no longer recommended for insomnia.

2. Barbiturates are habit forming, they have a low therapeutic index, and severe withdrawal effects may occur when the medication is stopped. Other drugs are now recommended for treatment of insomnia.

3. Other CNS depressants, especially alcohol, should be avoided. There may also be an additive effect when the herbal products kava or valerian is used.

4. Zaleplon is indicated for the short-term treatment of insomnia; it is not approved for long-term use. It has a very short half-life, so the patient should be taught that if sleep difficulties include early awakenings, a dose can be taken as long as it is at least 4 hours before the patient must arise. In addition, the patient should explore other nonpharmacologic options for the treatment of insomnia and try to find the cause of the sleep problems. See Box 12-1 for information on nonpharmacologic measures to promote sleep.

## CHAPTER 13

**Central Nervous System Stimulants and Related Drugs**

**Chapter Review and NCLEX® Examination Preparation/Critical Thinking and Application**
1. b
2. b, c, e
3. a
4. d
5. b
6. b
7. b, c, d
8. a
9. 100 mg (See Overview of Dosage Calculations, Section IV.)
10. 37.5 mg (See Overview of Dosage Calculations, Section IV.)
11. a. Stacey probably has narcolepsy.
    b. Methylphenidate (an amphetamine) or modafinil (a nonamphetamine) may be ordered.
    c. These drugs boost mental alertness, increase motor activity, and diminish the patient's sense of fatigue by stimulating the cerebral cortex and possibly the reticular activating system.
    d. Stacey should avoid other central nervous system stimulants, in particular, caffeine-containing products (e.g., coffee, tea, colas, and chocolate). She should check with her physician before taking any over-the-counter drug or herbal product, and she should not consume any substance that contains alcohol. In addition, she should keep a journal to document her response to the medication.
12. Weight loss caused by anorexia is associated with these drugs, so it is important to monitor for weight gain or loss in children who are taking drugs for attention-deficit/hyperactivity disorder. Height and weight should be measured and recorded before therapy is initiated, and growth rate should be plotted during therapy. Nutritional status should be assessed, with attention to daily dietary intake and the amount eaten before drug therapy and after therapy is initiated.
13. With orlistat, patients need to watch dietary fat intake. Restricting the intake of fat to less than 30% of total caloric intake may help decrease the occurrence of gastrointestinal side effects. Supplementation with fat-soluble vitamins may be indicated.
14. These drugs work to reduce the severity of the headaches but do not prevent headaches.
15. Specialists sometimes recommend periodic "drug holidays" (e.g., 1 day per week without medication) to diminish the addictive tendencies of the stimulant drugs. School-aged children often do not take these drugs on weekends and school vacations.

**Case Study**
1. Serotonin receptor agonists work by stimulating 5-HT1 receptors in the brain; this stimulation results in constriction of dilated blood vessels in the brain and decreased release of inflammatory neuropeptides.
2. Orally administered medications may not be tolerated because of the nausea and vomiting that often accompany the headaches. Alternative formulations such as subcutaneous self-injections, sublingual forms, and nasal sprays are advantageous. They also typically have a more rapid onset of action, producing relief in some patients in 10 to 15 minutes compared with 1 to 2 hours with tablets.
3. Use of sumatriptan is contraindicated in patients with drug allergy and the presence of serious cardiovascular disease because of the vasoconstrictive potential of these medications.
4. Foods containing tyramine should be avoided because tyramine is known to precipitate severe headaches. Tyramine-containing foods include beer, wine, aged cheese, food additives, preservatives, artificial sweeteners, chocolate, and caffeine.
5. Keeping a journal of the occurrence of headaches, precipitating factors, and response to drug therapy is also encouraged so that the patient's progress and response to drug therapy can be followed.

## CHAPTER 14

**Antiepileptic Drugs**

**Critical Thinking Crossword**
*Across*
2. Emergency
6. Primary
10. Hepatotoxicity
11. Seizure
12. Slowly
*Down*
1. Secondary
3. Convulsion
4. Benzodiazepines
5. Idiopathic
6. Phenobarbital
7. Autoinduction
8. Epilepsy
9. Phenytoin

**Chapter Review and NCLEX® Examination Preparation/Critical Thinking and Application**
1. d
2. a
3. b, c, d
4. c
5. b

6. c
7. a, b, c
8. b
9. b
10. a. 450 mg/day; 150 mg per dose
    b. 3 mL per dose
11.

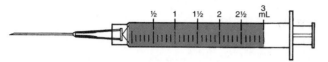

12. Carbamazepine undergoes autoinduction, the process by which the metabolism of a drug increases over time, which leads to lower-than-expected drug concentrations.
13. Jeremy's mother needs to be told that topiramate must be taken whole, not crushed, broken in half, or chewed. It does have a very bitter taste and seems to be better tolerated when taken with food. She can still give it with gelatin as long as the dosage form remains whole.
14. Although it is true that pregnancy is a common contraindication to antiepileptic drugs, the prescriber will consider the risks to the mother and infant of untreated maternal epilepsy and the increased risks for seizure activity. The newer-generation antiepileptic drugs appear to be safer in pregnancy than the traditional drugs; many women take these drugs throughout their pregnancies. However, women with epilepsy need to be monitored closely by both an obstetrician and a neurologist during pregnancy. Birth defects in infants of mothers with epilepsy are higher than normal regardless of whether the mother was receiving drug therapy.

## Case Study

1. The signs and symptoms that Mattie is experiencing are typical of absence seizures. These are most often seen in children.
2. She needs to be sure to measure the dose carefully with an exact graduated device or oral syringe, rather than using a household teaspoon, and to give the medication at the same time daily. She needs to report excessive sedation, confusion, lethargy, or decreased movement. See the Patient Teaching Tips in your textbook for more information.
3. Encourage her to keep a journal to record Mattie's signs and symptoms before, during, and after any seizure activity to measure the therapeutic effectiveness of the medication.
4. A therapeutic response to antiepileptic drugs does not mean that the patient has been cured of the seizures but only that seizure activity is decreased or absent. Further evaluation will be needed before a decision is made to stop the medication. Treatment may need to last for years or may be lifelong.

## CHAPTER 15

## Antiparkinson Drugs

### Chapter Review and NCLEX® Examination Preparation/Critical Thinking and Application
1. b
2. a
3. d
4. c
5. d
6. a, b, c, e
7. b
8. a, c, e
9. d
10. 2.5 tablets
11. a. Dopamine must be given in this form because exogenously administered dopamine cannot pass through the blood–brain barrier; levodopa can.
    b. The addition of carbidopa avoids the high peripheral levels of dopamine and unwanted side effects induced by the very large dosages of levodopa necessary when the drug is given alone.
    c. Carbidopa does not cross the blood–brain barrier and thus prevents levodopa breakdown in the periphery. This, in turn, allows levodopa to reach and cross the blood–brain barrier. In the brain, the levodopa is then broken down to dopamine, which can be used directly.
    d. Meat, fish and cheese should not be taken concurrently with levodopa.
12. The nurse must ask whether Mrs. R. is lactating; if so, use of amantadine is contraindicated. In addition, pregnancy may be a contraindication to many antiparkinson drugs.
13. Older patients, especially men with benign prostatic hyperplasia, are at risk for urinary retention. Jane's neighbor may or may not have that condition, but his age is a major factor. Jane's age is not a concern at this time. This drug may also cause palpitations.
14. The "on–off phenomenon" occurs because of rapid swings in the patient's response to levodopa. The result is worsening of the disease when too little dopamine is present, or dyskinesias when too much is present. In contrast, the "wearing-off phenomenon" occurs when antiparkinson medications begin to lose their effectiveness, despite maximal dosing, as the disease progresses.

## Case Study

1. The primary cause of Parkinson's disease is an imbalance in the two neurotransmitters dopamine and acetylcholine (ACh) in the basal ganglia of the brain. This imbalance is caused by a failure of the nerve terminals in the substantia nigra to produce dopamine, which acts in the basal ganglia to control body movements. A correct balance between dopamine and ACh is needed for the proper regulation of posture,

muscle tone, and voluntary movement. The deficiency of dopamine can also lead to excessive ACh activity because of the lack of dopamine's normal balancing effect. Symptoms of Parkinson's disease do not appear until approximately 80% of the dopamine store in the substantia nigra of the basal ganglia has been depleted.

2. Drug therapy is aimed at increasing the levels of dopamine at the remaining functioning nerve terminals. It is also aimed at blocking the effects of ACh and slowing the progression of the disease.

3. Amantadine causes the release of dopamine from nerve endings that are still intact. The result is higher levels of dopamine in the central nervous system.

4. It is most effective in the early stages of Parkinson's disease, but as the disease progresses and the number of functioning nerves diminishes, amantadine's effect is also reduced. Amantadine is usually effective for only 6 to 12 months.

5. Patients with Parkinson's disease often experience rapid swings in response to levodopa; this fluctuating response is known as the "on–off phenomenon." This phenomenon is seen in patients who take levodopa for a long time. Such patients may experience periods when they have good control ("on" time) and periods when they have bad control or breakthrough Parkinson's disease ("off" time). Carbidopa is a peripheral decarboxylase inhibitor that does not cross the blood–brain barrier. As a result, carbidopa is able to prevent levodopa from breaking down in the periphery and allows more levodopa to reach and cross the blood–brain barrier. Levodopa–carbidopa combinations, such as Sinemet CR, may help decrease the "off" time.

## CHAPTER 16

### Psychotherapeutic Drugs

**Chapter Review and NCLEX® Examination Preparation/Critical Thinking and Application**
1. b, c, e
2. a
3. c
4. a, c, d
5. d
6. c
7. d
8. c
9. 3 tablets (See Overview of Dosage Calculations, Section II.)
10. 900 mg; 3 capsules (See Overview of Dosage Calculations, Section II.)
11. l
12. f
13. g
14. o
15. b
16. i
17. j
18. k
19. c
20. n
21. a
22. d
23. h
24. e
25. m
26. a. Carl may have taken an overdose of the benzodiazepine.
    b. If an overdose of the benzodiazepine is suspected, flumazenil (Romazicon) may be given to reverse the effect of the benzodiazepine overdose. The treatment for benzodiazepine overdose is generally supportive.
27. a. Mr. D. needs to be aware of the foods and drinks, including red wine, that he can no longer have because they contain tyramine.
    b. It appears that Mr. D. may have inadvertently ingested something containing tyramine, which has caused a hypertensive crisis.
28. Second-generation antidepressants offer an advantage over other antidepressants because they have fewer and less severe side effects.
29. If the antidepressant taken is a first-generation (tricyclic) antidepressant, excessive dosages could result in lethal cardiac dysrhythmias and seizures. These dysrhythmias are responsible for most of the deaths caused by tricyclic antidepressant overdoses.

### Case Study

1. See Table 16-2 for potential adverse effects of benzodiazepines. Most are related to their effects on the central nervous system (CNS). Patient teaching includes warning the patient to avoid driving or operating heavy equipment or machinery until he becomes accustomed to the side effects of the medication. In addition, measures should be taken to avoid orthostatic hypotension. Finally, he should avoid alcohol and other CNS depressants while taking this medication.

2. If he is experiencing life-altering anxiety, then he should also consider obtaining psychotherapy to assist him at this time.

3. Benzodiazepines are potentially habit forming and addictive, with possible withdrawal symptoms such as anxiety, panic attacks, convulsions, nausea, and vomiting. The medication should not be withdrawn abruptly. Patients should always be advised to take the medication as directed and never to stop taking the medicine abruptly. Benzodiazepines should be withdrawn gradually.

4. There is a potential for benzodiazepines to cause serious, life-threatening toxicities, but when taken alone in normal dosages in otherwise healthy patients, they are very safe and effective anxiolytics. When

they are taken with other sedating medications or with alcohol, however, life-threatening respiratory depression or arrest can occur. An overdose of benzodiazepines may result in one or more of the following symptoms: somnolence, confusion, coma, and respiratory depression. Overdose may be treated with the benzodiazepine-specific antidote flumazenil (Romazicon) or administration of activated charcoal.

5. Buspirone has the advantages of being both nonsedating and non–habit-forming compared with the benzodiazepines.

## CHAPTER 17

### Substance Use Disorder

### Chapter Review and NCLEX® Examination Preparation/Critical Thinking and Application

1. h
2. i
3. f
4. e
5. g
6. d
7. j
8. a
9. c
10. b
11. a, c, f
12. d
13. b, c, e
14. c
15. b
16. a, b
17. 2 mL (See Overview of Dosage Calculations, Section IV.)
18. The nicotine transdermal system (patch) and nicotine polacrilex (gum) can be used to supply nicotine without the carcinogens in tobacco. The patches provide a stepwise reduction in delivery and work by gradually reducing the nicotine dose over time. With the gum, rapid chewing releases an immediate dose of nicotine, but this dose is about half of what the average smoker receives from one cigarette, and the onset of action is longer than with smoking. Therefore the reinforcement and self-reward effects of smoking are minimized. Zyban is a sustained-release form of the antidepressant bupropion and was the first nicotine-free prescription medicine used to treat nicotine dependence. Varenicline (Chantix) both activates and antagonizes the alpha-4-beta-2 nicotinic receptors in the brain. This effect provides some stimulation to nicotine receptors while also reducing the pleasurable effects of nicotine from smoking. This drug has demonstrated greater efficacy than bupropion.

19. Benzodiazepines are used for all three levels of ethanol withdrawal. Lower dosages are used for mild symptoms, and higher dosages are needed for severe withdrawal. The oral route is preferred; however, it is often necessary to use the intravenous route for patients experiencing severe withdrawal. Patients who are experiencing severe withdrawal often require monitoring in an intensive care unit for cardiac and respiratory function, fluid and nutrition replacement, vital signs, and mental status. Restraints are indicated for a patient who is confused or agitated to protect the patient from self-harm and to protect others (delirium tremens can be a terrifying and life-threatening state). Thiamine administration, hydration, and magnesium replacement may be indicated depending on the severity of the withdrawal state.

20. Dextromethorphan is an ingredient in several over-the-counter products, including Robitussin DM cough syrup and Mucinex DM tablets. Some adolescents have discovered that taking dextromethorphan in large amounts leads to a "high" that is accompanied by hallucinations. The hallucinations have been documented to be similar to those associated with the street drug phencyclidine (PCP). In addition, it has been found that teens who abuse dextromethorphan may also abuse other drugs such as lysergic acid diethylamide (LSD), PCP, ecstasy, and inhalants. The hazardous short- or long-term effects that may occur with these drugs include nausea, hot flashes, reduced mental status, dizziness, seizures, loss of coordination and balance, brain damage, and death.

21. Methamphetamine is a chemical class of amphetamine, but it has a much stronger effect on the central nervous system (CNS) than the other classes of amphetamine. Crystallized methamphetamine, known as *ice, crystal*, or *crystal meth*, is a smokable and more powerful form of the drug. The over-the-counter decongestant pseudoephedrine is commonly used to synthesize methamphetamine in secret drug laboratories, often in private homes. This practice has led to dramatic increases in the abuse of this drug. In 2005, the Combat Methamphetamine Epidemic Act required restricted retail sales of all nonprescription drug products containing pseudoephedrine. Specific restrictions include allowing sales only from *behind* the pharmacy counter, requiring photo identification and electronic or paper recordkeeping of purchasers (which must remain on file for 2 years), and setting maximum allowable amount (in grams) of pseudoephedrine that can be sold per consumer per month.

## Case Study

1. Ethanol is a CNS depressant.
2. Acute severe alcoholic intoxication may cause cardiovascular depression, and long-term excessive use has largely irreversible effects on the heart. Moderate amounts may either stimulate or depress respiration, but large amounts produce lethal respiratory depression.
3. First, you should monitor the patient's respiratory and cardiovascular status and prevent injury from falling or aspiration from vomiting. In addition, you should be alert to the patient's behavior and mental status to identify changes in his condition. Withdrawal from alcohol can lead to serious conditions such as delirium tremens. Careful assessment of vital signs and mental status is imperative at this time because early withdrawal symptoms may be an increase in blood pressure and pulse with an altered mental status.
4. Mr. C. should stay in the hospital for observation for and possible treatment of delirium tremens, which may begin with tremors and agitation and progress to hallucinations and sometimes death. See Box 17-6 for information on treatment of ethanol withdrawal.
5. Chronic excessive ingestion of ethanol is directly associated with several serious mental and neurologic disorders. Nutritional and vitamin B deficiencies can occur, which result in conditions such as Wernicke's encephalopathy, Korsakoff's psychosis, polyneuritis, and nicotinic acid deficiency encephalopathy. Seizures may also occur. In addition, long-term ingestion of ethanol may result in alcoholic hepatitis or liver cirrhosis.

## CHAPTER 18

### Adrenergic Drugs

### Chapter Review and NCLEX® Examination Preparation/Critical Thinking and Application

1. d
2. b
3. a, b, d
4. a
5. c
6. b
7. a, b, e
8. a, c, e
9. c
10. 50 mcg per dose (See Overview of Dosage Calculations, Section IV.)
11. 0.5 mL (See Overview of Dosage Calculations, Section III.)
12.

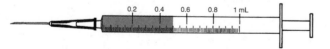

13. a. The alpha-adrenergic activity of this drug causes vasoconstriction in the nasal mucosa. This produces shrinkage of the mucosa and promotes easier nasal breathing.
    b. Perhaps she administered the spray too often. Excessive use of nasal decongestants can lead to greater congestion because of a rebound phenomenon.
14. Use of the drug is contraindicated in patients who have a tumor that secretes catecholamines, such as a pheochromocytoma.
15. The action of dopamine depends on the dosage. At low dosages, it can dilate blood vessels in the brain, heart, kidneys, and mesentery, increasing blood flow to these areas. Increased renal flow may help remove excess fluid volume. At higher infusion rates, dopamine can improve contractility and cardiac output.
16. The toxic effects of adrenergic drugs are mainly an extension of their common adverse effects, such as seizures, hypotension or hypertension, dysrhythmias, and other effects, but the two most life-threatening toxic effects involve the central nervous system and cardiovascular system. Seizures can be managed effectively with diazepam. An extreme elevation in blood pressure poses the risk for hemorrhage in the brain and elsewhere in the body. To lower the blood pressure quickly, a rapid-acting beta-adrenergic blocking drug can be used to reverse the adrenergic effects. Most of the adrenergic drugs have very short half-lives; therefore their effects are relatively short-lived. Stopping the drug should quickly cause the toxic symptoms to subside. The treatment of overdoses often focuses on treating the symptoms and supporting the patient's respiratory and cardiac functions.
17. a. He is probably having an anaphylactic reaction to the penicillin.
    b. First, the nurse must stop the medication! Then she will have someone else notify the physician while she stays with the patient to monitor and support the ABCs (airway, breathing, and circulation).
    c. Epinephrine is the drug of choice for anaphylactic reactions.

## Case Study

1. Before giving this medication, you should assess for hypersensitivity to albuterol and assess breath sounds and vital signs (blood pressure, pulse rate, respiratory rate) to obtain a baseline for comparative purposes. Because this medication may cause tachycardia and cardiac dysrhythmias, the patient's pulse rate and rhythm should be monitored during the treatment. Afterward, you should assess the patient's vital signs and breath sounds again and assess for therapeutic response to the medication.

2. The onset of inhaled albuterol is almost immediate; it would take more time for orally administered albuterol to be absorbed and to become effective. Therefore the inhaled form will take effect faster than the oral form.

3. These are expected side effects of the albuterol and will soon wear off.

4. Salmeterol is indicated for asthma and prevention of bronchospasms in patients who may need long-term maintenance therapy for their asthma. Patients should be taught that salmeterol is not to be used for relief of acute symptoms, and education about its dosing is important. Dosing of salmeterol is usually 1 puff twice daily 12 hours apart for maintenance. For prevention of exercise-induced asthma, the recommendation is 2 puffs 1/2 to 1 hour before exercise and no additional dosing for 12 hours. If Maureen is still taking the inhaled steroid, then the bronchodilator should be taken first, and she should wait approximately 5 minutes before using the steroid inhaler. She will need to rinse her mouth with warm water after taking the inhaled corticosteroid. All equipment should be cleaned regularly.

## CHAPTER 19

### Adrenergic-Blocking Drugs

### Chapter Review and NCLEX® Examination Preparation/Critical Thinking and Application

1. a, b, d
2. a
3. c
4. b
5. d
6. c
7. d
8. b
9. a
10. 83 mL/hr (See Overview of Dosage Calculations, Section V.)
11. 4 mL
12. Extravasation can cause vasoconstriction and ultimately tissue death (necrosis). If the vasoconstriction is not reversed quickly, the whole limb can be lost. Phentolamine, an alpha blocker, can reverse this potent vasoconstriction and restore blood flow to the ischemic, vasoconstricted area. When phentolamine is injected subcutaneously in a circular fashion around the extravasation site, it causes alpha-adrenergic receptor blockade and vasodilation. This in turn increases blood flow to the ischemic tissue and thus prevents permanent damage.
13. Some beta blockers are considered cardioprotective because they inhibit stimulation by the circulating catecholamines that were released during muscle damage, such as that caused by a myocardial infarction. When a beta blocker occupies their

receptors, the circulating catecholamines cannot bind to their receptors. Thus the beta blockers "protect" the heart from being stimulated by these catecholamines, which would only further increase the heart rate and the contractile force and thereby increase myocardial oxygen demand.

14. She should take her apical pulse for 1 full minute and monitor her blood pressure because cardiac depression can occur with these drugs. If her systolic blood pressure decreases to lower than 100 mm Hg or her pulse decreases to fewer than 60 beats/min, she needs to contact her physician. She should also report any weight gain, especially 2 lb or more in a 24-hour period or 5 lb or more in 1 week, and any weakness, shortness of breath, or edema.

15. A common problem with the alpha blockers such as tamsulosin is that when patients first start taking these drugs, they may experience lightheadedness and orthostatic hypotension. Patients usually quickly develop a tolerance to this effect. He should be taught to take care when standing up to prevent falling if he gets lightheaded; taking the first dose at bedtime may help. In addition, other adverse effects of blurred vision, dizziness, and drowsiness may lead to injuries if he falls. Special care must be taken for safety until he knows how he responds to the medication.

### Case Study

1. Nonselective beta blockers (which block both $beta_1$ and $beta_2$ receptors) may precipitate bradycardia and hypotension; their use is contraindicated in patients with asthma. Therefore if the patient has heart disease and respiratory disease, a $beta_1$ blocker, or "cardioselective" drug, would be very beneficial because it would not produce constriction or increased airway resistance as would $beta_2$ blockers.

2. When a beta blocker is given, it occupies receptors and prevents circulating catecholamines (which are released when a myocardial infarction occurs) from binding to these receptors. The beta blocker thus prevents stimulation of the heart by these catecholamines, which would further increase heart rate, contractile force, and myocardial oxygen demand. In addition, cardioselective $beta_1$ blockers such as atenolol block the $beta_1$-adrenergic receptors on the surface of the heart. This reduces myocardial stimulation, which in turn reduces heart rate, slows conduction through the atrioventricular node, prolongs sinoatrial node recovery, and decreases myocardial oxygen demand by decreasing myocardial contractile force (contractility).

3. Table 19-4 lists beta blocker–induced adverse effects. Patient teaching should include instructions to monitor the apical pulse for 1 full minute and monitor blood pressure because of the cardiac depression that can occur and to notify the physician if systolic

blood pressure decreases to lower than 100 mm Hg or pulse decreases to fewer than 60 beats/min. In addition, patients need to report any weight gain, especially a gain of 2 lb or more in a 24-hour period or 5 lb or more in 1 week, and any weakness, shortness of breath, or edema. These symptoms may indicate the onset of heart failure. The patient should also be taught about orthostatic changes and cautioned to rise slowly when getting up to avoid syncope. For other teaching points, see Patient Teaching Tips in the text.

4. Make sure that patients are weaned off these medications slowly, if this is indicated, because of the possible rebound hypertension or chest pain that rapid withdrawal can precipitate. Beta blockers may cause impotence, which may be the reason Bruce wants to stop the medication, but the nurse needs to ask Bruce about his reason for wanting to stop atenolol.

## CHAPTER 20

**Cholinergic Drugs**

**Chapter Review and NCLEX® Examination Preparation/Critical Thinking and Application**

1. h
2. g
3. f
4. b
5. j
6. e
7. i
8. a
9. c
10. b
11. b
12. a, b, d
13. d
14. c
15. b, c, d, f
16. a
17. b
18. b, d
19. 17 gtt/min (16.7 rounds to 17) (See Overview of Dosage Calculations, Section V.)
20. 26.7 mg (See Overview of Dosage Calculations, Section IV.)
21. SLUDGE stands for salivation, lacrimation, urinary incontinence, diarrhea, gastrointestinal cramps, and emesis.
22. a. Bethanechol (Urecholine) is the drug of choice.
    b. None. Bethanechol use is contraindicated in patients with a genitourinary obstruction. The drug will be discontinued immediately.
23. a. Cholinergic crisis
    b. Ensure that atropine, the antidote, is readily available.

24. a. She should experience less eyelid drooping (ptosis), less double vision (diplopia), less difficulty swallowing and chewing, and less weakness.
    b. She needs to report any increased muscle weakness, abdominal cramps, diarrhea, or difficulty breathing.

## Case Study

1. There are no "cures" for Alzheimer's disease, but several drugs are available for management of symptoms. Their use can sometimes yield enough improvement in a patient's mental status to make a noticeable improvement in the quality of life for patients, caregivers, and family members. However, individual response to these medications does vary from patient to patient. Available drugs include donepezil (Aricept), tacrine (Cognex), galantamine (Razadyne, Reminyl), rivastigmine (Exelon), and memantine (Namenda).
2. Rivastigmine is also approved for treating dementia that is associated with Parkinson's disease.
3. Direct-acting cholinergic agonists bind to cholinergic receptors and activate them. Indirect-acting cholinergic agonists act by making more acetylcholine (ACh) available at the receptor site. As a result, ACh binds to and stimulates the receptors. It does this by inhibiting the action of cholinesterase, the enzyme responsible for breaking down ACh.
4. Adverse effects of rivastigmine include dizziness, headache, nausea and vomiting, diarrhea, and anorexia (loss of appetite). Administering this drug with meals helps decrease the gastrointestinal side effects, although absorption may also be decreased. Patients who become dizzy with the therapy must be assisted with ambulation. Doses are titrated carefully to help minimize adverse effects.
5. Rivastigmine is also available in rapid orally disintegrating tablets, which may be easier for Arthur to take.

## CHAPTER 21

**Cholinergic-Blocking Drugs**

**Chapter Review and NCLEX® Examination Preparation/Critical Thinking and Application**

1. a, c, f
2. a, c, d
3. b
4. c
5. b
6. a, b, d
7. d
8. 0.6 mL
9. a. 40 mcg (See Overview of Dosage Calculations, Section IV.)
    b. 0.2 mL

10. Atropine sulfate is used preoperatively to reduce salivation and excessive secretions in the respiratory and gastrointestinal tracts. Glycopyrrolate (Robinul) is also used for this purpose.

11. a. Initially, Mr. M. will be treated with hospitalization and close, continuous monitoring (including continuous electrocardiographic monitoring). Fluid therapy and other standard measures used to treat shock are instituted as needed. Activated charcoal may be effective in removing the drug that has not yet been absorbed.

    b. In the case of hallucinations, physostigmine has proven helpful, although its use as an antidote for cholinergic blocker overdose is controversial because it has the potential to produce severe adverse effects such as seizures and cardiac asystole and is usually reserved for the treatment of patients who show extreme delirium or agitation or who could inflict injury upon themselves.

12. Antihistamines can have additive effects with cholinergic blockers, resulting in increased anticholinergic effects.

13. a. In the treatment of symptomatic bradycardia, higher dosages of atropine result in an increase in heart rate because of the cholinergic-blocking effects on the heart's conduction system. Atropine blocks the inhibitory vagal (cholinergic) effects on the pacemaker cells of the sinoatrial and atrioventricular nodes, which will hopefully lead to an increased heart rate because of unopposed sympathetic stimulation.

    b. Atropine has a therapeutic effect in cases of exposure to organophosphate insecticides because it blocks cholinergic receptors.

## Case Study

1. Tolterodine should not be used in patients with narrow-angle glaucoma or urinary retention. If patients have a history of decreased liver function or are taking drugs that inhibit cytochrome P-450 enzyme 3A4, the tolterodine dose will be reduced. Mrs. W.'s "eye problems" need to be evaluated further to rule out glaucoma.

2. Tolterodine appears to be associated with a much lower incidence of dry mouth. This may be caused by tolterodine's specificity for the bladder as opposed to the salivary glands.

3. When these cholinergic-blocking drugs are used to treat urinary incontinence, the inability to sweat or perspire should be managed with an increase in fluids and avoidance of extreme heat. Mrs. W. needs to avoid overheating when working outside.

4. Although this drug may be associated with a lower incidence of dry mouth, it may still cause this unpleasant side effect because it is a cholinergic-blocking drug. Dry mouth may be managed best by drinking adequate fluids, chewing gum, performing frequent mouth care, sucking on sugar-free hard candy, and using saliva-substitute products.

## CHAPTER 22

### Antihypertensive Drugs

**Critical Thinking Crossword**
*Across*
1. Secondary
5. Idiopathic
7. Orthostatic
8. Vasodilators
*Down*
2. Essential
3. Primary
4. Diuretics
6. ACE

**Chapter Review and NCLEX® Examination Preparation/Critical Thinking and Application**
1. c
2. b, d, e
3. b
4. a
5. d
6. a, c
7. c
8. c
9. c
10. 2 tablets per dose (See Overview of Dosage Calculations, Section II.)
11. 4 mL (See Overview of Dosage Calculations, Section V.)
12. Because nitroprusside has a very short half-life (10 minutes), the nurse will first discontinue the infusion. Treatment for the hypotension is supportive; pressor drugs can be given to raise the blood pressure quickly if necessary.
13. a. Captopril is probably best for Irene. In critically ill patients, a drug with a short half-life (e.g., captopril) is better because if problems arise, they will be short-lived. Also, Irene has liver dysfunction, so captopril has an advantage because it is not a prodrug (a prodrug is inactive in its initial form and must be biotransformed in the liver to its active form to be effective).

    b. Because of his history of poor adherence, Kory would benefit from a drug with a long half-life and long duration of action, which he would need to take only once a day. Therefore one of the newer angiotensin-converting enzyme (ACE) inhibitors—benazepril, fosinopril, lisinopril, quinapril, or ramipril—would be best.
14. There is a first-dose effect with prazosin. This means that the patient will experience a considerable drop in blood pressure after taking the first dose, so he needs to take it if he will be lying down for a while or before bedtime and arise slowly. This effect decreases with time or with a reduction in the dosage, as ordered by the physician.
15. a. Beta blockers and ACE inhibitors
    b. Calcium channel blockers and diuretics

## Case Study

1. Initial drug therapy would include thiazide-type diuretics. Other drugs that may also be started include ACE inhibitors, angiotensin II receptor blockers, beta blockers, calcium channel blockers, or a combination. Because John is African American, calcium channel blockers and diuretics would most likely be chosen over beta blockers and ACE inhibitors.
2. Teach him about the possibility of orthostatic hypotension and instruct him to change positions slowly, especially after stooping or bending over or when rising from supine or sitting to standing.
3. Exercise is an important part of a healthy lifestyle. However, emphasize the importance of safety and the need to avoid excessive exercise, hot climates, saunas, hot tubs, and hot environments. Heat may precipitate vasodilation and lead to worsening of hypotension, with the risk for fainting and injury to himself.

## CHAPTER 23

### Antianginal Drugs

### Chapter Review and NCLEX® Examination Preparation/Critical Thinking and Application

1. c
2. c
3. a, c, d, e
4. d
5. a
6. a
7. a
8. b
9. a
10. b
11. 2 capsules
12. DO NOT cut the patch in half! The nurse needs to call the pharmacy to obtain the correct dosage of the transdermal patch, one that delivers 0.2 mg/hr.
13. The nurse will call 911 and assist the patient until the ambulance arrives. The nurse will check the ABCs (airway, breathing, and circulation) and administer cardiopulmonary resuscitation if it becomes necessary. At this time, the nurse does not know the man's condition and certainly cannot administer someone else's medication to him. Isordil is available in a sublingual form, but the nurse cannot administer one person's medication to another person, especially to someone with an undetermined condition.
14. Ms. V. might be taking a beta blocker. Fatigue and lethargy are the most common patient complaints with the use of beta blockers, and mental depression can be exacerbated, particularly in older adults. Also, one of the central nervous system adverse effects of beta blockers is the occurrence of unusual dreams.

15. Theresa has a good start, but she also needs to include in her journal a description of the activity she was performing at the time her angina occurred and the number of tablets she had to take before the pain subsided. Also, she must keep the tablets in an airtight, dark glass bottle away from sunlight because the active ingredient in nitroglycerin is easily destroyed. The fact that she had no adverse effects such as headache may indicate that the drug is no longer active and needs to be replaced.

## Case Study

1. Chronic stable angina, also known as *classic* or *effort angina*, can be triggered by either exertion or stress (cold temperature or emotions).
2. When experiencing an acute anginal attack, he needs to stop his activity and lie down immediately, take one sublingual tablet as soon as possible after the pain begins, remain calm, and rest.
3. If he obtains no relief after taking one sublingual tablet, his handball partner should call 911 immediately and have emergency response personnel take him to the hospital. The emergency response team would be better equipped to help him if further complications (e.g., a myocardial infarction) occur. The patient can take one more tablet while awaiting emergency care and a third tablet 5 minutes later but no more than three tablets total.
4. Beta blockers are most effective in the treatment of typical exertional angina.

## CHAPTER 24

### Heart Failure Drugs

### Chapter Review and NCLEX® Examination Preparation/Critical Thinking and Application

1. c
2. d
3. a
4. b
5. a
6. a, c, d, e, f
7. a, c, e, f
8. d
9. a, b, c, d, e
10. b
11. 2 mL
12.
13. 250 mcg

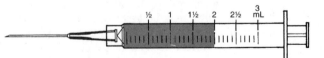

14. Vomiting, headache, fatigue, and dysrhythmia are adverse effects of cardiac glycosides. The presence of a serum potassium level of more than 5 mEq/L, along with these symptoms, means that administration of digoxin immune Fab is indicated for the treatment of severe digoxin toxicity.

15. At this time, nesiritide is generally used in the intensive care setting as a final effort to treat severe, life-threatening heart failure, often in combination with several other cardiostimulatory medications. It is no longer recommended as a first-line drug for heart failure. Instead, it is recommended that its use be strictly limited to treatment of patients with acutely decompensated heart failure who have dyspnea at rest. It should not be used to replace diuretics and should not be used repetitively or to improve renal function.

16. Increased urinary output and decreased dyspnea and fatigue are therapeutic effects of digoxin. The constipation needs to be assessed. Mr. F. should not consume large amounts of bran or other foods high in fiber because the bran will bind to the digitalis and make less of the drug available for absorption.

17. a. Milrinone increases the force of contraction (positive inotropic effect) and relaxes the blood vessels (vasodilation), causing a reduction in afterload, or the force against which the heart must pump to eject its volume.
    b. Additive inotropic effects may be seen with coadministration of digoxin.
    c. Ventricular cardiac dysrhythmias

## Case Study

1. a. Positive inotropic effect: Increases myocardial contractility
   b. Negative chronotropic effect: Decreases heart rate
   c. Negative dromotropic effect: Slows the conduction of electrical impulses in the heart
2. Effects on:
   a. Stroke volume: Increased
   b. Venous blood pressure and vein engorgement: Decreased
   c. Coronary circulation: Increased
   d. Diuresis: Increased because of improved circulation
3. First, complete your assessment by checking her apical pulse, heart and lung sounds, and blood pressure. In addition, check her potassium level because low levels of potassium may lead to digoxin toxicity. If you have not yet given the digoxin dose, hold it and call the physician immediately. Monitor her for signs of digoxin toxicity, especially dangerous dysrhythmias. The digoxin level of 3.5 ng/mL is above the therapeutic range.

## CHAPTER 25

### Antidysrhythmic Drugs

### Chapter Review and NCLEX® Examination Preparation/Critical Thinking and Application
1. d
2. c, d, e
3. a
4. a
5. b
6. d
7. a
8. b
9. b, c, e
10. b
11. 150 mg
12. 2 mL
13. a, (3); b, (1); c, (2)
14. a. Class II antidysrhythmics, or beta blockers, are indicated because they have been shown to significantly reduce the incidence of sudden cardiac death after myocardial infarction.
    b. If Mr. K. had asthma, cardioselective beta blockers would be indicated. Noncardioselective beta blockers block not only the beta₁-adrenergic receptors in the heart but also the beta₂-adrenergic receptors in the lungs. As a result, preexisting asthma could be worsened if a noncardioselective beta blocker is administered.
15. Amiodarone is indicated for the management of life-threatening ventricular tachycardia or ventricular fibrillation that is resistant to other drug therapy. Although it is very effective, amiodarone can penetrate and concentrate in the adipose tissue of any organ in the body, where it may have unwanted effects. It may cause either hypothyroidism or hyperthyroidism, corneal microdeposits, pulmonary toxicity (which is fatal in about 10% of patients), and even dysrhythmias. Amiodarone has a very long half-life, and the side effects may take months to subside.
16. a. Lidocaine must be injected intramuscularly or intravenously; when lidocaine is taken orally, the liver converts most of it to inactive metabolites.
    b. Lidocaine is extensively metabolized in the liver. For patients in liver failure or with a history of cirrhosis, a dosage reduction of 50% is recommended.
17. Alicia should not double up on her medication. The physician needs to be contacted about the missed dose and about Alicia's symptoms of diarrhea and lightheadedness, which are adverse effects of the quinidine.

## Case Study

1. Calcium channel blockers block the slow inward flow of calcium ions into the slow (calcium) channels in cardiac conduction tissue. The conduction effects of these drugs are limited to the atria and the atrioventricular node, where conduction is prolonged and the tissues are made more refractory to stimulation. As a result, they reduce the incidence of paroxysmal supraventricular tachycardia (PSVT). These drugs have little effect on the ventricular tissues.
2. Prevention or reduction of supraventricular rhythms
3. Calcium channel blockers are contraindicated in the presence of pulmonary congestion. A further assessment of his respiratory status must be performed before the medication is started.
4. The physician may prescribe adenosine (Adenocard), which is useful for the treatment of PSVT that has failed to respond to verapamil.

## CHAPTER 26

**Coagulation Modifier Drugs**

### Chapter Review and NCLEX® Examination Preparation/Critical Thinking and Application

1. k
2. n
3. j
4. l
5. m
6. b
7. a, c
8. c
9. i
10. h
11. e
12. g
13. a, c, d
14. b
15. b
16. a
17. c
18. b, c, d, e
19. d
20. c
21. d
22. b
23. b
24. 0.8 mL
25. 7.5 mg (patient weighs 75 kg)
26. Low-molecular-weight heparins (LMWHs) such as enoxaparin are contraindicated in patients with an indwelling epidural catheter. The medication can be given 2 hours after the epidural is removed. This is very important for nurses to remember because giving an LMWH with an epidural has been associated with epidural hematoma.

27. a. The anticoagulant effects of heparin can be reversed with protamine sulfate.
    b. In general, 1 mg of protamine sulfate can reverse the effects of 100 units of heparin.
    c. The activated partial thromboplastin time (aPTT) is the test most commonly used.
28. a. Vitamin K
    b. Current recommendations are to use the lowest amount of vitamin K possible based on the clinical situation.
    c. After the use of vitamin K for warfarin toxicity, warfarin resistance will occur for up to 7 days; thus the patient cannot be anticoagulated by warfarin during this period. In such cases, either heparin or an LMWH may need to be added to provide adequate anticoagulation if necessary.
29. The physician will probably prescribe one of the antifibrinolytic drugs, which are used to stop excessive oozing from surgical sites, such as chest tubes.
30. Desmopressin is used in patients with type I von Willebrand's disease; it increases the levels of clotting factor VIII.
31. The alteplase can be readministered because it has a very short half-life of 5 minutes. Because of its short half-life, it is given along with heparin to prevent reocclusion of the infarcted blood vessel.
32. a. They are possible indications of bleeding problems related to the anticoagulation therapy.
    b. Ursula might also be exhibiting a change in pulse rate or rhythm, blood pressure, or level of consciousness.
    c. The nurse will notify the physician immediately. She must not administer any other anticoagulants; if Ursula is receiving a continuous infusion of an anticoagulant, she must stop the infusion. The nurse will take Ursula's vital signs and stay with her. She will prepare to administer the appropriate antidote.
33. Heparin is commonly used for deep vein thrombosis prophylaxis in a dose of 5000 units two or three times a day given subcutaneously and does not need to be monitored when used for prophylaxis.

## Case Study

1. Use of aspirin is contraindicated in the presence of peptic ulcer disease. Doug has been started on the clopidogrel therapy to reduce the risk for stroke.
2. He should be taught to watch for signs of abnormal bleeding and should immediately report any of the following signs and symptoms to the health care provider: respiratory difficulty, back pain, skin rash, evidence of gastrointestinal bleeding, any other bleeding abnormality, diarrhea, acute severe headache, and change in vision (blurred vision or loss of vision).

3. He needs to take measures to prevent bleeding, such as using a soft toothbrush and an electric razor, and should take great care when trimming his nails, gardening, and participating in rough or contact sports. He needs to take precautions to protect himself from injury and subsequent bleeding or bruising, which can be extremely dangerous while he is taking antiplatelet drugs.
4. Herbal products that contain St. John's wort, garlic, ginger, ginseng, and ginkgo should be avoided because they have anticoagulant properties.

## CHAPTER 27

### Antilipemic Drugs

### Chapter Review and NCLEX® Examination Preparation/Critical Thinking and Application
1. d
2. a, c, d, e
3. a
4. b
5. d
6. c
7. a
8. a, b, e
9. a, c, d, e
10. c
11. 1.5 tablets
12. 750 mg per dose; 3 tablets per dose
13. a. Fibric acid derivative—it is believed that these drugs work by activating the lipoprotein lipase, an enzyme responsible for the breakdown of cholesterol.
    b. Lipid-lowering drug and vitamin—exact mechanism unknown; beneficial effects are believed to be related to its ability to inhibit lipolysis in adipose tissue, decrease esterification of triglycerides in the liver, and increase the activity of lipase.
    c. HMG–CoA reductase inhibitor—reduces blood cholesterol by decreasing the rate of cholesterol production
    d. Bile acid sequestrant—binds bile, preventing the resorption of the bile acids from the small intestine. The insoluble bile acid and resin (drug) complex that is formed is excreted in the feces.
14. Unless Mr. H. has additional risk factors, his high level of low-density lipoprotein (LDL) cholesterol alone does not warrant drug therapy at this time. He will be recommended for dietary therapy with an LDL goal of less than 160 mg/dL. All reasonable nonpharmacologic means of controlling Mr. H.'s LDL level need to be tried and found to fail before he is given drug therapy. Mr. H. needs to find time in his busy schedule to exercise and eat more wisely. See Table 27-3.
15. Mrs. K. is probably experiencing constipation and either belching or increased flatulence associated with cholestyramine use (she may also be experiencing heartburn, nausea, and bloating). Mrs. K. requires extra patient teaching and support to help her maintain compliance with the drug therapy; she should be assured that these adverse effects will probably diminish over time.
16. No. Justus is not a candidate for niacin therapy because niacin use is contraindicated in patients with peptic ulcer. Also, when niacin is taken with an HMG–CoA reductase inhibitor, the likelihood of myopathy development is greatly increased, although it is not uncommon to see these drugs used together.
17. Mrs. N. must take her antihypertensive and cholestyramine (Questran) at different times of the day because the bile acid sequestrant may interfere significantly with the absorption of other drugs taken at the same time. All other drugs should be taken at least 1 hour before or 4 to 6 hours after the administration of antilipemics.

### Case Study
1. No, he is not right. Dietary measures are a part of antilipemic therapy. Nonpharmacologic measures include consumption of a low-fat, low-cholesterol diet; supervised, moderate exercise; weight loss; cessation of smoking and drinking; and relaxation therapy.
2. This drug is used primarily to lower total and LDL cholesterol levels and triglyceride levels; it has been shown to raise the high-density lipoprotein (HDL) level as well.
3. Elevations in liver enzyme levels may also occur, and the patient will be monitored for excessive elevations, which may indicate the need for alternative drug therapy. In addition, total cholesterol level, LDL-to-HDL ratio, and triglyceride levels need to be monitored to evaluate therapeutic effect.
4. Myopathy (muscle pain) is an uncommon but clinically important side effect that may occur in some patients taking statins. It may progress to a serious condition known as *rhabdomyolysis* in which the breakdown of muscle protein occurs, leading to myoglobinuria and possible renal damage. Patients receiving statin therapy need to be taught to report unexplained muscle pain to their health care providers immediately.

## CHAPTER 28

### Diuretic Drugs

### Chapter Review and NCLEX® Examination Preparation/Critical Thinking and Application
1. c
2. f
3. e

**189**

**Answer Key**

4. i
5. g
6. j
7. h
8. a
9. d
10. b
11. a, c, d, e
12. c
13. a
14. d
15. b
16. a
17. a
18. d
19. b, e
20. 15 mL

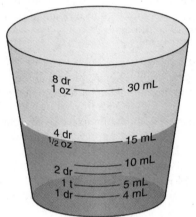

21. 150 mL (hint: 20% indicates 20 g per 100 mL)

$$\frac{20\,g}{100\,ml} = \frac{30\,g}{x\,mL}$$

(20 g)(x mL) = (100 mL)(30 g); 20x = 3000;
x = 150 mL
(See Overview of Dosage Calculations, Section III.)

22. a. Ms. A. was probably prescribed a carbonic anhydrase inhibitor (CAI).
   b. An undesirable effect of the CAIs is that they elevate the blood glucose level, causing glycosuria in diabetic patients. They may also interact with some oral antidiabetic drugs.

23. a. For mannitol to be effective in treating acute renal failure, enough renal blood flow and glomerular filtration must exist to enable the drug to reach the tubules.
   b. Mannitol is always administered intravenously through a filter because it can crystallize when exposed to low temperatures (which is more likely to occur when concentrations exceed 15%). In addition, inspect the fluid container visually for precipitants.
   c. Arthur's headache and chills are probably side effects of the mannitol therapy. At this time, the therapy should be continued, but Arthur needs to be monitored for the development of more serious adverse effects.

24. a. Mr. F. will probably be prescribed spironolactone in high doses; this drug is often used for the treatment of ascites associated with cirrhosis of the liver.
   b. His serum potassium level will need to be monitored frequently because he has impaired renal function. The spironolactone may cause hyperkalemia.

25. a. Impotence and decreased libido are among the side effects of thiazide. Brendan is possibly experiencing these effects.
   b. He needs to stop eating licorice because consuming it can lead to an additive hypokalemia in patients taking thiazide. Brendan's fatigue may be the result of severe hypokalemia and will be evaluated.

26. It is likely that Mrs. H.'s neighbor was prescribed one of the potassium-sparing diuretics and thus was not instructed to eat additional potassium-rich foods. Mrs. H. needs to follow the dietary recommendations provided for her, not for her neighbor.

27. Loop diuretics have a distinct advantage over thiazide diuretics in that their diuretic action continues even when creatinine clearance decreases below 25 mL/min. This means that even when kidney function diminishes, loop diuretics can still work. As renal function decreases, the efficacy of thiazides diminishes because delivery of the drug to the site of activity is impaired. Thiazides are not to be used if creatinine clearance is less than 30 to 50 mL/min. Normal creatinine clearance is 125 mL/min, depending on age of the patient. However, metolazone remains effective to a creatinine clearance of 10 mL/min and thus can be used in cases of renal failure.

## Case Study

1. These symptoms suggest hypokalemia. Furosemide causes potassium to be excreted along with sodium and water.
2. She could have eaten foods high in potassium, including bananas, oranges, apricots, dates, raisins, broccoli, green beans, potatoes, tomatoes, meats, fish, wheat bread, and legumes.
3. Spironolactone is a potassium-sparing diuretic; it causes sodium and water to be excreted, but potassium is retained.
4. The use of angiotensin-converting enzyme inhibitors or potassium supplements in combination with potassium-sparing diuretics can result in hyperkalemia. When taken together, lithium and potassium-sparing diuretics can result in lithium toxicity. The use of nonsteroidal antiinflammatory drugs with potassium-sparing diuretics can reduce the effectiveness of the diuretics.

## CHAPTER 29

**Fluids and Electrolytes**

**Chapter Review and NCLEX® Examination Preparation/Critical Thinking and Application**

1. a, b, d, e
2. c
3. d
4. c
5. b
6. b
7. b
8. a
9. d
10. b
11. a. 42 mL/hr
    b. 11 gtt/min (rounded up from 10.5) (See the Overview of Dosage Calculations, Section V.)
12. 100 mL/hr (50 mL : 0.5 hr :: $x$ mL : 1 hr; $x$ = 100 mL/hr)
13. **Advantages:** Crystalloids are less expensive than colloids and blood products for replacing fluids and better for emergency short-term plasma volume expansion. They also promote urinary flow. They do not carry the risk for transmission of viral diseases or anaphylaxis and do not promote bleeding.
    **Disadvantages:** The fluids can leak out of the plasma into the tissues and cells, which results in edema (e.g., peripheral edema or pulmonary edema). They may dilute plasma proteins, resulting in lower colloid oncotic pressure (COP), and dilute erythrocyte concentration, resulting in decreased oxygen tension. Large volumes are needed to be effective, but prolonged infusions and administration of large volumes may worsen acidosis or alkalosis. Last, their effects are relatively short-lived compared with those of colloids.
14. a. Blood products
    b. They are the only fluids that contain hemoglobin.
    c. They are natural products that require human donors, which means that they can be incompatible with a recipient's immune system. These products can also transmit pathogens from the donor to the recipient.
15. Tanya is exhibiting early symptoms of hypokalemia. Initial treatment will include potassium supplements, either intravenous or oral, until the laboratory results return to normal. At home, she needs to eat foods high in potassium, such as bananas, oranges, apricots, dates, raisins, broccoli, green beans, potatoes, tomatoes, meats, fish, wheat bread, and legumes. In addition, she will need therapy to address her eating disorder issues.

16. a. Hyponatremia
    b. Vomiting is a possible adverse effect of oral administration of sodium chloride; if vomiting occurs, he needs to be careful about monitoring for further fluid and electrolyte loss.
17. a. Signs of transfusion reaction include apprehension, restlessness, flushed skin, increased pulse and respiration rate, dyspnea, rash, joint or lower back pain, swelling, fever and chills, nausea, weakness, and jaundice.
    b. Although it is possible for pathogens such as that causing acquired immunodeficiency syndrome (AIDS) to be transmitted via blood products, reassure Victor's wife that techniques are now used that have drastically reduced the incidence of such problems.
    c. Victor's restlessness and increased pulse are signs of a reaction to the blood product. The nurse will stop the transfusion immediately and change the infusion to normal saline. The nurse will stay with Victor and assess his vital signs and have another nurse notify the physician immediately; the facility's protocol for transfusion reactions will be followed.

**Case Study**

1. The normal total protein level is in the range of 7.4 g/dL. If the level drops below 5.3 g/dL, the COP becomes less than the hydrostatic pressure, and fluid shifts into the tissues, which results in edema.
2. The albumin will increase the COP and move fluid from outside the blood vessels to inside the blood vessels, thus reducing the edema.
3. Colloids such as albumin are the choice for this patient. Crystalloids can leak out of the plasma into the tissues and cells, resulting in edema anywhere in the body. Crystalloids also dilute the proteins in the plasma, further reducing the COP. Finally, crystalloids are more likely to cause edema because of the larger volumes needed to achieve the desired clinical effect. Colloids reduce edema and expand plasma volume by pulling fluid from the extravascular space into the blood vessels.
4. Colloids can alter the coagulation system, which results in impaired coagulation and possibly bleeding. They have no oxygen-carrying ability and contain no clotting factors, and they may also dilute the plasma protein concentration, which may impair the function of platelets.

## CHAPTER 30

## Pituitary Drugs

### Chapter Review and NCLEX® Examination Preparation/Critical Thinking and Application

1. a. Glucocorticoids, mineralocorticoids, androgens
   b. Cosyntropin
   c. Regulates anabolic processes related to growth and adaptation to stressors; promotes skeletal and muscle growth; increases protein synthesis; increases liver glycogenolysis; increases fat mobilization
   d. Somatropin and somatrem
   e. Antidiuretic hormone
   f. Vasopressin and desmopressin
   g. Promotes uterine contractions
   h. Pitocin
2. d
3. c
4. b
5. a
6. c
7. a
8. a
9. d
10. a. The total dose per week for this child (44 lb = 20 kg) is 6 mg.
    b. Dose per injection (6 daily injections) = 1 mg per dose per day for 6 days
11. 0.5 mL

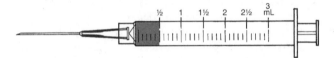

12. In addition to information about proper subcutaneous injection techniques, the teaching plan needs to include a reminder of the dosage form and amount, the importance of compliance with therapy, and keeping the follow-up appointments. The nurse will show the parents how to keep a journal of Patricia's growth measurements.
13. Cosyntropin (Cortrosyn) is used for the diagnosis of adrenocortical insufficiency, not for treatment. After a diagnosis is made, the actual drug treatment generally involves replacement hormonal therapy using drug forms of the deficient corticosteroid hormones.

### Case Study

1. Vasopressin or desmopressin
2. Vasopressin should be given cautiously in patients with migraine headaches, seizures, cardiovascular disease, renal disease, and asthma.
3. Treatment will be injections, either intramuscular or subcutaneous, two to four times a day. This drug therapy will increase water resorption in the distal tubules and collecting ducts of the nephron, performing all the physiologic functions of antidiuretic hormone. As a result, water excretion is diminished.
4. Therapy should eliminate his severe thirst and decrease his urinary output.

## CHAPTER 31

## Thyroid and Antithyroid Drugs

### Critical Thinking Crossword
*Across*
3. Secondary
6. Thyroxine
7. Primary

*Down*
1. Levothyroxine
2. Hyperthyroidism
4. Propylthiouracil
5. Tertiary
6. Thyrotropin

### Chapter Review and NCLEX® Examination Preparation/Critical Thinking and Application

1. c
2. d
3. a
4. a, c, d
5. c
6. d
7. a
8. b
9. b
10. 0.088 mg
11. 1.5 mL
12. Mrs. W. probably has hypothyroidism, which may result in the formation of a goiter, an enlargement of the thyroid gland resulting from its overstimulation by elevated levels of thyroid-stimulating hormone. She may benefit from one of the thyroid drugs, including synthyroid, levothyroxine, liothyronine, or liotrix. Levothyroxine is generally preferred because, as a chemically pure formulation of 100% thyroxine, its hormonal content is standardized; therefore its effect is predictable.
13. Surgery to remove all or part of the thyroid gland is an effective way to treat hyperthyroidism, but as a result, lifelong hormone replacement is normally required.
14. There are two errors. (1) Levothyroxine is dosed in micrograms. A common medication error is to write the intended dose in milligrams instead of micrograms. If not caught, this error would result in a 1000-fold overdose. Doses higher than 200 mcg must be questioned in case this error occurred. (2) The route is not written. This drug would be administered orally.

15. The most damaging or serious adverse effects of propylthiouracil (PTU) medications are liver and bone marrow toxicity. Therefore it is important to assess liver function studies and a complete blood count (white blood cells, red blood cells, platelets). In addition, PTU is rated as a pregnancy category D drug; a pregnancy test will be needed.

## Case Study

1. Her symptoms suggest hypothyroidism, and a thyroid replacement hormone, such as levothyroxine, would be indicated for this condition.
2. The thyroid preparations are given to replace what the thyroid gland cannot itself produce to achieve normal thyroid levels, known as a "euthyroid" condition.
3. Thyroid preparations need to be taken at the same time every day to maintain constant blood levels. Taking the medication in the morning will help reduce problems with insomnia, which may result when the medication is taken later in the day or in the evening.

## CHAPTER 32

### Antidiabetic Drugs

### Chapter Review and NCLEX® Examination Preparation/Critical Thinking and Application

1. b
2. d
3. a
4. c
5. a
6. a
7. d
8. b
9. b
10. d
11. b
12. d
13. 4 units (238 − 150 = 88 ÷ 20 = 4.4). (The answer is 4 because 20 divides into 88 four whole times. The "leftover" 8 does not add up to 20, so it does not count toward the insulin dose.)
14. 37 units

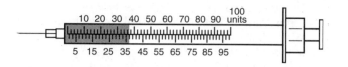

15. a. Pramlintide, an incretin mimetic, given by subcutaneous injection, works by mimicking the action of the natural pancreatic hormone amylin. Amylin is secreted along with insulin in response to food intake and influences postmeal glucose levels by slowing gastric emptying, suppressing glucagon secretion (which reduces the liver's glucose output), and increasing the sense of satiety. As a result, blood glucose levels are reduced.
   b. Metformin works primarily by inhibiting hepatic glucose production and increasing the sensitivity of peripheral tissue to insulin, thus lowering blood glucose levels.
16. a. Confusion, irritability, tremor, and sweating
   b. The brain needs a constant amount of glucose to function; thus the central nervous system manifestations of hypoglycemia (e.g., irritability and confusion) are often the first to appear.
   c. In the conscious person, oral forms of glucose are used, such as rapidly dissolving buccal tablets or semisolid gel forms designed for rapid mucosal absorption. She could also try corn syrup, honey, fruit juice, a nondiet soft drink, or a small snack such as crackers or half a sandwich.
17. a. The graduate nurse will check the order at least three times and then have another licensed nurse check the prepared injection to be sure it is in accordance with the prescriber's order. These second checks may vary with facilities.
   b. The graduate nurse's coworker is right. Novolin-R is regular insulin, and regular insulin is clear.
   c. If left at room temperature, the insulin in the vial must be discarded after 1 month.
18. Mrs. F. needs to make some significant lifestyle changes. She must stop smoking, lose weight, and exercise regularly, which will help with both the high blood glucose level and the hypertension. The American Diabetes Association also recommends that, in addition to lifestyle changes, the oral biguanide drug metformin (Glucophage) be started as initial therapy for lowering blood glucose levels.
19. a. Disulfiram-type reaction
   b. In addition to assessing vital signs, assess his blood glucose level immediately.
   c. Dennis may have been drinking alcohol. Sulfonylureas may interact with alcohol in a way that is similar to the interaction with disulfiram, which is used to deter alcohol ingestion in people with chronic alcoholism. This *disulfiram-type* reaction includes vomiting and hypertension. In addition, the alcohol taken with the sulfonylurea may enhance the action of the antidiabetic drug, causing increased hypoglycemia.

20. If the patient receiving metformin is to undergo diagnostic studies with contrast dye, the prescriber will need to discontinue the drug on the day of the test and restart it 48 hours after the tests. It may be necessary to reevaluate the patient's renal status.
21. a. Hypoglycemia
    b. Hyperglycemia
    c. Hyperglycemia
    d. Hypoglycemia
    e. Hypoglycemia

## Case Study

1. Glipizide works best if given 30 minutes before meals. This allows the timing of the insulin secretion induced by the glipizide to correspond with the elevation in blood glucose level induced by the meal in much the same way as endogenous insulin levels are raised in a person without diabetes. Its effect is much like the body's normal response to meals and will help to keep the blood glucose levels from becoming too high.
2. To provide a picture of the patient's adherence to the therapy regimen for the previous several months, hemoglobin A1C is measured. This value reflects how well the patient has been doing with diet and drug therapy.
3. Mr. D. should contact his provider immediately. He may require a change in his diabetic treatment while he is sick because vomiting and inability to eat can cause a change in his blood glucose levels. If he is unable to eat and yet takes the glipizide, he is at risk for experiencing severe hypoglycemia.

## CHAPTER 33

### Adrenal Drugs

#### Chapter Review and NCLEX® Examination Preparation/Critical Thinking and Application

1. a
2. c
3. a, b, c
4. b
5. d
6. c
7. b
8. b, c, e
9. b
10. 1/2 tablet
11. 3.2 mg per dose
12. Ms. R.'s glucocorticoid can interact with aspirin and other nonsteroidal antiinflammatory drugs (NSAIDs), producing additive effects and increasing the chance of gastric ulcer development. Also, she must avoid people with infections because her own immune system is suppressed. The children in the hospital may have infections. In addition, she needs to report any fever, increased weakness and lethargy, or sore throat.
13. a. The use of systemic glucocorticoids with anti-diabetic drugs may reduce the hypoglycemic effect of those drugs. Determine a baseline blood glucose level and monitor Peter for any problems.
    b. Oral dosage forms must be taken with milk or food to minimize gastrointestinal upset. Another option is for the provider to order a histamine-2 receptor antagonist or proton pump inhibitor to prevent ulcer formation (glucocorticoids may cause gastric ulcers). Patients must be instructed not to take the drug with alcohol, aspirin, or other NSAIDs to minimize gastric irritation and the chance for gastric bleeding.
14. The nurse should intervene. The student nurse needs to wear clean (nonsterile) gloves when applying the medication with a sterile tongue depressor or cotton-tipped applicator if the skin is intact. If the skin is not intact, a sterile technique should be used.
15. In addition to routine teaching about metered-dose inhaler administration technique, the nurse will instruct Nina to rinse out her mouth with lukewarm water after each use of the inhaler to prevent the development of an oral fungal infection.

## Case Study

1. One very important point about corticosteroids is that they must not be stopped abruptly. These drugs require a tapering of the daily dose because the administration of these drugs causes the endogenous (body's own) production of the hormones to stop. This is referred to as *hepato-pituitary-adrenal* or *adrenal suppression*. This suppression places the patient at risk for developing hypoadrenal crisis (shock, circulatory collapse) in times of increased stress (i.e., surgery, trauma). Tapering of daily doses allows the HPA axis the time to recover and to start stimulating the normal production of the endogenous hormones.
2. Short- or long-term therapy may cause steroid psychosis. In addition, long-term effects cause cushingoid symptoms, including moon face, weight gain, muscle wasting, and increased deposition of fat in the trunk area, leading to truncal obesity. (See Table 33-4.)
3. Oral contraceptives may increase the half-life of adrenal drugs. The prescriber will consider this when establishing the dose. She needs to be instructed not to use the NSAID ibuprofen while taking the prednisone because taking these drugs together may cause additive gastrointestinal effects and an increased chance of gastric ulcer development.
4. The best time is early in the morning (6:00 AM to 9:00 AM) because this follows the normal diurnal pattern of endogenous corticosteroid secretion and results in the least amount of adrenal suppression.

## CHAPTER 34

**Women's Health Drugs**

**Chapter Review and NCLEX® Examination Preparation/Critical Thinking and Application**
1. b, c, e
2. a
3. b
4. a
5. b
6. b
7. c, e, f
8. a, d
9. a
10. 1.3 mL (1.25 rounds to 1.3)

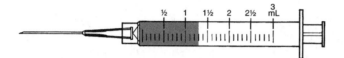

11. 10 mL
12. a. The nurse will ask Isabelle if she is taking medication for her depression. Estrogen therapy is indicated for the symptoms of menopause, but the use of estrogen with a tricyclic antidepressant may result in toxicity of the latter drug.
    b. The smallest dose of estrogen that alleviates the symptoms is used for the shortest possible time.
13. a. The nurse practitioner will probably prescribe medroxyprogesterone, which is indicated for the treatment of secondary amenorrhea.
    b. The progestin may cause a decrease in glucose tolerance when given with antidiabetic drugs. Ms. K. will need to carefully monitor her blood glucose levels.
14. a. Perhaps Jacklyn's prescription could be switched to a 28-day form of Ortho-Novum, which is taken for all 28 days of the menstrual cycle rather than for 3 weeks with 1 week off.
    b. One of the benefits of oral contraceptive use is decreased blood loss during menstruation.
15. These drugs work to promote fertility in two different ways. Clomiphene is given to cause ovarian follicle maturation. Choriogonadotropin alfa is then given to stimulate the rupture of the mature follicles and to develop the corpus luteum, which supports early pregnancy.
16. Mrs. I. needs to know that smoking can diminish the therapeutic effects of the estrogen she is taking and add to the risk for thrombosis. Also, she should be cautioned to wear sunscreen while in Aruba because estrogen makes the skin more susceptible to sunburn.
17. Mrs. S. is assuming that the medication is estrogen therapy. Alendronate (Fosamax) is indicated to prevent osteoporosis in postmenopausal women. The nurse will need to explain to her that it is a nonestrogen, nonhormonal medication used for prevention of bone loss in the postmenopausal period.
18. Megestrol is used in the management of anorexia, cachexia, or unexplained substantial weight loss in patients with acquired immunodeficiency syndrome (AIDS). In addition, it may be used to stimulate appetite and promote weight gain in patients (male or female) with cancer.

**Case Study**
1. It is essential to perform a pregnancy test to rule out pregnancy before J.Q. begins the oral contraceptive.
2. Smoking would increase J.Q.'s risk for thromboembolic events if she begins oral contraceptives that contain estrogen. In addition, the smoking may reduce the estrogenic effects. In addition, assess for a history of thromboembolic events such as myocardial infarction, venous thrombosis, pulmonary embolism, or stroke.
3. Oral contraceptive hormones must be taken at the same time every day and exactly as prescribed. If one dose is missed, advise the patient to take the dose as soon as it is remembered; however, if it is close to the next dose time, advise the patient not to double up and to use a backup form of contraception in these situations. Provide more specific instructions regarding the omission of more than one pill or 1 day's dose depending on the specific oral contraceptive drug prescribed.

CHAPTER 35

**Men's Health Drugs**

**Chapter Review and NCLEX® Examination Preparation/Critical Thinking and Application**
1. b
2. b, d, f
3. a
4. d
5. c
6. b
7. c
8. a
9. d
10. a, b, e
11. a. The nurse should use the 200-mg/mL strength. Using the 100-mg/mL strength would require 3 mL, which may require two separate injections.
    b. The nurse will administer 1.5 mL of the 200-mg/mL strength.

12. a. Testosterone's poor performance in the oral dosage form is a result of the fact that most of a dose is metabolized and destroyed by the liver before it can reach the circulation.

b. Methyltestosterone (Android) and fluoxymesterone (Halotestin) are both testosterone derivatives that are effective when given orally or buccally with the methyltestosterone.

c. With either drug, contraindications that could apply to Mr. M. include significant cardiac, hepatic, or renal disease; male breast cancer; genital bleeding; or prostate cancer.

13. a. No. The manufacturer's guidelines suggest that the patient not swallow, chew, or eat the buccal tablet but that it be completely absorbed in the mouth. The part of the drug that is swallowed will not reach the intended site of action because of heavy first-pass metabolism.

b. Patients taking any hormone-related drug should never abruptly stop the drug. The prescriber may consider whether a transdermal form is suitable for Mr. M.

14. With finasteride, education about the drug's therapeutic effects and adverse effects should be provided at the patient's educational level. Female family members, significant others, and caregivers who are pregnant or of childbearing age should be educated about the need to avoid exposure during handling of this drug, including *not* touching any broken or crushed tablets, which could result in exposure to the drug and the risk for teratogenic effects. Wearing gloves is recommended. Finasteride may be given orally without regard to meals. It should be protected from exposure to light and heat.

15. The Testoderm patch is applied only to the scrotal skin. The skin should be clean, dry scrotal skin that has been shaved for optimal skin contact. These patches are replaced every day. Androderm patches should be applied to clean, dry skin on the back, abdomen, upper arms, or thighs; the scrotum and bony areas (shoulder, hip) should be avoided. These patches are often ordered to be changed every 7 days. AndroGel is applied to the shoulders, arms, or abdominal skin daily.

## Case Study

1. Sildenafil (Viagra) is contraindicated in patients with cardiovascular disorders and is contraindicated if the patient is taking nitrates because of the potential for severe hypotensive effects.

2. Headache, flushing, and dyspepsia are the most common adverse effects reported. Priapism, an abnormally prolonged penile erection, is a rare occurrence, but if it occurs, it is a medical emergency, and he needs to seek care immediately. In addition, he should report any visual changes immediately.

3. Older individuals experience declining liver function, so drugs may not be metabolized as effectively as when they were younger. A decreased dosage of sildenafil is generally indicated for patients older than 65 years of age and for those with liver or renal impairment. In addition, there have been reports of vision loss in men who have been taking this class of drugs.

4. Sildenafil should be taken 1 hour before intercourse and no more than once a day.

## CHAPTER 36

### Antihistamines, Decongestants, Antitussives, and Expectorants

**Chapter Review and NCLEX® Examination Preparation/Critical Thinking and Application**

1. a, b, c, e
2. a
3. b, e
4. c
5. b
6. d
7. b, d, e
8. c
9. c
10. b
11. a. 15 mL (See Overview of Dosage Calculations, Section II.)

b.

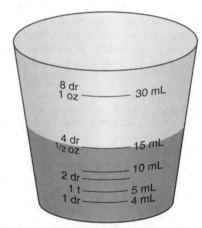

12. 2.5 mL
13. No. Mrs. L. is likely experiencing rebound congestion caused by sustained use of the naphazoline for several days.
14. Keith is exhibiting symptoms of the cardiovascular effects that can occur when a topically applied adrenergic nasal decongestant is absorbed into the bloodstream. Usually the amount absorbed is too small to cause systemic effects at normal dosages. Excessive dosages of these medications, however, are more likely to cause systemic effects elsewhere in the body. These may include cardiovascular effects such as hypertension and palpitations and central nervous system (CNS) effects such as headache, nervousness, and dizziness. These systemic

effects are the result of alpha-adrenergic stimulation of the heart, blood vessels, and CNS.

15. Benzonatate's mechanism of action is entirely different from that of the other drugs. It suppresses the cough reflex by numbing the stretch receptors, which keeps the cough reflex from being stimulated in the medulla. It is associated with fewer drug interactions than the opioid antitussives and dextromethorphan.

16. The nurse will ask Irene whether she is taking any thyroid medication or whether she has cardiac disease, glaucoma, or hypertension. A drug interaction can occur if she takes dextromethorphan (an antitussive) with an antithyroid drug. The other conditions listed are contraindications. Irene should call her health care provider before she goes to the drugstore.

17. First, Lisa's brother received Robitussin A-C, an opioid antitussive containing codeine, for his cough. Lisa has been prescribed Robitussin, an expectorant, for her nonproductive cough associated with bronchitis. Second, even if the two children were prescribed the same drug, Lisa is only 5 years old and requires a smaller dosage than her brother. Prescription medications should not be shared among family members.

18. Antihistamines should generally be used with caution in lactating mothers. The decision will be made by weighing the drug's potential effect on the baby versus the need for her to take the medication.

## Case Study

1. James's diabetes should not affect his treatment.
2. The topical diphenhydramine might come in combination with a drug such as calamine, camphor, or zinc oxide.
3. He should be informed that taking any of the sedating antihistamines may cause drowsiness, so he should be instructed to avoid driving or operating heavy machinery if these side effects occur or until he knows how he responds to the medication.
4. James should also be informed not to consume alcohol or take other CNS depressants because they may interact with the diphenhydramine to exacerbate drowsiness and sedation.

## CHAPTER 37

### Respiratory Drugs

### Chapter Review and NCLEX® Examination Preparation/Critical Thinking and Application

1. b, d, e, f
2. d
3. b
4. a
5. c

6. b
7. b
8. a
9. a, b
10. After 25 days (8 puffs per day, divided into 200 doses)
11. 3.6 mg
12. Tom is exhibiting some side effects of theophylline therapy, and the level in his blood is too high (the common therapeutic range for theophylline is a blood level of 10 to 20 mcg/dL). It is likely that the dosage will be decreased.
13. Sylvia is exhibiting dose-related adverse effects of the albuterol. If Sylvia is now using the albuterol more frequently as a rescue inhaler, the health care provider will need to review and adjust her medication regimen.
14. a. Anticholinergics, corticosteroids, and beta agonists
    b. Of concern is Mrs. V.'s glaucoma. Anticholinergics are to be used cautiously in patients with acute narrow-angle glaucoma.
15. a. The disadvantage of administering the corticosteroids orally is that they can then lead to systemic effects, such as increased susceptibility to infection, fluid and electrolyte disturbances, endocrine effects, dermatologic effects, and nervous system effects. They can also interact with other systemically administered drugs. The advantage of administering corticosteroids by inhalation is that they are delivered directly to the site of action—the lungs. This generally limits, but does not completely prevent, systemic effects.
    b. The use of an inhaled corticosteroid frequently allows for a reduction in the daily dose of the systemic corticosteroid. This reduction should be gradual to prevent Addisonian crisis because of suppression of the adrenal gland.
16. Albuterol is a beta agonist that can be used to treat acute bronchospasms. Fluticasone is a corticosteroid and is not effective for acute bronchospasm. Fluticasone is useful for long-term management of asthma and works to reduce inflammation.
17. He needs to be reminded to avoid foods and beverages that contain caffeine (e.g., chocolate, coffee, cola, cocoa, tea) because their consumption can exacerbate central nervous system stimulation.

## Case Study

1. Montelukast, a leukotriene receptor antagonist, works to reduce the inflammatory response in the lungs but does not have the adverse effects that corticosteroids have.
2. Leukotriene receptor antagonists are primarily used for prophylaxis and chronic management of asthma and are not appropriate for treatment of acute asthma attacks; however, they should decrease the frequency of the attacks.

3. You should tell Jennie that she needs to check with her health care provider before taking any over-the-counter medications.
4. These drugs should be taken every night on a continuous schedule even if symptoms improve.

## CHAPTER 38

### Antibiotics Part 1

### Critical Thinking Crossword
*Across*
3. Prophylactic
6. Tetracycline
7. Penicillin
8. Bactericidal
9. Cephalosporin
*Down*
1. Macrolide
2. Sulfonamide
4. Bacteriostatic
5. Superinfection

### Chapter Review and NCLEX® Examination Preparation/Critical Thinking and Application
1. b, d, e
2. a
3. b
4. c
5. d
6. d
7. c
8. b
9. b, c, d
10. 25 mL per dose. Each dose will contain 500,000 units (every 6 hours will be 4 doses per day; divide 2 million units per day by 4 to get 500,000 units per dose). (See Overview of Dosage Calculations, Section III.)
11. 10 mL
12. Imipenem–cilastatin (Primaxin) does contain two drugs, but one of the drugs (cilastatin) works to prevent the antibiotic (imipenem) from being destroyed by bacterial enzymes that can make the antibiotic ineffective.
13. Cefoxitin (Mefoxin) is frequently used in patients undergoing abdominal surgeries because it can effectively kill intestinal bacteria, including anaerobic bacteria.
14. a. Sean must not take doxycycline with milk because that can result in a significant reduction in the absorption of the drug. Also, Sean needs to be aware that tetracyclines can cause photosensitivity; he needs to avoid direct exposure to sunlight and use sunscreen or protective clothing.
    b. The diarrhea is probably the result of alteration of the intestinal flora caused by the drug therapy.

15. She is experiencing a superinfection because the antibiotics she has been taking for bronchitis have reduced the normal vaginal bacterial flora, and the yeast that is usually kept in balance by this normal flora has an opportunity to grow and cause an infection.

## Case Study
1. He needs to be assessed for renal problems and blood dyscrasias. Also, the use of co-trimoxazole is contraindicated in cases of known drug allergy to sulfonamides or chemically related drugs such as sulfonylureas (used for diabetes), thiazide and loop diuretics, and carbonic anhydrase inhibitors.
2. If he is taking a sulfonylurea for his type 2 diabetes, close monitoring is needed because sulfonamides can potentiate the hypoglycemic effects of sulfonylureas in patients with diabetes. In addition, although he is currently receiving intravenous heparin and not warfarin, he may be switched to oral anticoagulants soon, so keep in mind that sulfonamides can potentiate the anticoagulant effects of warfarin and lead to hemorrhage.
3. These antibiotics achieve very high concentrations in the kidneys, through which they are eliminated. Therefore they are primarily used in the treatment of urinary tract infections.
4. Sulfonamides do not actually destroy bacteria but inhibit their growth. For this reason, they are considered bacteriostatic antibiotics. Bactericidal antibiotics kill bacteria.

## CHAPTER 39

### Antibiotics Part 2

### Chapter Review and NCLEX® Examination Preparation/Critical Thinking and Application
1. c
2. b
3. a
4. a, b, c
5. c
6. c
7. a, b, e
8. b, c, d
9. d
10. 40 mL (See Overview of Dosage Calculations, Section II.)
11. 187.5 mg
12. The current practice is once-a-day aminoglycoside dosing. The nurse can tell her that studies have shown that once-daily dosing provides a sufficient plasma drug concentration to kill bacteria and has either an equal or lower risk for toxicity compared with multiple daily dosing. Hopefully, this type of dosing will be safer and more effective for her.

13. A blood sample for measurement of "trough" level is drawn at least 8 to 12 hours after completion of dose administration. The therapeutic goal is a trough level at or below 1 mcg/mL. If the trough level is above 2 mcg/mL, then the patient is at greater risk for ototoxicity and nephrotoxicity. Trough levels are normally monitored initially and then once every 5 to 7 days until the drug therapy is discontinued. The patient's serum creatinine level will also be measured at least every 3 days as an index of renal function, and drug dosages will be adjusted as needed for any changes in renal function.

14. Yes. In patients who receive amiodarone therapy, dangerous cardiac dysrhythmias are more likely to occur when quinolones are taken. Hopefully, another drug besides levofloxacin has shown effectiveness against the bacteria that is causing his infection.

15. Nitrofurantoin is used primarily to treat urinary tract infections because it is renally excreted and concentrates in the urine.

## Case Study

1. You will monitor for ototoxicity and nephrotoxicity. Symptoms of ototoxicity include dizziness, tinnitus, and hearing loss. Symptoms of nephrotoxicity include urinary casts, proteinuria, and increased blood urea nitrogen and serum creatinine levels. Monitoring the drug's trough levels and renal function studies can help prevent those toxicities.

2. The aminoglycosides and penicillins are often used together because they have a synergistic effect; that is, the combined effect of the two drugs is greater than that of either drug alone.

3. Yes, there is a concern! The desired trough level is 1 mcg/mL, so a level of 3 mcg/mL could mean that he is receiving a dose that is too high. The increased serum creatinine level is also a concern because it could be an indication of impaired renal function. The physician must be notified immediately and doses of the aminoglycoside withheld until the physician responds.

## CHAPTER 40

### Antiviral Drugs

### Chapter Review and NCLEX® Examination Preparation/Critical Thinking and Application
1. d
2. d
3. a
4. c
5. a, b
6. b
7. a
8. a, b, c
9. d

10. 5 mL
11. 22 mg
12. It is possible to treat both Amy and the fetus. Zidovudine, one of the few anti–human immunodeficiency virus (HIV) drugs known to prolong patient survival, can be used for maternal and fetal treatment. During the pregnancy, Amy can receive the oral form of the drug. During labor, she can receive the drug intravenously. Drug therapy for the infant can begin within 12 hours of delivery and continue for 6 weeks.

13. a. Acyclovir (Zovirax) is indicated for herpes zoster (shingles).
    b. Bailey will be treated with acyclovir again; it is the drug of choice for treatment of both initial and recurrent episodes of shingles.

14. a. Ribavirin is used to treat infections caused by respiratory syncytial virus.
    b. Yes. Brenda's treatment will last at least 3 days but not longer than 7 days.

15. The patient may be experiencing zidovudine's major dose-limiting adverse effect, which is bone marrow suppression.

16. No. The nurse's coworker is doing fine. Acyclovir administered by intravenous infusion is first diluted in the solution recommended by the manufacturer and is administered slowly over at least 1 hour to prevent renal damage.

17. No. Therapy with oseltamivir (Tamiflu) needs to begin within 2 days of the onset of influenza. It is probably too late for this medication to be effective for Stacy.

18. Ganciclovir may be administered to *prevent* cytomegalovirus disease (generalized infection) in high-risk patients, such as those receiving organ transplants.

## Case Study

1. Mr. C. needs to use a glove when applying topical acyclovir (Zovirax) to the affected area, which should be kept clean and dry. Also, he should not use any other creams or ointments on the area.

2. Mr. C.'s herpes infection cannot be "cured," although the acyclovir will help to manage the symptoms.

3. Stress the importance of treatment for Mr. C. and his sexual partner and discuss with him how to prevent transmission of the virus.

4. There are several viruses in the *Herpesviridae* family, including herpes simplex type 1, which causes mucocutaneous herpes—usually blisters around the mouth; varicella-zoster virus (herpes simplex type 3), which causes both chickenpox and shingles; herpesvirus type 4 (also called Epstein-Barr virus); and herpesvirus type 8, which is believed by some to cause Kaposi's sarcoma, a cancer associated with acquired immunodeficiency syndrome (AIDS).

## CHAPTER 41

### Antitubercular Drugs

**Chapter Review and NCLEX® Examination Preparation/Critical Thinking and Application**

1. a
2. b
3. a, b, c
4. c
5. a
6. a
7. c
8. a, d, e
9. a, b, c
10. 3 tablets (See Overview of Dosage Calculations, Sections I and II.)
11. 1800 mg; yes, the maximum dose is 2 g (2000 mg)
12. a. Liver function studies should be performed because isoniazid can cause hepatic impairment. In addition, an eye examination is important because the drug may cause visual disturbances.
    b. Diane may be a slow acetylator. Acetylation, the process by which isoniazid is metabolized in the liver, requires certain enzymes to break down the isoniazid. In slow acetylators, who have a genetic deficiency of these enzymes, isoniazid accumulates. The dosage of isoniazid may need to be adjusted downward in these patients.
13. a. Streptomycin is administered intramuscularly, deep into a large muscle mass, and the sites are rotated.
    b. Although it may not be a concern in terms of Ms. I.'s streptomycin therapy, oral contraceptives become ineffective when given with rifampin. If rifampin is part of her therapy, Ms. I. should switch to another form of birth control.
14. A thorough eye examination may be called for before therapy is initiated because ethambutol can cause a decrease in visual acuity resulting from optic neuritis, which is also a contraindication to the use of ethambutol. In addition, isoniazid may cause optic neuritis and visual disturbances.
15. a. Mr. F. needs to know that his compliance with therapy is essential for achieving a cure. Although he is keeping his follow-up appointments, Mr. F. also needs to take his medication as ordered. He should be warned not to consume alcohol because the antitubercular drugs may cause liver toxicity, and he should be encouraged to take care of himself by ensuring adequate nutrition, rest, and relaxation.
    b. The therapeutic response can be confirmed by results of laboratory studies (sputum culture and sensitivity tests) and chest radiographic findings.
16. a. Frannie, similar to all patients taking antitubercular drugs, needs to be compliant with the therapy regimen and keep her follow-up appointments. She should be reminded that she can spread the disease (during the initial period of the illness); she should wash her hands frequently and cover her mouth when coughing or sneezing. Frannie also needs adequate nutrition and rest.
    b. It is likely that Frannie is on rifampin therapy. She should be told that her urine, stool, saliva, sputum, sweat, and tears may become red-orange-brown in color and that this is an effect of rifampin therapy.

### Case Study

1. George's gout is a consideration; pyrazinamide can cause hyperuricemia, so gout or flare-ups of gout can occur in susceptible patients. His diabetes is a concern, too; ethambutol should be used cautiously in patients with diabetes. A baseline hearing test should be performed if streptomycin is considered because this drug may cause ototoxicity. In addition, liver function studies are needed because his heavy alcohol use may have caused liver damage.
2. An individual with a genetic deficiency of the liver enzymes that metabolize drugs can be classified as a "slow acetylator." When isoniazid is taken by slow acetylators, the drug accumulates because there are not enough of the enzymes to break down the isoniazid. As a result, the dosage of isoniazid may need to be reduced.
3. Results of liver function studies should be assessed carefully before therapy is initiated because some drugs (isoniazid, pyrazinamide) are hepatotoxic. Liver function test results should be monitored closely during therapy as well.
4. Isoniazid can cause a pyridoxine (vitamin $B_6$) deficiency. Patients should take pyridoxine as prescribed by the physician to prevent some of the neurologic effects of vitamin $B_6$ deficiency, such as numbness and tingling of the extremities (peripheral neuritis).

## CHAPTER 42

### Antifungal Drugs

**Chapter Review and NCLEX® Examination Preparation/Critical Thinking and Application**

1. j
2. e
3. f
4. g
5. a
6. c
7. h
8. i
9. d
10. b
11. c
12. a, b, c, e

13. d
14. b
15. a
16. d
17. a, e
18. a, c
19. 50 mL/hr (See Overview of Dosage Calculations, Section V.)
20. 660 mg; 440 mg
21. a. Fluconazole (Diflucan), unlike itraconazole and other -azoles, can pass into the cerebrospinal fluid (CSF), which makes it useful in the treatment of cryptococcal meningitis.
    b. Unfortunately, Mr. K. will need to remain on the medication (at a reduced dosage) for 10 to 12 weeks after the negative results on his CSF culture.
22. a. Amphotericin B needs to be diluted according to the manufacturer's guidelines and administered using an infusion pump. The nurse must not use solutions that are cloudy or that have visible precipitates. Before administration, the nurse will check for an order to premedicate the patient with an antiemetic, antihistamine, antipyretic, or corticosteroid to prevent or minimize infusion-related reactions.
    b. The nurse will monitor closely for expected adverse effects such as cardiac dysrhythmias, visual disturbances, paresthesias (numbness or tingling of the hands or feet), respiratory difficulty, pain, fever, chills, and nausea.
    c. No, unless a severe reaction occurs (e.g., exacerbation of adverse effects or a decline in vital signs). To decrease the severity of expected adverse effects, the patient may be pretreated with an antipyretic (e.g., acetaminophen), antihistamines, and antiemetics.
23. Nystatin oral troches or lozenges are to be dissolved slowly and completely in the mouth for the best effects and should not be chewed or swallowed. Chrissie needs a review of how to use this medication.
24. Lipid formulations of amphotericin B have been developed in an attempt to decrease the incidence of its adverse effects and increase its efficacy. The disadvantage is that they are more expensive than conventional amphotericin B.

## Case Study

1. Voriconazole is used to treat major fungal infections in patients who do not tolerate or respond to other antifungal drugs. The physician probably tried other drugs first.
2. Use of voriconazole is contraindicated in patients taking other drugs that are metabolized by cytochrome P-450 enzyme 3A4 (e.g., quinidine) because of the risk for inducing serious cardiac dysrhythmias.

3. Careful cardiac monitoring is needed if Sally is also taking quinidine while taking this antifungal drug.

## CHAPTER 43

### Antimalarial, Antiprotozoal, and Anthelmintic Drugs

**Chapter Review and NCLEX® Examination Preparation/Critical Thinking and Application**

1. a
2. a
3. c
4. b, c, d, e
5. c
6. b, e
7. d
8. a, c
9. The dose is 280 mg (4 mg/kg × 70 kg); the nurse will draw up 4.7 mL of the diluted solution for the infusion. (See Overview of Dosage Calculations, Section III.)
10. 5 tablets
11. Malaria is caused by *Plasmodium* organisms. During the asexual stage of the *Plasmodium* life cycle, which occurs in the human host, the parasite resides for a while outside the erythrocyte; this is called the *exoerythrocytic phase*. The most effective drug for eradicating the parasite during this phase is primaquine.
12. Before primaquine is administered, Professor H. will be given a pregnancy test. This is a pregnancy category C drug, so the nurse will need to know if certain precautions are needed in Professor H.'s case. She will also be assessed for hypersensitivity and any disease states that cause granulocytopenia (rheumatoid arthritis, systemic lupus erythematosus). In addition, primaquine must be used with caution in patients with methemoglobinemia, porphyria, methemoglobin reductase deficiency, and glucose-6-phosphate dehydrogenase (G6PD) deficiency.
13. Mefloquine is indicated for the treatment of chloroquine-resistant malaria. Quinine, an older drug, may also be used. Quinine can be used alone but is more commonly given in combination with pyrimethamine, a sulfonamide, or a tetracycline (e.g., doxycycline).
14. Each of these three patients has a protozoal infection. The patient with the intestinal disorder has giardiasis. The patient with acquired immunodeficiency syndrome (AIDS) has pneumocystosis. The patient with the sexually transmitted infection has trichomoniasis. See Table 43-3 for specific drugs used to treat these diseases.

## Case Study

1. Intestinal roundworms are diagnosed based on symptoms and examination of stool specimens.
2. Contraindications include allergy to the medication and pregnancy. Even though she is only 15 years old, she will be assessed for possible pregnancy before this medication is given. In addition, her liver function test results will be assessed because use of pyrantel is contraindicated in patients with liver disease.
3. It paralyzes intestinal worms so that the body is able to remove them via the feces.
4. Based on her weight of 57 kg, the dose for her would be 627 mg (11 mg × 57 kg).
5. Adverse effects of pyrantel therapy include headache, dizziness, insomnia, skin rashes, anorexia, cramps, diarrhea, nausea, and vomiting.

## CHAPTER 44

### Antiinflammatory and Antigout Drugs

### Chapter Review and NCLEX® Examination Preparation/Critical Thinking and Application

1. b
2. b
3. a, b, d, e
4. c
5. a, c, d
6. a
7. b
8. c
9. a
10. No. The child weighs 15 kg, and the appropriate dose for that weight is 50 mg orally twice daily, not 100 mg.
11. 1.3 mL

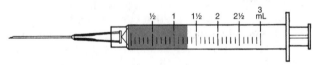

12. Chronic salicylate intoxication, which occurs as a result of either high dosages or prolonged therapy with high dosages of aspirin
13. Mr. C. has an acute overdose of a nonsalicylate nonsteroidal antiinflammatory drug (NSAID). If the condition progresses, symptoms can include intense headache, dizziness, cerebral edema, cardiac arrest, and even death in extreme cases.
14. Mr. H. needs to know that compliance with the entire medical regimen is important for the success of his treatment for gout. Allopurinol needs to be taken with meals to help prevent the occurrence of gastrointestinal symptoms such as nausea, vomiting, and anorexia. Fluids should be increased to 3 L/day, and hazardous activities must be avoided if dizziness or drowsiness occurs with the medication. Also, alcohol and caffeine need to be avoided because these drugs increase uric acid levels and decrease the levels of allopurinol.

15. a. Ketorolac (Toradol) is indicated for the short-term management (up to 5 days) of moderate to severe acute pain that requires analgesia at the opioid level. It is not indicated for the treatment of minor or chronic painful conditions.
    b. The main adverse effects of ketorolac (Toradol) include renal impairment, gastrointestinal pain, dyspepsia, and nausea. These problems limit the length of time that the medication can be used.
16. The vinegary odor means that the aspirin has experienced some chemical breakdown, and she should not use it! She needs to discard it safely and purchase a new bottle.
17. Febuxostat is indicated for the treatment of acute gout but may pose a risk for cardiovascular events. Randy's history of hypertension and coronary artery disease may be of concern.

## Case Study

1. The specific cyclooxygenase-2 selectivity of these drugs allows them to control the inflammation and pain without producing some of the toxicity associated with NSAID therapy.
2. The most common adverse effects include fatigue, dizziness, lower extremity edema, hypertension, dyspepsia, nausea, heartburn, and epigastric discomfort. Any stomach pain, unusual bleeding, or blood in vomit or stool must be reported to the physician immediately. Chest pain, palpitations, and any gastrointestinal problems need to be reported as well.
3. Celecoxib is not used in patients with known sulfa allergy.
4. She needs to avoid alcohol and aspirin while taking this medication and check with her provider before taking any over-the-counter medications.

## CHAPTER 45

### Antineoplastic Drugs Part 1: Cancer Overview and Cell Cycle–Specific Drugs

### Critical Thinking Crossword
*Across*
3. Spread
4. Folic
7. Extravasation
8. Nadir
9. Limiting
10. Leukemia
*Down*
1. Malignant
2. Leucovorin
5. Nonspecific
6. Benign
7. Emetic

**Chapter Review and NCLEX® Examination Preparation**

1. a, b, c, e, f
2. d
3. a
4. b
5. c
6. d
7. d
8. c
9. a, e
10. 25,000 units; yes
11. a. 8.2 mg
    b. 8.2 mL

## Case Study

1. Methotrexate is an antimetabolite—specifically, a folate antagonist. It inhibits the action of an enzyme that is responsible for converting folic acid to a substance used by the cell to synthesize DNA for cell reproduction. As a result, the cell dies.
2. Laboratory test results should be checked for white blood cell and red blood cell counts, hemoglobin level and hematocrit, platelet counts, and renal and liver function studies.
3. The concurrent administration of nonsteroidal anti-inflammatory drugs (NSAIDs) and methotrexate may lead to possible reduced renal elimination of methotrexate with potentially fatal hematologic and gastrointestinal toxicity. Allen should be instructed to avoid all NSAIDs, including aspirin, while taking methotrexate.
4. Antiemetic therapy will be needed to decrease nausea and vomiting. Leucovorin may be used to protect the patient from potentially fatal bone marrow suppression, a toxic effect of methotrexate.

### CHAPTER 46

**Antineoplastic Drugs Part 2: Cell Cycle–Nonspecific and Miscellaneous Drugs**

**Chapter Review and NCLEX® Examination Preparation/Critical Thinking and Application**

1. c
2. a
3. b
4. a, c, e, f
5. b
6. d
7. a
8. b, c, e
9. d
10. 125 mL/hr
11. 46 mL/hr (rounded up from 45.5) (See Overview of Dosage Calculations, Section V.)

12. Cytoprotective drugs help to reduce the toxicity of various antineoplastics. As a result, the adverse effects may be reduced, so increased dosages of the antineoplastic medication may be tolerated, which allows greater destruction of cancer cells. Examples include the following:
    - Amifostine (Ethyol), used during therapy with cisplatin to reduce renal toxicity
    - Dexrazoxane (Zinecard), used during therapy with doxorubicin to reduce cardiac toxicity
13. The nurse will not agree. The nurse recognizes that the most likely cause of the patient's respiratory problems is the development of pulmonary toxicity (pulmonary fibrosis and pneumonitis) secondary to therapy with bleomycin.
14. No! In most facilities, institutional guidelines direct that the pharmacy department mix these drugs. Special requirements must be met for the safety of those working with these drugs, including the use of a laminar airflow hood and appropriate personal protective equipment (e.g., gown, mask, and gloves). It would not be safe for the nurse or for those around the nurse to mix the chemotherapy drug on the nursing unit.
15. The nurse will stop the infusion immediately but won't pull out the intravenous catheter quite yet. The physician must be notified immediately, and the nurse will expect to receive orders to treat this extravasation of mechlorethamine by injecting a solution of 10% sodium thiosulfate and sterile water (see Table 46-2) through the existing line into the extravasated site (and then remove the line) and through multiple subcutaneous injections into the site. Over the next few hours, the patient will receive repeated subcutaneous injections into the area, and cold compresses will be applied to the site.

## Case Study

1. Nephrotoxicity (possible damage to the kidneys), peripheral neuropathy (possible damage to peripheral nerves), and ototoxicity (possible damage to hearing and vestibular function)
2. Baseline renal studies need to be performed because this drug is highly nephrotoxic. If Dottie is receiving any other drugs that are potentially nephrotoxic (e.g., aminoglycoside therapy), dosage changes will need to be considered. If she has gout, concurrent use of cisplatin may result in hyperuricemia or worsening of the gout. Baseline auditory studies, baseline liver function studies, measurement of white blood cell count, hemoglobin level, hematocrit, and platelet level are needed because of the anticipated bone marrow suppression.
3. Because peripheral neuropathies may occur, numbness, tingling, or pain in the extremities must be reported to the physician immediately to prevent complications and enhance comfort.

4. Yes, this is a concern because dehydration while taking cisplatin may lead to renal damage. Patients who are at home after treatment with this drug need to be reminded of the importance of hydration and need to be told to contact a physician if they experience dry mucous membranes, very dark amber urine, little or no urinary output, or vomiting of large amounts over a period of 8 hours or less. It may be a challenge, but she needs to try to take in 3000 mL of fluid per day to prevent dehydration.

## CHAPTER 47

### Biologic Response–Modifying and Antirheumatic Drugs

**Chapter Review and NCLEX® Examination Preparation/Critical Thinking and Application**
1. e
2. a
3. g
4. b
5. h
6. d
7. c
8. c
9. a, b, c, d, e
10. c
11. c
12. a, b, d, e
13. a. 2.5 mg
   b. 0.5 mL

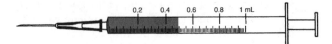

14. 1.3 mL (See Overview of Dosage Calculations, Section III.)
15. The major dose-limiting side effect of interferons is fatigue. Patients taking high dosages become so exhausted that they are often confined to bed. Sonja needs to know this before she starts the therapy.
16. Colony-stimulating factors (CSFs) such as filgrastim (Neupogen), pegfilgrastim (Neulasta), and sargramostim (Leukine) can be given for chemotherapy-induced leukopenia. These drugs should be administered 24 hours after the chemotherapy drugs have been given because the myelosuppressive effects of the chemotherapy drugs tend to cancel out the therapeutic benefits of the CSFs.
17. She will receive oprelvekin (Neumega), which is given via subcutaneous injections daily for up to 21 days. Because she has severe thrombocytopenia, however, the nurse must be careful to prevent excessive bleeding and bruising at the injection

sites and to teach Brittany measures to reduce bleeding risks.
18. Methotrexate is given *weekly*, not daily!
   The nurse needs to clarify and correct this mistranscribed order. It is very important to note that the drug is given once per week, not once per day. Serious medication errors, including deaths, have occurred when the drug was given daily instead of once a week.

### Case Study
1. Oprelvekin has a dual classification as both an interleukin (interleukin-11 [IL-11]) and hematopoietic drug.
2. A complete blood count will be monitored, specifically, to note the platelet counts, to monitor the therapeutic effects of the oprelvekin, and to watch for decreasing levels of hemoglobin or hematocrit, which may indicate that blood loss is occurring.
3. Treatment may be ordered to begin within 6 to 24 hours after completion of antineoplastic therapy. She will receive daily subcutaneous dosing for up to 21 days. The injection sites will be rotated in areas, including the thigh, abdomen, hip, and upper arm.
4. Donna will need teaching about ways to reduce risk for bleeding, such as using a soft toothbrush, not flossing her teeth, and not using a razor if she shaves her underarms or legs. In addition, she needs to be aware that any cuts or wounds, including injection sites, may bleed longer. Direct pressure should be applied to control bleeding. The site will require close monitoring until bleeding has stopped. She needs to report any abnormal bleeding from her gums, from her nose, or in her stool or urine to her physician immediately.

## CHAPTER 48

### Immunosuppressant Drugs

**Chapter Review and NCLEX® Examination Preparation/Critical Thinking and Application**
1. b
2. c
3. c
4. a
5. a, c, d, e
6. b
7. a, e
8. a, c, f
9. 4 capsules
10. a. 750 mg for this dose
    b. 15 mL (See Overview of Dosage Calculations, Section II.)

11. a. Sirolimus (Rapamune) can help prevent organ rejection. If Mrs. F.'s immune system cannot recognize the new kidney as foreign, it will not mount an immune response against it. This promotes success of the transplant.
    b. The antifungal drug is added several days before surgery as prophylaxis for oral candidiasis.
12. Encourage the patient to take the drug with meals or mixed with chocolate milk, milk, or orange juice to prevent stomach upset.
13. Styrofoam containers or cups should be avoided because the drug has been found to adhere to the inside wall of such containers. The nurse needs to find a glass or cup that is not made of Styrofoam. After the drug is mixed, the patient needs to drink it immediately.
14. Tess is experiencing symptoms consistent with adverse effects of muromonab-CD3. The nurse will need to monitor her closely for signs of fluid retention and pulmonary edema and for an allergy-like reaction known as *cytokine release syndrome*, which can be severe. Patients are often premedicated with corticosteroids (e.g., intravenous methylprednisolone) in an effort to avoid or alleviate this problem.
15. Fingolimod (Gilenya) and glatiramer acetate (Copaxone) are immunosuppressants that are indicated for reduction of the frequency of relapses (exacerbations) in a type of multiple sclerosis known as *relapsing-remitting multiple sclerosis*.

## Case Study

1. Yes, immunosuppressant therapy will be lifelong.
2. White patches on the tongue, mucous membranes, and oral pharynx would be indicative of candidiasis.
3. Mr. K. needs to be seen by a physician immediately. These symptoms could indicate that he has a severe infection.
4. Patients taking immunosuppressant drugs need to avoid live vaccines because of the immunosuppressant therapy. There may be a risk for an infection developing because of the administration of a live vaccine to a person with lowered immunity.

## CHAPTER 49

### Immunizing Drugs

### Chapter Review and NCLEX® Examination Preparation/Critical Thinking and Application
1. a. Zoster vaccine (Zostavax)
   b. Active
   c. Active
   d. *Haemophilus influenzae* type b prophylaxis
   e. Hepatitis B virus vaccine (inactivated)
   f. Rh$_O$(D) immunoglobulin (RhoGAM)
   g. Passive
   h. Active
   i. Tuberculosis prophylaxis

j. Active
k. Diphtheria, tetanus, and pertussis prophylaxis, pediatric
l. Passive
m. Postexposure passive tetanus prophylaxis
n. Active
o. Diphtheria and tetanus prophylaxis (pediatric [older than age 7 years] and adult)
2. b
3. d
4. c
5. a
6. c
7. a, c
8. b
9. c
10. 0.005 mg (See Overview of Dosage Calculations, Section I.)
11.

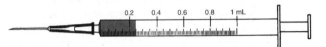

12. She will most likely receive the DTaP (diphtheria, tetanus, and acellular pertussis vaccine [Adacel]). With the recent increase in cases of pertussis, DTaP is recommended for adults in place of tetanus-diphtheria, which lacks the pertussis component.
13. Sometimes, after vaccination, the levels of antibodies against a particular pathogen decline over time, and a second dose of the vaccine is given to restore the antibody titers to a level that can protect the person against the infection. This second dose is referred to as a *booster shot*.
14. Each year a new influenza vaccine is developed that contains three influenza virus strains that represent the strains most likely to circulate in the United States in the upcoming winter. The vaccination from the previous year may not be effective for the influenza virus strains occurring in the current year.
15. Carl may experience localized swelling, redness, discomfort, and warmth at the injection site. Acetaminophen and rest are recommended for the relief of these side effects, and application of warm compresses to the injection site may also help ease some of the discomfort.
16. There are three types of anthrax based on the routes of inoculation: cutaneous, inhalational, and gastrointestinal. Of the three, anthrax contracted by inhalation of the bacterial spores is the most deadly and has a mortality rate of more than 80%.
17. Paul is experiencing more than the expected adverse effects of his vaccinations. He is probably experiencing "serum sickness," which may occur after repeated injections of equine-derived immunizing drugs. Because his symptoms may indicate

respiratory impairment, he needs to be taken to the hospital for evaluation and monitoring; he needs to call 911 rather than try to drive himself to the hospital. He may receive analgesics, antihistamines, epinephrine, or corticosteroids (or a combination of these drugs) to treat this reaction.

## Case Study

1. Rabies is a very potent virus.
2. Those at high risk for rabies exposure, such as veterinarians, will receive the rabies virus vaccine (Imovax, RabAvert) as preexposure prophylaxis, followed by booster shots every 2 to 5 years based on blood titers. This is a type of active immunization.
3. You will receive drugs that give both active and passive immunization. Postexposure prophylaxis consists of injections of the rabies virus vaccine (see the answer to Question 2) and rabies immune globulin (Imogam Rabies-HT). Because rabies can progress so rapidly, the body does not have time to mount an adequate immune defense—death occurs before it can do so. The passive immunization confers temporary protection that is usually sufficient to keep the invading organism from causing death even though it does not stimulate an antibody response. The active immunization you receive will stimulate an antibody response.

## CHAPTER 50

### Acid-Controlling Drugs

### Chapter Review and NCLEX® Examination Preparation/Critical Thinking and Application

1. h
2. e
3. i
4. k
5. c
6. a, b
7. f
8. d
9. b
10. g
11. b
12. c
13. d
14. b, d, e
15. b
16. b, c
17. c
18. c
19. 2 mL
20. 200 mL/hr (See Overview of Dosage Calculations, Section V.)
21. You need to let him know that long-term self-medication with antacids may mask symptoms of serious underlying diseases. He needs to be evaluated for possible bleeding ulcer or even a malignancy, but

you may not want to scare him with those possibilities! If his current self-treatment is no longer working, he needs a medical evaluation. Advise him not to take the baking soda but to instead see his provider.
22. Omeprazole must be taken 30 to 60 minutes before meals, and the capsule must be taken whole, not crushed, opened, or chewed. Omeprazole may also be given with antacids, if ordered.
23. Patients with heart failure or hypertension need to use antacids that are low in sodium. Suggest an aluminum-based antacid. Instruct patients to take the antacid alone, not at the same time as other medications (unless specifically instructed to do so) because the antacid will interfere with the absorption of the other medications. Antacids should be taken 1 hour before or 1 to 2 hours after other medications. If symptoms continue or worsen, consult the health care provider.
24. Antacids may promote premature dissolving of the enteric coating; if the coating is destroyed early in the stomach, gastrointestinal (GI) upset may occur. He needs to take the aspirin tablets with food, not with antacids.
25. Stress ulcer prophylaxis (or therapy to prevent severe GI damage) is undertaken in almost every critically ill patient in an intensive care unit and for many patients on general medical-surgical units.

## Case Study

1. Although histamine-2 ($H_2$) antagonists are available over the counter, the dose of the over-the-counter preparation will not be the same strength as the usual dose of the prescription formulation.
2. The drug effects of the $H_2$ blockers are limited to specific blocking actions on the parietal cells of the gastric glands in the stomach. As a result, hydrogen ion production is decreased, which leads to an increase in the pH of the stomach (i.e., decreased stomach acid).
3. Use of $H_2$ receptor antagonists is contraindicated in patients with known drug allergy or impaired renal function or liver disease. Cautious use is recommended in patients who are confused, disoriented, or older. Interactions may occur with drugs that have a narrow therapeutic range. Caution must be used if she is taking theophylline for her asthma. Patients requiring these medications must avoid aspirin and other nonsteroidal antiinflammatory drugs, alcohol, and caffeine because of their ulcerogenic or GI tract–irritating effects.
4. Smoking has been shown to decrease the effectiveness of $H_2$ blockers because the absorption of $H_2$ antagonists is impaired in individuals who smoke. Hopefully, if she is not smoking, this will not be a problem for her, but spending several hours in a smoke-filled room may have an effect. Also, the beer and possibly spicy pizza may aggravate the underlying condition.

## CHAPTER 51

**Bowel Disorder Drugs**

**Critical Thinking Crossword**

*Across*

6. Emollient
7. Probiotic
8. Saline
9. Bulk-forming

*Down*

1. Adsorbent
2. Opiates
3. Hyperosmotic
4. Stimulant
5. Anticholinergic

**Chapter Review and NCLEX® Examination Preparation/Critical Thinking and Application**

1. d
2. a
3. d
4. c
5. c
6. c
7. a, d
8. d
9. a
10. a. 1.5 mg per dose (6 mg/day)
    b. 3 mL per dose
11. 7.5 mL (See Overview of Dosage Calculations, Section II.)
12. Darkening of the tongue or stool is a temporary and harmless side effect associated with the use of bismuth subsalicylate (Pepto-Bismol).
13. Use of the belladonna alkaloid preparations, such as Donnatal, is contraindicated in patients with narrow-angle glaucoma. She should not use this drug.
14. Several factors may be causing Hillary's constipation, including lack of proper exercise, poor diet (which might involve inadequate roughage and an excess of dairy products), use of aluminum-containing antacids, and stress.
15. a. The bulk-forming laxatives tend to produce normal stools, have few systemic effects, and are among the safest available.
    b. Ira needs to mix the medication with at least 6 to 8oz of fluid and drink it immediately. He should never take it dry.
16. a. Because glycerin is very mild, it is often used in children.
    b. Abdominal bloating and rectal irritation

## Case Study

1. Antibiotic therapy destroys the balance of normal flora in the intestines, and diarrhea-causing bacteria proliferate.
2. *Lactobacillus acidophilus,* a probiotic, is indicated for diarrhea caused by antibiotic treatment that has destroyed the normal intestinal flora.
3. Supplying *Lactobacillus acidophilus* bacteria helps restore the balance of normal flora and suppress the growth of diarrhea-causing bacteria.
4. It is considered a dietary supplement. It is often used to treat uncomplicated diarrhea, although this is an off-label use (not approved by the Food and Drug Administration).

## CHAPTER 52

**Antiemetic and Antinausea Drugs**

**Chapter Review and NCLEX® Examination Preparation/Critical Thinking and Application**

1. a, b, d, e
2. c, e
3. d
4. c
5. b
6. d
7. c
8. c
9. c
10. 2 mL

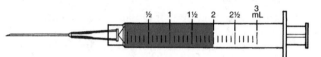

11. 30 mL (See Overview of Dosage Calculations, Section II.)
12. a. Petra should take the metoclopramide 30 minutes before meals and at bedtime.
    b. Combining metoclopramide with alcohol can result in additive central nervous system depression. Petra needs to be instructed not to take the medication with alcohol.
13. This drug comes in oral, intramuscular, intravenous, and rectal forms, but because she was on "nothing-by-mouth" status and has no intravenous access, the intramuscular route was ordered. The nurse can call Nellie's health care provider to obtain an order for an alternate route but cannot change the route without an order because the dosage may also be different.
14. Dronabinol is a synthetic derivative of the major active substance in marijuana. The nurse explains to him that it is used to stimulate appetite and weight gain in patients with acquired immunodeficiency syndrome (AIDS).

## Case Study

1. The only listed contraindication is drug allergy.
2. Antiemetics are often administered before a chemotherapy drug is given, frequently ½ hour to 3 hours before treatment.
3. The headache is caused by the ondansetron and can be relieved with acetaminophen.

## CHAPTER 53

## Vitamins and Minerals

### Chapter Review and NCLEX® Examination Preparation/Critical Thinking and Application

1. c
2. g
3. b
4. h
5. e
6. k
7. i
8. d
9. j
10. a
11. l
12. f
13. a, d, e
14. b
15. d
16. c
17. d
18. d
19. c
20. 100 mL/hr
21. 1 mL (See Overview of Dosage Calculations, Section III.)
22. Broad-spectrum antibiotics can inhibit the intestinal flora, which provide the body with vitamin $K_2$. As a result, a deficiency may occur. Vitamin K can be given either orally or by injection in adults.
23. Dietary sources of vitamin D include fish oils, salmon, sardines, and herring; fortified milk, bread, and cereals; and animal livers, tuna, eggs, and butter. In addition, vitamin D is synthesized in the skin through exposure to ultraviolet radiation (sunshine).
24. a. Pernicious anemia
    b. The absorption of cyanocobalamin (vitamin $B_{12}$, or extrinsic factor) requires the presence of intrinsic factor, which is a glycoprotein secreted by gastric parietal cells. After the binding takes place, the complex is absorbed in the small intestine. Because an ileal resection removes a portion of the small intestine, malabsorption of cyanocobalamin can occur.
    c. Cyanocobalamin injections are used to treat pernicious anemia caused by a lack of intrinsic factor.
25. To avoid venous irritation, give intravenous (IV) calcium via an IV infusion pump and with proper dilution. Giving IV calcium too rapidly may precipitate severe hypercalcemia, with subsequent cardiac irregularities, delirium, and coma. Administer IV calcium slowly, as ordered, and within the manufacturer guidelines (e.g., usually less than 1 mL/min). Patients need to remain recumbent for 15 minutes after the infusion to prevent further problems. If extravasation of the IV calcium solution occurs, discontinue the infusion immediately but leave the IV catheter in place for antidote administration. The prescriber may then order an injection of 1% procaine or other antidotes or fluids to reduce vasospasm at the site and dilute the irritating effects of calcium on surrounding tissue. However, follow all facility policies and procedural guidelines and manufacturer insert information as deemed appropriate.

### Case Study

1. Normal serum magnesium levels are 1.7 to 2.2 mg/dL.
2. During intravenous magnesium infusion, monitor the patient's electrocardiographic and vital signs, and rate patellar or knee-jerk reflexes. Impaired reflexes are used as an indication of drug-related central nervous system (CNS) depressant effects. CNS depression may quickly lead to respiratory or cardiac depression; thus perform frequent monitoring. Document the infusion and infusion site and record each set of vital sign measurements and ratings of reflexes appropriately. Other signs that require immediate attention are confusion, irregular heart rhythm, cramping, unusual fatigue, lightheadedness, and dizziness.
3. Contact the prescriber immediately, stop the infusion, and monitor the patient.
4. Calcium gluconate must be readily accessible for use as an antidote to magnesium toxicity.

## CHAPTER 54

## Anemia Drugs

### Chapter Review and NCLEX® Examination Preparation/Critical Thinking and Application

1. d
2. b, c, f
3. c
4. b, c
5. b, c, d, e
6. c
7. a
8. a
9. b
10. 0.75 mL

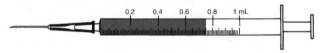

11. 26 mg (rounded up from 25.9) (See Overview of Dosage Calculations, Section III.)
12. Anyone who is about to receive a first dose of iron dextran is at risk for fatal anaphylaxis. Because of this, a test dose of 25 mg of iron dextran should be administered by the chosen route and appropriate method. An anaphylactic reaction may occur within a few moments, although waiting at least 1 hour